Renal Pathophysiology

Renal Pathophysiology

SECOND EDITION

Alexander Leaf, M.D.
Chief of Medical Services
Massachusetts General Hospital
Jackson Professor of Clinical Medicine
Harvard Medical School

Ramzi S. Cotran, M.D.
Pathologist-in-Chief
Peter Bent Brigham Hospital
F. B. Mallory Professor of Pathology
Harvard Medical School

New York / Oxford
OXFORD UNIVERSITY PRESS
1980

Library of Congress Cataloging in Publication Data

Leaf, Alexander.
   Renal pathophysiology.

   Includes bibliographical references and index.
   1. Kidneys—Diseases. 2. Kidneys. 3. Water-
electrolyte balance (Physiology)   I.   Cotran, Ramzi S.,
joint author. II. Title. [DNLM 1. Kidney—
Physiopathology.   WJ300 L434r]
RC903.L37 1980   616.6'1   80-11839
ISBN 0-19-502688-8   ISBN 0-19-502689-6 (pbk.)

Printed in the United States of America

Preface to the First Edition

This book developed during the teaching of renal pathophysiology to Harvard medical students. When an attempt was made to teach a shortened "core curriculum," it seemed desirable to put down explicitly what our students were expected to know. These chapters afforded a syllabus to be used as a focus for discussions in small groups, and the number of didactic lectures was sharply reduced. Putting the material in writing was deemed essential in this complex and ever-growing field to save the students time in seeking and assimilating the available knowledge, and it was expected also to allow for independent reading on topics of particular interest to them. Whether it achieved any such exalted educational goal remains debatable. Nevertheless, this book should serve the beginner as an introduction to an area of pathophysiology that is being continuously acted out by our patients on the stage of clinical medicine and surgery. It should also be a useful reference and review for the medical graduate who has not pursued training directly in this specialty.

The Appendix was added to provide a somewhat more basic background for the membrane transport phenomena upon which all kidney and body fluid physiology is based. Skipping this Appendix will not inhibit comprehension of the book. However, it seemed desirable to include some more rigorous view of the basis of the phenomena dealt with for the student who has appropriate interests and background. By contrast, Chapter 10, The Clinical and Physiological Significance of the Serum Sodium Concentration, has been included to bring aspects of the earlier chapters directly into clinical focus. The physician who assimilates the information in this book will discover, if he has not already, that good clinical practice is the appropriate application of the principles of pathophysiology to the management of the patient.

No attempt has been made to be comprehensive or to document exhaustively the statements made in the text. Rather, the reader is referred to reviews or general discussions from which further detailed references may be obtained. Only in the discussion of controversial, unsettled issues are references sprinkled more liberally so that the reader can easily check statements in the text if he desires. The authors apologize, therefore, to all their friends and colleagues whose original and important contributions have not been cited.

We wish to express thanks to Barbara Leaf for her secretarial assistance and to the many students over the past seven years who have used, and tempered, earlier versions of this syllabus. Our thanks go also to Drs. Cecil H. Coggins and Norman Lichtenstein for invaluable discussions and editorial assistance, and to Dr. Eleanora Galvanek for providing some of the illustrations.

Boston, Massachusetts   A.L.
December 1975   R.C.

Preface to the Second Edition

The second edition of *Renal Pathophysiology* retains the educational goals, format, and chapter sequence of the first edition and updates the rather significant advances in renal physiology and pathophysiology of the past five years. We are thankful for the warm reception given the first edition, but are also indebted to the many students and teachers who have offered suggestions and criticisms and, in various ways, served to improve the present version.

A considerable number of changes and additions have been made in this new edition. Recent advances in the understanding of the regulation of extracellular fluid volume have been included. New aspects of hormonal modulation of the renal circulation and filtration, and of control of sodium and water excretion, have been added. The discussion of the pathogenesis of acute renal failure has been rewritten, as have portions of the chapter on acid–base regulation, to clarify questions raised by the presentations in the first edition. New concepts concerning immunopathogenesis of glomerulonephritis have been introduced in the chapter on glomerular injury, and a new section on the glomerular manifestations of systemic diseases has been included. In

the chapter on interstitial diseases, the important role of vesicoureteral reflux is discussed and a new section on the microangiopathic
renal disorders completes the discussion of vascular diseases of the
kidney.

We wish to renew our thanks to our colleagues and students for invaluable discussions that have clarified our understanding of renal
pathophysiology and, it is hoped, our ability to transmit it in this text.

Harvard Medical School   A.L.
Boston, Massachusetts   R.C.
April 1980

Contents

3

Regulation of the Volume and Concentration of the Body Fluids, 54

4

Acid–Base Regulation, 81

5

Pathophysiology of Potassium Excess and Deficiency, 111

6

Edema, 136

7

Diuretics, 145

√8

Acute Renal Failure, 162

9

Chronic Renal Failure, 184

10

The Clinical and Physiological Significance of the Serum Sodium Concentration, 210

11

Calcium, Magnesium, and Phosphate, 247

✓ 12

Glomerulonephritis, 274

13

Vascular Diseases of the Kidney and Hypertension, 332

14

Pyelonephritis and Other Tubulointerstitial Diseases, 357

Appendix: Membrane Transport, 382

Index, 403

Renal Pathophysiology

Renal Pathophysiology

1

Renal Circulation

INTRODUCTION

The kidneys are highly vascularized organs. The two kidneys, with a combined weight of some 300 gm in man, receive 25% of the cardiac output; the arrangement of the blood vessels in the kidneys is highly specialized and adapted to the function of this organ. Thus, the interdependence of blood supply and function is of an unusually high degree. Figure 1-1 shows the relationships of the kidneys to the large vessels.

Figure 1-2 shows the organization of blood vessels in a rat kidney injected with silicone rubber. Here the separate zones of the kidney—from outside in cortical, subcortical, outer medullary, inner medullary, and apical tip or papilla—are readily discerned. This orderly arrangement is typical of kidneys with a single papilla in animals that can elaborate a very concentrated urine (> 2500 mOsm/liter). In man these zones are not so readily distinguished, and the multilobar structure of the kidney adds further confusion to the pattern; cortex (comprising some 80% of the tissue) and medulla, however, are easily seen in the normal kidney.

The main renal artery (usually single, but double in some 25% of the population, an important factor in renal transplant surgery) di-

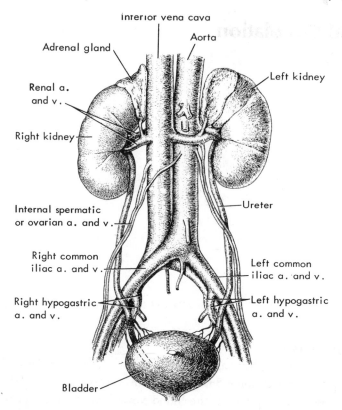

interior vena cava

Adrenal gland

Aorta

Renal a.
and v.

Left kidney

Right kidney

Internal spermatic
or ovarian a. and v.

Ureter

Right common
iliac a. and v.

Left common
iliac a. and v.

Right hypogastric
a. and v.

Left hypogastric
a. and v.

Bladder

Fig. 1-1 Vascular relationships of the kidneys in man.

vides in the pelvic region to form true interlobar arteries that run between adjacent lobes to the junction of cortex and medulla, where they branch to form the arcuate arteries. These course along beneath the cortex parallel to the capsular surface, and may subdivide further. The existing evidence indicates that the arcuate arteries are end arteries that do not anastomose with similar vessels arising from adjacent interlobar arteries. Figure 1-3 shows the renal arterial supply (1) schematically.

The arcuate arteries terminate by turning up into the cortex to form interlobular arteries. Other interlobular arteries from the convex surface of the arcuate vessels run parallel to one another outward through the cortical tissue. Because the human kidney is a compound organ, in which each lobe or portion drained by a papilla forms a vas-

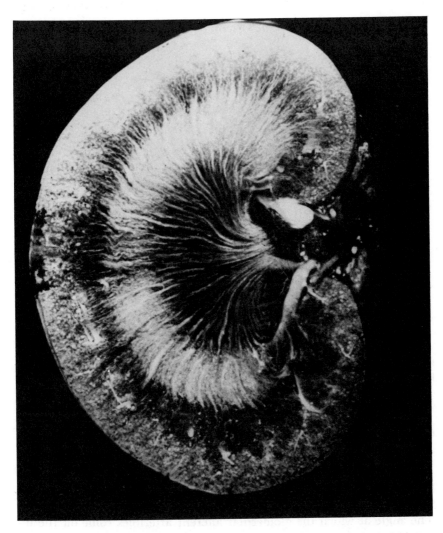

Fig. 1-2 The vascular pattern of a normal rat kidney as visualized by arterial injection of silicone rubber. The outermost layer is the cortex, the granular appearance resulting from the filling of the glomerular capillary tufts with the white silicone rubber; below are the subcortical zone, outer medulla, inner medulla, and finally, the single papilla pointing toward the renal hilum.

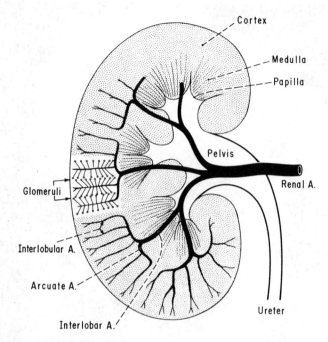

Fig. 1-3 Schematic representation of arterial supply to multilobed mammalian kidney.

cular unit, there is some interdigitation of vessels at the periphery of adjacent lobes where the lobes are in contact.

Although a few interlobular arteries pass through the cortex as perforating arteries that anastomose with the vessels of the renal capsule, the great majority give off smaller glomerular afferent arterioles. The angle at which the glomerular afferent arterioles come off the interlobular arteries is acutely recurrent at first, directing them back toward the medulla, then more at right angles, and finally, the interlobular vessels terminate in glomerular afferent arteries directed toward the surface of the kidney. This characteristic arrangement of proximal drooping branches, then perpendicular branches, and finally, vertical distal branches probably serves to distribute blood pressure and flow appropriately to the glomeruli that these afferents supply. A few glomerular afferent arteries arise directly from arcuate or even interlobar arteries. These vessels, together with the most proximal and recurrent branches of the interlobular arteries, supply juxtamedullary glomer-

uli. A few aglomerular branches are present in both cortex and juxtamedullary zones, but these are thought to be afferent glomerular arterioles whose associated glomerular tufts have atrophied.

At the glomerulus the afferent arteriole breaks up into a compact
anastomosing network of capillaries. A distinct basement membrane is
sandwiched between the fenestrated endothelial cells of these capillaries and the branching epithelial cells (podocytes) that cover the visceral surface of Bowman's capsule on the outer surface of the capillaries.

The network of capillaries comprising the glomerular tuft rejoin to
form the glomerular efferent arteriole. In man there are two types of
nephrons: cortical, with short loops of Henle, and juxtamedullary,
with long loops. Figure 1-4 shows the vascular patterns associated with
cortical and juxtamedullary glomeruli schematically. There are two
corresponding types of glomerular efferent arterioles. The efferent arterioles from the cortical glomeruli are fine and short and break up
into the capillary plexus that lies between the interlobular arteries,
enmeshing renal tubules. The efferent arterioles of the juxtamedullary
glomeruli, in contrast, after giving off a number of fine branches to
the adjacent capillary plexus, divide into a dozen or so descending
vasa recta that enter the medulla. Some juxtamedullary glomeruli
have two efferent arterioles, one going to the nearby capillary plexus
and the other supplying the vasa recta directly. But many of the glomeruli that give rise to vasa recta lie in the middle zone of the cortex
rather than in the juxtamedullary zone.

The descending vasa recta run in bundles into the medulla. These
bundles are largest in the outer portions of the medulla, but attenuate
as single vessels branch to serve the medullary capillary plexus at various levels within the medulla. Toward the tip of the papilla only a
single vessel may remain. The ascending vasa recta reform from the
medullary capillary plexus and are slightly more numerous than the
descending vasa recta. They form a countercurrent exchange system
with their closely associated descending vasa recta as well as with the
descending and ascending limbs of the loops of Henle. Since the vasa
recta break up into plexuses of capillary beds surrounding the loops
of Henle at varying depths in the inner medulla, and the loops of
Henle also penetrate this zone to varying depths, it appears that the
blood supply per length of nephron remains fairly constant all the
way to the tip of the papillae; loops of Henle and their associated vascular bundles penetrate the inner medulla to similar depths.

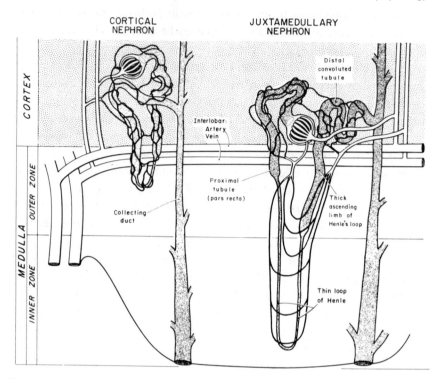

Fig. 1-4 Comparison of postglomerular circulation in cortical and juxtamedullary glomeruli.

A unique aspect of the renal circulation is that it involves two serial capillary circulations. The first consists of the glomerular capillary tufts, which are perfused at high pressure favoring filtration; the second includes the low-pressure "reabsorbing" capillary plexuses of cortex and medulla, which arise from the branching of the efferent glomerular arterioles. It had been thought that the efferent glomerular arteriole broke up into a capillary plexus surrounding, and limited to, its own renal tubule, but it is now evident that the peritubular capillary plexus of other neighboring nephrons may also be supplied.

The potential for regulation of the renal circulation by independent modulation of tone of the afferent and efferent glomerular arterioles is obvious. But there is little evidence to support the idea, often advanced, that direct arteriovenous shunts exist. Almost all the blood returns to the venous system from postglomerular capillaries. Separate regulation of cortical and medullary circulations may, however, permit these to vary independently. It seems possible that short circuits that appear to occur within the renal parenchyma result from a rapid flow of blood through a low-pressure system composed of widely dilated normal channels. If such a dilatation should occur in the vessels in one zone of the kidney, such as the juxtamedullary zone, it could preempt the major portion of the renal blood flow, leaving other zones relatively or absolutely underperfused. There is now considerable doubt that such redistribution of blood flow occurs within the kidneys.

Single veins accompany the larger arteries throughout the kidney. Interlobular veins receive blood directly from the cortical capillary plexus. Blood from the medulla enters short, stout, thin-walled veins that run roughly parallel to the arcuate arteries and collect the blood from the bundles of ascending vasa recta. In addition, single ascending vasa recta may pass the arcuate vessels, enter the cortex, and terminate in the interlobular veins. There are no large venous anastomoses within the kidneys, but there are small anastomoses between the arcuate veins that differ, therefore, from the corresponding arteries.

THE JUXTAGLOMERULAR APPARATUS

A functionally important component of the renal vasculature is the juxtaglomerular apparatus. This is usually described as including the afferent and efferent arterioles adjacent to their respective glomerulus, the macula densa of the corresponding distal tubule, and a collection of cells that lie near the glomerular hilus between the afferent and efferent glomerular arterioles.

The juxtaglomerular apparatus begins some 30 to 50 μ proximal to the glomerulus, where the elastic tissue in the wall of the afferent arteriole gradually diminishes and its smooth muscle cells become more rounded and epitheloid in form. Many of these myoepitheloid cells have granules containing the enzyme renin, which activates the angiotensin system. The distal tubule cells, or macula densa, touching the juxtaglomerular cells and afferent arteriole are taller and narrower with fewer mitochondria than the neighboring tubular epithelial cells. From its position and arrangement, this complex seems capable of monitoring the blood in the afferent and efferent arterioles, as well as the urine in this portion of the distal tubule, and of modifying arteriolar tone. These aspects of the function of the juxtaglomerular apparatus are under intensive study. It is known that the myoepithelial cells are the major source of renin and thus play an important role in circulatory and body fluid homeostasis. Evidence is accumulating that they effect an intranephron feedback by which rates of chloride reabsorption in the macula densa cells may modulate the filtration rate of the respective glomerulus (2). With renin substrate (an α_2-globulin) provided to the kidneys via the blood supply, the remainder of the elements required to synthesize the active angiotensin are all present within the kidney (17) and can produce angiotensin II from renin substrate during a single transit of the latter through the kidney.

MEASUREMENT OF RENAL BLOOD FLOW

In the intact animal or human being the clearance techniques devised by Homer W. Smith and his associates remain the standard approach to the measurement of renal blood flow. This methodology is described in Chapter 2. As it is generally applied, the clearance technique using the renal excretion of p-aminohippurate (PAH) at low plasma concentrations (approximately 1.0 mg/dl plasma) suffers from two limitations. The first is that it is assumed that all the PAH is cleared by the kidney on a single transit through that organ or, since the actual extraction averages about 90%, the calculated blood flow is corrected for this mean value of extraction. Whether this incomplete extraction is caused by a failure of all the tubules to extract and secrete all the PAH bathing their peritubular surfaces or by some blood supplying nonfunctioning renal tissue is not known. To correct for possible variations in extraction, the Fick principle may be applied. By catheterization of a renal vein the actual arteriovenous difference in concentration of PAH may be obtained and used to calculate the renal clearance, thus correcting for the incomplete extraction of PAH regardless of its cause.

$$RPF = \frac{UV}{a - v}$$

in which RPF is the renal plasma flow (ml/minute), U is urine concentration of PAH (mg/ml), V is the urine flow (ml/minute), and a and v are arterial and renal venous plasma concentration (mg/ml) of

PAH, respectively. This method of calculating total renal blood flow entails the inconvenience of renal vein catheterization and is, therefore, of very limited usefulness.

A more serious limitation of the renal clearance technique, however, is that it provides no information regarding the distribution of blood flow within the kidneys. It has been suggested repeatedly that alterations in the distribution of blood flow may occur and influence renal function. The classic concept that all nephrons are always perfused (provided adequate perfusion pressure is maintained in the renal arteries), which was based largely on the constancy of the maximal rate of glucose reabsorption, is being challenged, and methods of measuring alterations in the pattern of blood flow within the kidneys in intact subjects are being explored. The startling clinical observation that a kidney removed from a patient dying of hepatorenal syndrome with advanced renal failure may show almost no pathologic changes when examined and may resume function promptly on transplantation into an appropriate subject has heightened the suspicion that the renal failure must be the result of an internal adjustment of the blood flowing through the kidneys.

A method developed by Thorburn, Barger, and co-workers (3) that can be applied to the intact animal or human is the inert gas wash-out technique. In this method a bolus of saline saturated with xenon-133 is injected into the aorta or renal artery via an intraarterial catheter, and the time course of retention of radioactivity in the tissue is monitored by external counting of gamma radiations over the kidneys. Since the radioactive xenon circulating through the kidneys is removed by a process that is blood flow limited, the rate of disappearance of radioactivity from the kidneys is determined by the rate of blood flow through the kidneys. When the counts over the kidney (ordinate) are plotted against time (abscissa), an exponential decay curve is obtained (see Fig. 1-5). This decay curve has several components. Barger and co-workers have shown that the fastest component (or first component) is a measure of cortical blood flow, the second component of outer medullary blood flow, the third of inner medullary and papillary tip blood flow, and the fourth of blood flow to the perihilar structures and renal fat. Because of the uncertainties of fitting exponential curves, the third and fourth components are generally not regarded with much confidence, but the first and second most likely are valid, at least for the normal kidney.

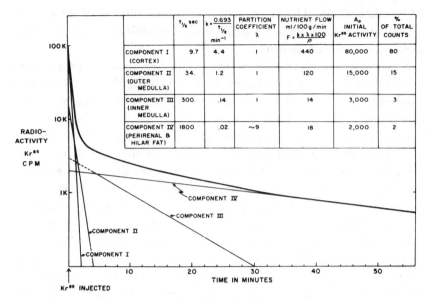

	$t_{1/2}$ sec	$k = \frac{0.693}{t_{1/2}}$ min^{-1}	PARTITION COEFFICIENT λ	NUTRIENT FLOW ml/100g/min $F = \frac{k \times \lambda \times 100}{\rho}$	A_0 INITIAL Kr^{85} ACTIVITY	% OF TOTAL COUNTS
COMPONENT I (CORTEX)	9.7	4.4	1	440	80,000	80
COMPONENT II (OUTER MEDULLA)	34.	1.2	1	120	15,000	15
COMPONENT III (INNER MEDULLA)	300.	.14	1	14	3,000	3
COMPONENT IV (PERIRENAL & HILAR FAT)	1800.	.02	~9	18	2,000	2

Fig. 1-5 The kinetics of "washout" from the kidney of krypton-85 injected into the renal artery (3). Reprinted from ref. 3 by permission of the American Heart Association.

Although interesting changes in these two components in a variety of states of altered renal function have been reported (4) the findings have not been confirmed with other methods. The gas wash-out technique has the great advantage that it can be used in the intact animal; the findings, however, must be interpreted most cautiously, in view of the mutually contradictory reports that have appeared. Attempts have been made to measure alterations in regional blood flow and in nephron filtration rates following physiologic and pharmacologic manipulation. With the use of other methods, including single-nephron filtration rates from cortical and juxtamedullary glomeruli (5, 6), microspheres (7, 8), glomerular basement membrane antibodies (9, 10), Hansen's technique (11, 12, 13), radiolabeled frog red blood cells (14), and angiography (15, 16)—all but the last mentioned requiring sacrifice of the animal—different and often contradictory findings have been reported, some confirming and others denying the occurrence of intrarenal changes in perfusion or filtration. Writing this paragraph for the 1st Edition with 52 articles on the subject in front of me, all of which appeared in 4 years' time—and a limited sample at that—from many highly reputable laboratories, I can only conclude that confusion reigns in this important area of renal physiology. Reviewing the situation at the time of preparing the 2nd Edition, I find that the state of confusion still persists. Clearly, when the truth is known, a major advance will be made in our understanding of the operation of the kidneys, where circulation and function are so closely integrated.

References

1. Fourman, J. and Moffat, D. B. The blood vessels of the kidney, Blackwell, Oxford pp. 1–161, 1971.
2. Thurau, K., Dahlheim, H., Grüner, A., Mason, J., and Granger, P. Activation of renin in the single juxtaglomerular apparatus by sodium chloride in the tubular fluid at the macula densa. Circ. Res. 30–31, Suppl. II, 182–198, 1972.
3. Thorburn, G. D., Kopald, H. H., Herd, A. J., Hollenberg, M., O'Morchoe, C. C., and Barger, A. D. Intrarenal distribution of nutrient blood flow determined with krypton^{85} in the unanesthetized dog. Circ. Res. 13:290–307, 1963.
4. Barger, A. C. and Herd, J. A. The renal circulation. New Eng. J. Med. 284: 482–490, 1971.
5. Mandin, H., Israelit, A. H., Rector, F. C., Jr., and Seldin, D. W. Effect of saline infusions in intrarenal distribution of glomerular filtrate and proximal reabsorption in the dog. J. Clin. Invest. 50:514–522, 1971.
6. Rouffignac, C. de. Do similar factors control the glomerular filtration rate of superficial and juxtamedullary nephrons? Proc. VIth Int. Cong. Nephrol., Abs. of Symposia, pp. 47–48, 1975.
7. Stein, J. H., Boonjaren, S., Wilson, C. B., and Ferris, T. F. Alterations in intrarenal blood flow distribution. Methods of measurement and relationship to sodium balance. Circ. Res. 32 & 33:61–71, 1973.
8. Katz, M. A., Blantz, R. D., Rector, F. C., Jr., and Seldin, D. W. Measurement of intrarenal blood flow: I. Analysis of microsphere method. Am. J. Physiol. 220:1903–1913, 1971.
9. Wallin, J. D., Rector, F. C., Jr., and Seldin, D. W. Effect of volume expansion on intrarenal distribution of plasma flow in the dog. Am. J. Physiol. 223:125–129, 1972.
10. Blantz, R. C., Wallin, J. D., Rector, F. C., Jr., and Seldin, D. W. Effect of variation in dietary NaCl intake on the intrarenal distribution of plasma flow in the rat. J. Clin. Invest. 51:2790–2395, 1972.
11. Hansen, O. E. The relationship between glomerular filtration rate and length of the proximal convoluted tubule in mice. Acta Pathol. Microbiol. Scand. 53: 265, 1961.
12. Bruns, F. J., Alexander, E. A., Riley, A. L., and Levinsky, N. G. Superficial and juxtamedullary nephron function during saline loading in the dog. J. Clin. Invest. 53:971–979, 1974.
13. Davis, J. M., Brechtelsbauer, H., Prucksunand, P., Weigl, J. Schnermann, J., and Kramer, W. Relationship between salt loading and distribution of nephron filtration rates in the dog. Plügers Arch. 350:259–272, 1974.
14. Baehler, R. W., Catanzaro, A. J., Stein, J. H., and Hunter, W. The radio-

labeled frog red blood cell. A new marker of cortical blood flow distribution in the kidney of the dog. Circ. Res. 32:718–724, 1973.

15. Sherwood, J. and Lavender, J. P. Renal medulla perfusion. Direct observations by fine detail angiography in the dog. Nephron 8:317–328, 1971.

16. Thind, G. S., Biery, D. N., Baum, S., Blakemore, W. S., and Zinsser, H. F. Use of *in vivo* magnification renal arteriography to study cadmium effects on vasoactive responses. Radiology 99:279–286, 1971.

17. Davalos, M., Frega, N. S., Saker, B., and Leaf, A. Effect of exogenous and endogenous angiotensin II in the isolated perfused rat kidney. Am. J. Physiol: Renal Fluid Electrolyte Physiol. 4(6):F605–F610, 1978.

2
Renal Physiology: An Introduction

INTRODUCTION

The kidney has many functions in addition to excreting the waste products of metabolism. Claude Bernard, the great nineteenth-century French physiologist, was the first to appreciate that higher animals "have really two environments: a *milieu extérieur* in which the organism is situated, and a *milieu intérieur* in which the tissue elements live." The latter is the extracellular fluid that bathes the cells of the body and is the true milieu of life; the kidney is the organ par excellence for maintaining the constancy of this internal environment, regulating the quantity of water, sodium, chloride, and numerous other ions and solutes in the body through excretion and retention.

In the last analysis, as Homer Smith indicated, the composition of the "internal environment" is determined, not by what the body takes in, but by what is retained and what is excreted. Waste products must be excreted to avoid autointoxication. The acid–base balance of the body is ultimately regulated by the kidneys; hydrogen ions are excreted or retained to maintain the normal pH of body fluids. But the kidney does more than this. It is also an endocrine gland secreting at least two important hormones. One is erythropoietin, which stimulates red cell production in the bone marrow. The other hormone, angiotensin, plays a dual role in regulating the blood pressure directly and indirectly by stimulating the adrenal cortex to secrete aldosterone, which in turn activates the kidneys to retain sodium. Vitamin D is now known to possess the characteristics of a hormone rather than of a dietary factor, and the last step in its synthesis occurs in the kidney. The kidney is also a major producer of prostaglandins.

It is generally thought that life on our planet had its origins in the brackish waters of the primeval oceans. When the first metazoan established itself on dry land, it took with it a bit of this primitive ocean to carry about as its extracellular fluid. The kidneys have succeeded in preserving the salinity of the primeval oceans, while modern ocean waters became much more concentrated as salts and minerals were leached from the land.

The kidney appears to function in a roundabout way. It first filters out from the plasma a large volume of protein-free filtrate (in the glomeruli) and then reabsorbs from this filtrate all the constituents the body needs (1). Since approximately one-fourth of the cardiac output perfuses the two kidneys, the fluid and solute exchanges in the kidney are enormous. In a normal 80-kg male, a glomerular filtration rate of 180 liters/24 hours would be a usual value; this is more than 10 times the volume of the subject's total extracellular fluid. Since the 24-hour urine output is approximately 1 liter, some 179 liters of glomerular filtrate must be reabsorbed by the renal tubules daily. The normal sodium concentration in plasma is approximately 140 mEq/liter. Thus, approximately 25,200 mEq of sodium are filtered per day at the glomeruli. Since sodium excretion must, on the average, be equal to the dietary salt intake for a steady state to exist, only some 100 to 200 mEq of sodium are excreted in the daily urine; thus 25,000 mEq of sodium must be reabsorbed to preserve body composition. This apparently extravagant function is highly effective in removing from the body the waste products of metabolism that are also filtered through the glomeruli. If tubular reabsorption of such wastes is limited, they are excreted efficiently in large amounts in the urine and their concentration in the body is kept very low. A kidney that began its development in the watery abundance of primeval lakes and rivers could afford to be extravagant in its handling of water, provided it effectively rid itself of waste products. A large volume of glomerular filtrate serves this purpose.

As animal life spread to land, to fresh water, and to modern oceans of high salinity, modifications in the kidney were required. On land the need is for the kidneys to conserve both salt and water. Higher animals, as will be discussed, developed a means of conserving water so effectively that some species can live in the most arid regions and maintain their water balance. Fish living in fresh water, on the other hand, are never short of water, but must conserve sodium effectively. Amphibia can absorb sodium chloride through their skins from very low concentrations of salt in freshwater ponds, and excrete a urine free of salt. Saltwater fish compensate for the inability of their kidneys to excrete a concentrated urine by ridding themselves through their gills of the excess sodium chloride they ingest. In a few species of salt-water fish, the glomeruli have actually atrophied. Such aglomerular fish secrete waste products into their tubules without risking the potential hazard of dehydration by loss of glomerular filtrate. With a variety of such adjustments the kidney has successfully surmounted environmental obstacles to allow animal species to populate all parts of our globe.

FUNCTIONAL AND MORPHOLOGIC DIFFERENTIATION IN THE NEPHRON

Figure 2-1 depicts a typical nephron schematically. Figure 2-2 compares a cortical nephron with a juxtamedullary nephron. Juxtamedullary nephrons, with their long loops of Henle, play a major role in concentrating the urine. In man the ratio of short cortical to long juxtamedullary nephrons is estimated as 7 to 1.

The glomerulus

The glomerulus consists of a capillary tuft that has invaginated Bowman's capsule. Thus, the membrane across which ultrafiltration occurs has several layers. By electron microscopy, the glomerular capillary wall is seen to consist of three structural layers; from inside out, these are the endothelial cells, the basement membrane, and the visceral epithelial cells. The endothelial cells are perforated by fenestrae, 500 to 1000 Å wide, through which solute and water readily pass. The basement membrane, between the endothelial and epithelial cells, is a continuous, nonporous structure about 1500 Å in thickness. The basement membrane, in turn, consists of an inner lucent layer, the lamina rara interna; a middle amorphous dense layer, the lamina densa; and

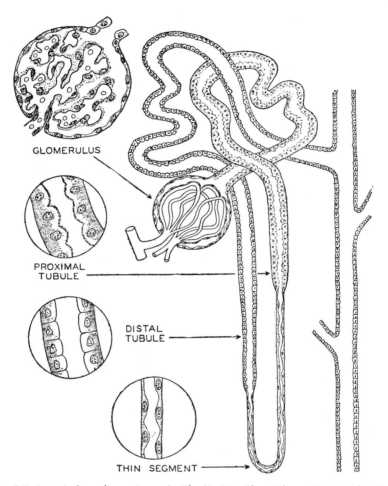

Fig. 2-1 A typical nephron. From Smith, H. W., *The Kidney* (New York: Oxford University Press, 1935) by permission of the publisher.

an external lucent layer, the lamina rara externa. The epithelial cells lining the visceral surface of Bowman's space possess interdigitating "foot processes" that rest on the basement membrane; these foot processes are separated by the so-called filtration slits, which are bridged by a thin diaphragm (Fig. 2-3). Since albumin, with a molecular weight of about 68,000, does not normally appear in the urine in more than trace amounts (30–120 mg/24 hours), the size of the albumin molecule was once thought to exceed the critical dimensions for filtration. Actually, the porosity of the glomerular capillary wall is not so refined, and some albumin normally escapes through the glomerular membranes only to be largely reabsorbed by the proximal tubular epithelium. In disease states affecting the glomeruli, the quantities of albumin filtered may be in excess of the limited reabsorptive capacity of the proximal tubule, and then large amounts of albumin will appear in the urine.

Physiologic data indicate that filtration of macromolecules (includ-

Fig. 2-2 A short cortical nephron compared with a longer juxtamedullary nephron. From Smith, H. W., *The Kidney* (New York: Oxford University Press, 1935) by permission of the publisher.

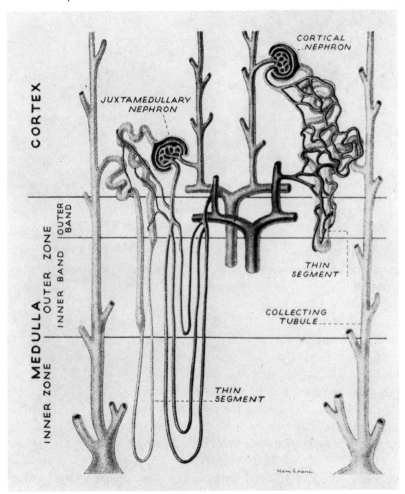

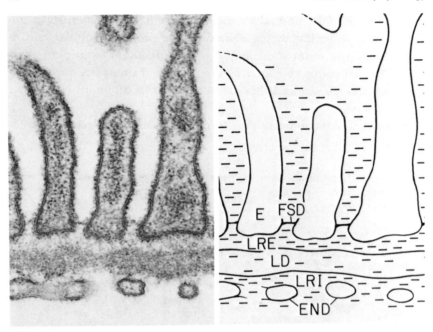

Fig. 2-3 Electron micrograph (left) and schematic drawing (right) of the components of the glomerular capillary wall. END, endothelium; LRI, lamina rara interna; LD, lamina densa; LRE, lamina rara externa; E, foot processes of the visceral epithelium; FSD, filtration slit diaphragm. Note that the negatively charged polyanion is present along the endothelium, lamina rara interna, and lamina rara externa and covers the epithelial cells (courtesy of Dr. M. A. Venkatachalam).

ing plasma proteins) across the glomerular wall decreases with increasing effective molecular radius, approaching zero at a radius of approximately 35 Å, which is the size of serum albumin (2). From electron microscopic studies with tracer particles (for example, ferritin, dextrans, and peroxidases of differing molecular weights) it has been concluded that the basement membrane at the level of the lamina rara interna is the principal structure responsible for this size discrimination (3–5), although pores of appropriate dimensions (35 Å) have not been demonstrated. But in addition to size, it has recently been shown that the electrical charge of the filtering molecules, as well as the electrophysical characteristics of the glomerular capillary wall, are important determinants of the permeability to proteins (4–6). The glomerular capillary wall contains abundant sialoproteins and is negatively charged. Passage of molecules that bear a net positive charge (cationic) will thus be facilitated, whereas anionic molecules will be hindered by the fixed negative charges in the membrane. These conclusions come from physiologic studies, in which dextrans (6, 7) and horseradish peroxidase (4) of equal size but different net charges were used; ultrastructural studies also show increased filtration of cationic ferritin molecules as compared to anionic molecules of the same size (3, 8). This charge discrimination is important in the virtual complete exclusion of albumin from the filtrate, since albumin is an anionic molecule with its isoelectric point at a pH of 4.5. Loss of fixed negative charges of the glomerular wall is now believed to be an important cause of both the proteinuria and the characteristic epithelial changes in some forms of human glomerulonephritis (7).

The role of the epithelial slit diaphragm in glomerular permeability is unclear. Rodewald and Karnovsky (7) showed that this fine membrane, which stretches between the foot processes of the epithelial cells, forms a continuous junctional band 300 to 450 Å wide. The membrane exhibits a zipper-like substructure, with alternating periodic cross-bridges extending from the plasma membranes to a central filament that runs between and parallel to the cell membranes. This substructure defines a uniform population of rectangular pores approximately 40×140 Å in cross section, and 70 Å apart. The measured pores occupy an area about 2 to 3% of the total surface area of the glomerular capillary, a figure that is remarkably close to that calculated for the total filtration surface by hydraulic conductivity data. In addition, tracer experiments with peroxidases of various molecular weights (8, 9) and cationic ferritin (5) suggest that the epithelial slits may also present an additional barrier to the proteins that pass through the basement membrane.

Although the individual glomeruli are microscopic, there are some 2 million nephrons in the two kidneys of the adult human, and the total glomerular capillary surface is estimated to be some 1.6 m², an area nearly as large as the total body surface. Filtration through this large surface is enhanced by the relatively large fraction of the surface through which filtration may occur: 2 to 3% of glomerular capillary surface compared with 0.1% of muscle capillaries (10). It is this large filtration surface that accommodates the huge volume of glomerular filtration—about 180 liters/day. The contribution of each glomerulus, however, to this initial step in urine formation is a filtration, on the average, of only 90 μl/day.

   Conditions in the glomerulus are optimal for promoting filtration. The large endothelial surface is subject to hydrostatic pressures that are normally about 60% of the mean arterial pressure. This hydrostatic pressure, favoring filtration from the glomerular capillaries, is opposed by the oncotic pressure of proteins and macromolecules in the blood plasma (about 25 mm Hg) and by renal tubular pressure. Dilatation of the afferent arteriole transmits a higher fraction of mean arterial pressure to the filtering surface, as does constriction of the efferent glomerular arteriole. Constriction of the afferent arteriole or dilatation of the efferent arteriole or both lowers the effective filtration pressure in the glomerulus. Thus, within the limts of usual arterial pressures, the filtration rate can be stabilized. Urine flow ceases, however, at a mean arterial pressure of about 60 mm Hg, which indicates that filtration stops at approximately this arterial pressure.

   Using a strain of rats with glomeruli situated directly on the renal cortical surface, Brenner and associates (11, 12, 13) have characterized the dynamics of glomerular ultrafiltration. Directly measured, glomerular transcapillary hydraulic pressure differences averaged about 35 mm Hg, or approximately 50% of mean systemic arterial values. From similar direct estimates of hydrostatic pressure in the proximal tubules and colloid osmotic pressures in systemic and efferent glomerular arteriolar plasma, these authors calculated the average net driving force for ultrafiltration in the glomerulus to be about 15 mm Hg at the afferent end of the glomerular capillary network. Knowing the driving force for filtration in a glomerulus and the single-nephron glomerular filtration rate, they were able to calculate the glomerular capillary ultrafiltration coefficient, which averaged 0.08 nl $(sec)^{-1}$ $(cm\ H_2O)^{-1}$ $(glomerulus)^{-1}$, or approximately 40 nl $(sec)^{-1}$ $(mm\ Hg)^{-1}\ cm^{-2}$; that is, one to two orders of magnitude larger than values reported for other capillaries. The high value of filtration permeability allows filtration pressure equilibrium to occur at the usual rates of glomerular capillary plasma flow in this species. That is, the filtration process at the afferent end of the glomerular capillary bed causes a rise in plasma protein concentration within the glomerular capillaries such that the increase in oncotic pressure opposing filtration nullifies the hydrostatic filtration pressure, and filtration ceases before the plasma enters the efferent glomerular capillary. Only under conditions involving high rates of glomerular capillary plasma flow [> 150 nl $(glomerulus)^{-1}$ $(min)^{-1}$ in the rat, a value approximately double the normal flow rate

in a hydropenic rat] was filtration disequilibrium achieved in Brenner's studies. It appears that filtration equilibrium may be the exception, however, and that disequilibrium exists in most species.

The Proximal Tubule

The proximal tubule extends from the glomerulus to the loop of Henle. It is easily recognized histologically by its large epithelial cells with brush borders nearly occluding the tubular lumens in fixed sections.

The function of this segment of the nephron is to reabsorb from the copious glomerular filtrate solutes and water that are essential to the body. The term *tubular reabsorption* refers to the direction of transport from tubular lumen across or between tubular epithelial cells, through the peritubular interstitium, and into the blood. We know from micropuncture studies that some 60 to 80% of the glomerular filtrate is reabsorbed by the proximal tubule and that this reabsorption takes place isotonically. In mammals the concentration of chloride increases along the proximal tubule. Since the osmolarity remains unchanged and the volume decreases, it could be surmised that bicarbonate must be reabsorbed in the proximal tubule. We know today that most hydrogen ion secretion by the kidney (about 90%) occurs in the proximal tubule. This is the means by which most of the filtered bicarbonate is recovered to preserve acid–base balance, a process discussed in detail in Chapter 4.

The structure of the proximal tubule is adapted to its function of reabsorbing large amounts of the filtered sodium chloride and water. The luminal surface shows many microvilli creating a brush border. Adjacent tubular cells are attached near their apical ends. This configuration has been likened to a "beer six-pack," with the intercellular attachments corresponding to the plastic rings holding the six-pack together (43). The peritubular side has a labyrinthian configuration created by extensive interdigitations of adjacent cells. This can be seen in Fig. 2-4. Both the luminal brush border and the labyrinthine basolateral infoldings of these cells greatly increase the surfaces available for reabsorption. As estimated from the morphometric analysis of the Wellings (44), there is between 50 and 100 m of junction/cm^2 of tissue surface in the proximal nephron.

The layer of cells lining the proximal tubule is a "leaky" epithelium; that is it accommodates a large flow of solute and water in the

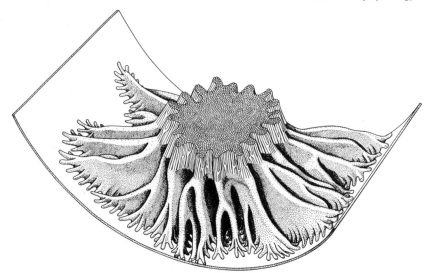

Fig. 2-4 Diagrammatic representation of a single, proximal, convoluted tubular cell resting on the basement membrane. Note the luminal microvilli and labyrinthine basal lateral infoldings of these cells, which greatly increase the surfaces available for reabsorption. From ref. 44, courtesy of Dr. L. W. Welling.

process of tubular reabsorption. The cell junctions are near their luminal surface and though traditionally they have been referred to as "tight" junctions, this is a misnomer as they are now recognized as important pathways for fluid and solute transport. Electrical resistance between lumen and peritubular fluid is much less than across the plasma membrane of individual cells, confirming that the intercellular channels constitute low resistance pathways across the proximal tubules. Thus, typical cell membrane resistances are of the order of 10^3 to 10^4 ohm-cm^2. An epithelium of tightly sealed cells would require an imposed transepithelial electric current to cross two plasma membranes and should have a resistance of this order. By contrast, mammalian proximal tubules give a transepithelial ohmic resistance of only some 5 ohm-cm^2, indicating that the intercellular junctions are leaky and provide a paracellular pathway for the flow of water, small molecules, and ions.

The transport system for sodium and chloride across the epithelial cells has a high capacity. The sodium chloride pumped out of the cells through their basolateral walls create local hypertonicity in the intercellular spaces, according to the hypothesis of Diamond (16). Since the apical (luminal) surfaces of these cells are highly permeable to water, water follows the sodium chloride from the tubular fluid into the intercellular spaces. With lower resistance to flow toward the base of the cells than toward the apex, the hydrostatic pressures created in the intercellular spaces force the fluid into the peritubular interstitium. By the time the reabsorbed fluid emerges from the tortuous intercellular spaces, the fluid has become isotonic with the luminal fluid. This arrangement, depicted in Fig. 2-5, would ensure reabsorption of a fluid isotonic with the luminal fluid. Whether the dimensions of the intercellular spaces and the distribution of sodium pump sites along the basolateral plasma membranes are such as to support this hypothesis is still controversial (45, 46). Another view is that the permeability of the tubular epithelium to water is so high that even gradients of reabsorbed solutes, which are too small to be measured across the tubular cells, will allow water to be reabsorbed osmotically (47). This latter view verges on an efficient "solute drag" mechanism, in which the reabsorbed solute sweeps water along with it in the proportion of water to solute that exists in the luminal fluid.

The proximal tubule reabsorbs large amounts of sodium chloride,

Fig. 2-5 Schematic representation of pathways of fluid reabsorption in the proximal tubule; to illustrate the postulated role of lateral intercellular spaces.

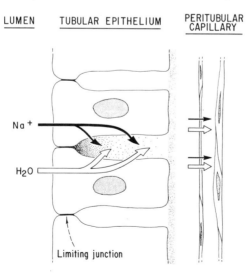

LUMEN   TUBULAR EPITHELIUM   PERITUBULAR
                                   CAPILLARY

Na$^+$

H$_2$O

Limiting junction

and this is, quantitatively, its major function. Although this salt re-absorption normally occurs in the absence of concentration gradients for sodium and with only small electrical gradients across the proxi-mal tubular epithelium, it is thought to be an active, energy-requiring process. When mannitol, or another poorly reabsorbed solute, is added to the urine in the proximal tubule, net reabsorption of sodium (and of fluid) continues until the sodium concentration in tubular fluid has fallen to some 70% of its concentration in plasma (17). This evidence of "uphill" transport of sodium, albeit modest when compared with the gradients established in the distal nephron, establishes that the transport processes are thermodynamically "active." The proximal tu-bule has a large capacity for sodium chloride reabsorption, while wa-ter moves passively and secondarily to the movement of this major solute.

Several mechanisms seem to participate in the reabsorption of large amounts of sodium chloride in the proximal tubule:

1. In the earliest portion of the proximal tubule, sodium is reab-sorbed by cotransport with glucose, amino acids, phosphate, and probably other essential small molecules. That is, sodium, main-tained at low concentrations within the proximal tubule cells by being pumped across the basolateral plasma membranes, moves on a carrier down its concentration and electrical gradient from the luminal fluid to the cell interior with a glucose, an amino acid or some other molecule coupled to the same carrier. The free energy available to move sodium from the luminal fluid into the cell across the brush border is sufficient to carry along a cotransported glucose or other molecule, which may actually be concentrated within the tubular cell thereby. The sodium ion is subsequently pumped into the peritubular fluid by the energy-requiring sodium, potassium-dependent adenosinetriphosphatase (Na, K-ATPase) to complete its reabsorption from the glomerular filtrate. Glucose or amino acid can passively cross the basolateral plasma membrane into the peritubular fluid moving down its concentration gradient (see Fig. 2-6). Such cotransport with sodium accommodates the re-absorption of glucose, amino acids, phosphate, and probably other important solutes, all at the expense of the energy provided for the extrusion of sodium from the cell interior across the basolat-eral plasma membrane. The cotransported molecules depend upon the simultaneous transport of sodium ions for their reabsorption

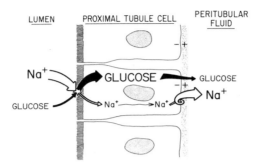

Fig. 2-6 Schematic representation of cotransport of glucose with sodium ions from the tubular lumen across the brush border into the cell. Sodium is subsequently actively "pumped" out of the cell across the basolateral plasma membrane, and glucose reabsorption is completed passively across this cell membrane.

and, in turn, sodium cannot be reabsorbed on these specialized carriers in their absence; a mutual interdependence exists between sodium and its cotransported molecules in this initial step of entry from tubular lumen into the renal tubular cells.

2. The secretion of hydrogen ions into the proximal tubule, which results in bicarbonate reabsorption, is in effect an ion exchange whreby a sodium ion is reabsorbed for each hydronium secreted (see Chapter 4).

3. The effect of bicarbonate reabsorption in the proximal tubule of mammals is to increase the intraluminal concentration of chloride ion relative to its concentration in the peritubular fluid. This creates a diffusion gradient for chloride ion that favors its reabsorption, and positive sodium ions are pulled along by the weak electrical forces so generated across the permeable proximal tubular epithelium. In fact, experimental removal of bicarbonate from the perfused proximal tubule reduces salt and water reabsorption in the proximal tubule by about one-third.

4. The fact that the cardiac glycoside ouabain, a potent inhibitor of Na, K-ATPase, can block 50% or more of sodium chloride reabsorption in the proximal tubule *in vitro* is regarded as evidence that much of the sodium reabsorption occurs via "conventional" sodium transport mechanisms.

Thus, the large isotonic reabsorption of sodium chloride across the highly permeable proximal tubule is accomplished by several different mechanisms, each contributing an unknown, but perhaps variable amount to the total process. It is probably correct that ions transported actively move *through* the transporting epithelial cells while their counterions move via low-resistance shunt pathways *between* the cells.

Measurements of the electrical potential across proximal tubular epithelium have yielded conflicting results. It now seems established, however, that the potentials are very small (18, 19). In one careful micropuncture study *in vivo,* in the rat (19), low potentials were found, and they varied and even changed polarity when measured along the length of the proximal tubule. In the first proximal loops, the transtubular potential was found to be negative (lumen relative to peritubular fluid), averaging − 0.8 mV. In more distal portions of the proximal tubules, the polarity reversed and the potential was positive, averaging + 1.6 mV. A consistent profile of potential difference was thus established under normal conditions with the first segments having negative, in contrast to subsequent segments with positive potential differences.

The potential differences observed relate to the dominant reabsorptive activities in the first as contrasted with subsequent segments of the proximal tubules. Cotransport of glucose with sodium occurs throughout the proximal tubule, but normally glucose reabsorption is completed in the first 15 to 20% of the proximal tubule. Sodium reabsorption is "electrogenic" in that it creates separation of electrical charge, leaving the lumen slightly negative to the peritubular fluid, and thus is responsible for the small negative potentials measured in the first segment of the proximal tubule.

Sodium reabsorption in ion exchange for secreted hydronium also occurs along the length of the proximal tubule. This is an electrically neutral exchange of positive ions at the luminal brush border and an electrically neutral movement of sodium bicarbonate from cell interior to peritubular fluid. Since it causes the reabsorption of sodium bicarbonate from the luminal fluid, the concentration of chloride in this fluid rises to that of sodium. The electrochemical gradients for sodium and chloride ions are, however, unequal. Chloride diffuses down its concentration gradient from luminal to peritubular fluid, creating the small positive transtubular potential difference that dominates subsequent segments of the proximal tubule and provides the driving force for further sodium reabsorption.

The reabsorption of sodium and chloride by these processes presumably establishes a small osmotic gradient across the highly permeable proximal tubular epithelium, which causes bulk flow via intercellular channels. By solvent drag a further moiety of sodium chloride reabsorption will occur.

Finally, as bicarbonate reabsorption progresses, its concentration in tubular fluid falls to very low levels, so that now a diffusion gradient is established for bicarbonate secretion. The bicarbonate that diffuses from peritubular fluid back into the lumen of the tubule will be reabsorbed again by further hydronium secretion in exchange for sodium reabsorption.

It is by these several processes in the proximal tubule that some 65% of filtered sodium and chloride are reabsorbed together with all the glucose, amino acids, and bicarbonate in the glomerular filtrate. Active sodium transport accounts for the negative potentials measured in the early proximal tubule and the small positive potentials through the later segments are attributable to chloride diffusion potentials.

Our understanding of the factors that regulate proximal tubular reabsorption of sodium is incomplete. Aldosterone and vasopressin, which so profoundly affect the distal reabsorption of salt and water, respectively, have no demonstrable effect on proximal tubular reabsorption. de Wardener and associates (20) demonstrated, however, that expansion of extracellular fluid volume by the infusion of saline solutions diminished the fraction of glomerular filtrate volume reabsorbed in the proximal tubule. The factor (or more likely, factors) involved are referred to as "third factor." The phenomenon can be demonstrated to occur even when the glomerular filtration rate is reduced by renal artery constriction and when an excess of hormones known to affect sodium and water reabsorption is present. An intensive search has thus far failed to establish humoral factors as regulators of this phenomenon although the likelihood that one or more natriuretic factors exists becomes increasingly probable.

One factor that seems to be important, however, is the oncotic pressure of serum proteins in the peritubular capillaries (21). Saline infusions expand extracellular fluid volume and dilute the serum proteins. This reduces the oncotic pressure, drawing fluid from the renal interstitium back into the peritubular capillaries. The resulting accumulation of salt and water in the renal interstitium enhances diffusion of sodium back from the intercellular spaces to the tubular lumen (22) and thus depresses the net reabsorption of sodium and water, leading to rejection of an increased fraction of the glomerular filtrate by the proximal tubule.

It is thought that the oncotic pressure within the peritubular capillaries does not actually provide the driving forces for reabsorption of tubular contents. The ability of the proximal tubule to produce a small gradient of sodium chloride concentration when the presence of nonreabsorbable solute prevents water reabsorption, as described above, is evidence that sodium chloride is reabsorbed actively. Furthermore, when protein was added by micropuncture to the proximal tubular fluid so that the oncotic pressure within the tubule equaled that within the peritubular capillaries net reabsorption of salt and water from tubular lumen still occurred (23). Though salt reabsorption is considered an active, energy-requiring process in the proximal tubule, the oncotic pressure within peritubular capillaries can apparently modify the rate of reabsorption.

In addition to reabsorbing sodium, chloride, and water and secreting hydrogen ions to effect the reabsorption of bicarbonate, the proximal tubule has other important functions. Glucose, amino acids, phosphate, uric acid, proteins, and potassium—to name a few important body constituents—are reabsorbed from the glomerular filtrate in the proximal tubule. In addition to hydrogen ions, other substances are secreted in the proximal tubule. Thus, organic acids, p-aminohippurate, phenol red, penicillin, and certain iodinated compounds useful as contrast material for visualizing the kidneys by x-ray are added to the urine by transport from the peritubular capillaries to the luminal fluid across the renal tubular epithelial cells as well as by filtration at the glomerulus. It is most interesting that the substances secreted by the tubules are largely foreign to the body; they compete with each other for the secretory transport system. Probenecid blocks the common secretory mechanism for this seemingly diverse group of substances. In certain diseases of the kidneys individual proximal tubular functions are impaired. In renal glycosuria, for instance, impairment of glucose reabsorption alone occurs. In other diseases more than one function may be lost; the extreme case is the Fanconi syndrome, characterized by partial or complete loss of all proximal tubular functions.

The loop of Henle

The loop of Henle commences where the pars recta of the proximal tubule dips downward into the renal medulla. In man the nephrons with outer cortical glomeruli have only short loops of Henle, whereas the glomeruli situated deep in the cortex, of the juxtamedullary nephrons, connect through their proximal tubules with very long loops of Henle that penetrate deep into the medulla and the pyramidal tip of the kidney. In fact, the inner zone of the medulla consists only of loops of Henle with their associated peritubular portal capillary system and collecting ducts. The loops of Henle and the capillaries make hairpin turns back toward the cortex, emerging close to their respective glomeruli. The loop of Henle has two anatomically and functionally distinct segments. From the end of the proximal tubule past the hairpin turn is the "thin segment." This becomes the thicker "ascending segment" in the outer medulla, which terminates at the macula densa of its respective juxtaglomerular apparatus in the cortex.

Although anatomists were long aware of the presence of the loop of Henle, its function was discovered only in the early 1950s. Before then physiologists had observed that only in the kidneys of birds and mammals did the loop of Henle exist and that these were the only members of the animal kingdom capable of excreting a urine hypertonic to the serum. In 1951 two physical chemists, Hargitay and Kuhn (24), working in Switzerland, pointed out the similarity between the anatomic arrangements of the loops of Henle and the design of countercurrent systems, well known to engineers.

Unlike all other tissues of the body, which were isosmotic with extracellular fluid ($\sim$280–290 mOsm/kg tissue water), the renal medulla is hypertonic. Following the suggestion of Kuhn, Wirz (25) established this hypertonicity of the renal medulla by measuring the melting temperature of frozen sections of various parts of the kidney. All the components of the medulla—tubular urine, tubular cells, interstitial fluid, capillaries, and blood—show this increased tonicity (total solute concentration). There is a tonicity gradient throughout the inner medulla, increasing to maximal values at the tips of the pyramids. This gradient of concentration from the isotonic renal cortex to maximal values at the tip of the renal papillae is the result of the activity of the renal countercurrent systems; the loops of Henle serve as countercurrent multipliers and the capillaries as simple countercurrent exchangers.

It has long been appreciated that the human kidney can excrete urinary solutes in a small volume of very concentrated urine (about 1000 mOsm/liter) under conditions of water deprivation or in a very dilute (approximately 50 mOsm/liter), copious urine when an abundance of water has been ingested. Man has not evolved mechanisms for the active transport of water; instead, gradients of water concentration (or of solute concentration) are produced by the active transport of solute. Water moves passively and secondarily to solute transport. Thus, how urine is concentrated or diluted must depend on how solute is transported and compartmentalized in the kidney.

The concept of countercurrent exchangers and countercurrent multipliers has long been known and used by engineers; its application to biology has only recently been appreciated. Figure 2-7 illustrates the general principle. A straight tube accommodating a flow of water at 10 ml/minute passes over a heat source that yields 100 cal/minute. If the water flowing into the tube has a temperature of 30° C, and all the heat is absorbed, the temperature of the effluent would be 40° C. The lower part of Figure 2-7 depicts what might occur if the tube were bent back upon itself in a hairpin curve. With the same flow rate and heat source the effluent would again emerge 10° C warmer than the entering fluid. But the efficient transfer of heat from the warmer fluid leaving the heat source to the cooler entering water might result in much higher temperatures at the tip of the hairpin turn, as depicted.

A biological example of passive countercurrent exchange can be cited. Physiologists had wondered how wading birds sustain their body temperatures when standing long hours in near-freezing water. An anatomic study of the relation of the arteries and veins to the feet revealed that they are organized as a countercurrent exchange system (26). The arteries carrying warm blood to the extremities are surrounded by a net of veins bringing cold blood from the feet back to the body. This arrangement allows transfer of heat from arterial to venous blood so that the blood finally reaching the immersed feet is cold and loses little further heat to the frigid water. The venous blood, thus warmed, does not cool the body excessively upon its return.

The juxtaposition and counterflow in the descending and ascending limbs of this heat exchanger permit an efficient but entirely passive transfer of heat. By contrast, a countercurrent multiplier requires energy to transfer heat or matter from one limb to the other and thus is capable of generating gradients of heat or of matter. Exchangers and multipliers are both present in the kidneys. The blood supply through the vasa recta to the inner medulla and pyramids protects and preserves the gradient of osmolality, which increases progressively from the cortex to the tips of the papillae, by countercurrent exchange. The source

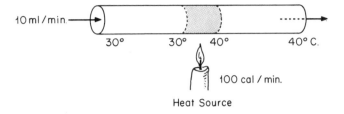

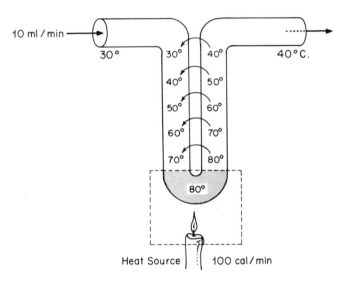

Fig. 2-7 Countercurrent principle.

of the solute gradient is, however, the result of countercurrent multipliers, the loops of Henle.

As described earlier, approximately 35% of the glomerular filtrate escapes reabsorption in the proximal tubule and enters the loop of Henle. How this fluid is modified in the countercurrent multiplier is shown schematically in Figure 2-8 (2). In this figure the process by which solute is concentrated some four times over isotonic is divided into two steps: column advancement and gradient formation. An ability to transport solute to a maximal gradient of 200 mOsm/liter between efferent and afferent limbs of the loop is assumed, and stepwise

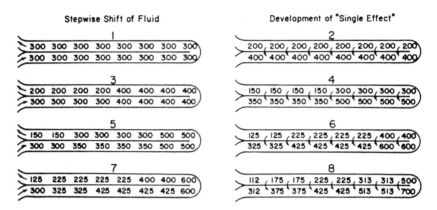

Fig. 2-8 Schematic operation of a countercurrent multiplier. From Pitts, Robert F.: *Physiology of the Kidney and Body Fluids.* Copyright © 1974 by Year Book Medical Publishers, Inc., Chicago. Used by permission.

changes are indicated. Gradient formation is shown (Step 2) as resulting in a concentration of 200 and 400 mOsm/liter in efferent and afferent limbs, respectively. Column advancement (Step 3) then brings the more concentrated fluid into the ascending limb so that the next step of gradient formation results in concentrations of 300 mOsm/liter in efferent and 500 mOsm/liter in afferent limbs near the hairpin turn, while the effluent becomes progressively more dilute (Step 4). Repetition of column advancement and gradient formation thus creates, by means of a relatively small gradient of transport from efferent to afferent limbs, a very large gradient along the longitudinal axis of the hairpin loop.

In the renal medulla, sodium chloride is the solute that undergoes transport. This salt is pumped from the ascending limb of the loop of Henle into the interstitium. The resulting increased osmolality of the interstitium draws water from the descending limb, so that its contents rises progressively toward the hairpin turn. By contrast, the ascending limb is impermeable to water, so that outward transport of sodium chloride progressively dilutes the tubular fluid, as it returns to the renal cortex to enter the distal convoluted tubule. This fluid may emerge at less than one-half the solute concentration of body fluids. More salt may be reabsorbed in the collecting ducts, making the fluid even more dilute. This is the free water, unobligated by solutes, that is excreted during a water diuresis when a state of water excess exists (Fig. 2-9).

Although operation of the countercurrent multiplier described above leads in man to concentrations of solute as high as 1200 mOsm/liter in the tip of the papilla, this gradient cannot be used to concentrate the total volume of tubular fluid that leaves the ascending limb of the loop of Henle. Absorption of this amount of water from the fluid in the collecting ducts as it passes back through the hypertonic inner medulla would simply reunite the water with the solute originally separated from it in the loop and thus reconstitute the original isotonic fluid. A reduction in the volume of fluid presented to the distal collecting ducts must occur, permitting the medullary gradient to be expended effectively in concentrating the urine. The reduction in volume occurs chiefly in the cortical portion of the collecting duct. The dilute fluid emerging from the ascending limb of the loop of Henle passes with little change in volume or concentration through the distal convoluted tubule (Fig. 2-9). During antidiuresis, however, vasopressin renders the epithelium of the collecting tubule highly permeable to

Fig. 2-9 Schematic representation of a juxtamedullary nephron illustrating the changes in solute concentration of tubular fluid during production of a dilute and a concentrated urine. The horizontal broken line separates the cortex, above, from the medulla. The heavier the shading the higher the concentration.

DIURESIS   ANTIDIURESIS

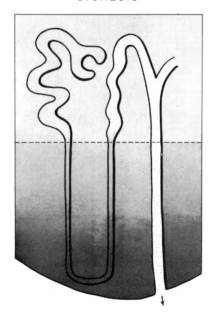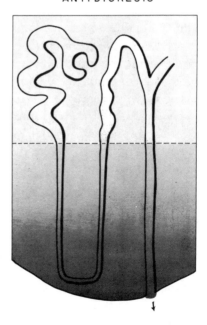

water. In the cortex the interstitium is maintained at approximately 280 mOsm/liter by continuous equilibration with the large volume of cortical blood flow. The osmotic gradient between the dilute luminal fluid in the cortical portion of the collecting duct and the isotonic interstitium causes, in the presence of vasopressin, a large transport of water out of the ducts, reducing the volume of fluid entering the hypertonic renal medulla. The high solute tonicity in the medullary interstitium is able to concentrate this remaining small volume effectively to levels of 1000 to 1200 mOsm/liter by the extraction of additional water equivalent to only a fraction of the original volume of fluid that passed through the loop of Henle and contributed its solute to the medullary interstitium.

What is the fate of the final moiety of water that is reabsorbed from the medullary portion of the collecting ducts during antidiuresis? That a steady state exists indicates that it is removed from the medulla; the vasa recta, the long vascular loops parallel to the loops of Henle, provide the only exit. These blood vessels operate as countercurrent exchangers, that is, passive conduits permeable to both solutes and water within which the blood becomes concentrated, as it passes down into the papilla, and diluted, as it flows back toward the cortex. The hairpin configuration of the vessels markedly reduces the tendency of the blood flow to dissipate the medullary gradient, but still permits it to supply nutrient to the medulla and to carry off the water entering the medulla from the collecting ducts during antidiuresis.

Under normal circumstances, only about one-half the total concentration in the medulla is made up of sodium salts derived from the countercurrent multiplier. Much of the remainder is urea, which reaches high concentrations within the medullary interstitium. This is a consequence of a cyclic trapping process involving the medullary interstitium, the loops of Henle, and the cortical and medullary portions of the collecting ducts (see Fig. 2-10). Urea diffuses from the medullary interstitium into the loops of Henle and is then carried through the distal convoluted tubule to the cortical portion of the collecting ducts. During antidiuresis, this segment of the collecting system is rendered permeable to water, but not to urea, by antidiuretic hormone. The loss of water increases the concentration of the urea within the luminal fluid that passes down the collecting duct toward the papillary tip. But vasopressin increases the permeability of the medullary portion of the collecting ducts to both urea and water (28).

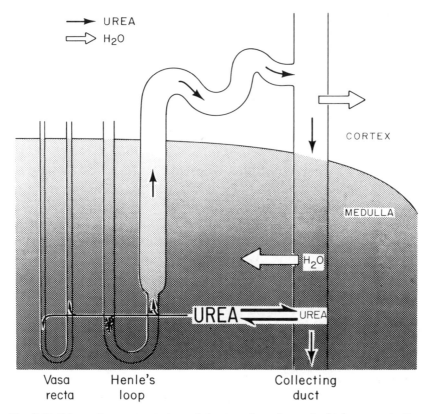

Fig. 2-10 Schematic representation of the trapping of urea in high concentrations within the medullary interstitium by recycling of urea through the interstitium, the ascending limb of Henle's loop, and the cortical and medullary segments of the collecting ducts.

There is controversy about the effect of vasopressin on the permeability of the medullary portion of the collecting duct to urea, but in any case the medullary collecting duct is more permeable to urea than its cortical segment is (29), which is necessary for the recycling of urea, as shown in Figure 2-10. Urea thus diffuses from the collecting tubule to the interstitium until its concentration in the luminal urine and the interstitium is equal. The urea in the interstitium diffuses into the ascending limb of the loop of Henle, and the cycle is repeated.

Because urea concentration on both sides of the epithelium of the collecting duct is nearly equal, it exerts almost no restraining influence on the reabsorption of water and thus permits the high salt concentrations in the medullary interstitium to balance osmotically the nonurea solute of the urine; urea in the urine "concentrates itself."

The technique developed by Burg for perfusing isolated segments of rabbit nephrons has led to a number of new insights into tubular function. Among the surprises was the discovery (30, 31) that, at least in the rabbit, the vigorous sodium chloride reabsorption in the thick ascending segment of the loop of Henle is accomplished by a primary active transport of chloride. The electrical potential difference across the epithelium of this segment of tubule was found to be 6 to 7 mV, with the lumen positive to the peritubular fluid. Since chloride reabsorption opposes the electrical gradient, it is considered to be active, and if chloride ions are replaced by sulfate ions, the potential difference is reduced to zero. Sodium, by contrast, appears to be reabsorbed passively, moving down the electrical gradient established by the active transport of chloride. As sodium and chloride are reabsorbed in this manner, the low osmotic water permeability of this segment allows their concentration in the luminal fluid to decrease to a minimal attainable value of about 50 mEq/liter. The potential difference at this steady state becomes maximal at about + 20 mV (lumen positive). This segment of the ascending limb is rich in Na, K-ATPase, and ouabain, which inhibits this enzyme, also blocks the active chloride transport process.

It was mentioned that the thin portion of the loop of Henle includes not only the descending limb, but also extends past the hairpin turn in the inner medulla or pyramid back up to the outer medulla, where its flat epithelial cells expand into the thick ascending segment. It has been a puzzling feature of the countercurrent multiplier that the gradient of solute concentration increases progressively to a maximal value at the tip of the pyramid, whereas the active transport of sodium and chloride is limited to the thick ascending segment in the outer cortex. Direct perfusion of the thin ascending segment has in fact shown that it is not engaged in active sodium chloride reabsorption (32).

How can the increasing concentration of solutes extend into the medullary interstitium deeper than the active transport systems do? Kokko and Rector (33) seem to have answered this question by proposing a scheme for countercurrent multiplication to the tip of the papillae that requires no active transport of sodium chloride in the *thin* ascending limb of Henle. In their scheme the energy generated by the active transport of salt in the thick ascending segment is efficiently transmitted to the papilla, the tip of the pyramid, via the role of urea. They point out that the isotonic fluid entering the thin descending limb of Henle's loop is rich in sodium chloride, but has a very low concentration of urea. This fluid becomes progressively more concentrated as it moves down the thin descending limb into the medulla, where the hypertonic interstitium osmotically sucks water, but not solutes, from its luminal content. At the hairpin turn a high sodium chloride concentration exists within the loop, whereas in the surrounding interstitium approximately one-half of the high osmolality is contributed by urea that is trapped in this area, by the mechanisms described earlier. This must mean that the concentration of sodium chloride in the luminal fluids exceeds its concentration in the interstitial fluid and that there is a gradient for its outward passive movement. All that is required, according to Kokko and Rector's scheme, is a change in permeability of the epithelium in the ascending thin limb such that, in contrast to the thin descending limb, it is permeable to sodium chloride, which can diffuse outward into the interstitium, and moderately permeable to urea, which can move to a lesser extent in the opposite direction, from the interstitium to the lumen (32). This scheme is a likely explanation for the progressive increase in concentration of sodium chloride during hydropenia, all the way to the tip of the renal pyramid. An active chloride reabsorptive process, restricted to the thick ascending segment in the outer medulla does the work.

The distal convoluted tubule

When the ascending limb of Henle's loop has reached the cortex and become the distal convoluted tubule, its contents may be well below isotonic (100 to 200 mOsm/kg of water). In the primate this dilute urine passes through the distal convoluted tubule (34), and its composition is modified by further reabsorption of sodium ions and by secretion of hydrogen ions, depending on the physiological state of the body. This is also the major site for potassium secretion.

The collecting ducts

From the distal convoluted tubule the dilute urine enters the collecting ducts that plunge down through the medulla and empty their contents at the tip of the renal pyramid, the papilla, into the pelvis of the kidney. Urine flows from the pelvis down the ureters into the bladder with little if any further modification, except some passive diffusion from urine across the pelvic, ureteral, and bladder mucosa.

The fate of the dilute urine entering the collecting ducts from the distal convoluted tubule is determined by the state of hydration of the subject. In a well-hydrated subject, the copious hypotonic fluid leaving the distal convoluted tubule flows down the collecting ducts with little further change in concentration and emerges in the renal pelvis as dilute urine. Water diuresis occurs. In the dehydrated or hydropenic individual, antidiuretic hormone is released from the posterior pituitary gland and increases the permeability of the collecting ducts to water so that the dilute fluid entering these ducts now equilibrates with the hypertonic interstitium as it passes down to the papillary tip. Highly concentrated urine, in small amounts, enters the renal pelvis on its way toward excretion; water is thereby conserved.

Antidiuretic hormone makes the epithelium of the distal collecting ducts permeable to urea as well as to water. This allows the major solute of the urine to equilibrate with itself in the medullary interstitium. The result is that the high sodium chloride concentrations in the interstitium concentrate nonurea solutes in the urine, whereas urea balances itself across the tubular epithelium. In fact, in animals on a low-protein diet it has been found that the urea concentration in the renal interstitium may be higher than in the urine, suggesting that, in addition to the recycling from the collecting ducts to the medullary interstitium described above, another process contributes to this accumulation. Ruminants, in which the ability to conserve urea on a low protein diet is most pronounced, have a highly developed renal pelvis with extensions running back up the pyramids to bathe the inner and outer medulla. Urea can diffuse from the pelvic urine back into the medullary interstitium, thus allowing further recycling and conservation (48).

Comparative studies on animals from different habitats have shown striking differences in the degree of development of the medullary countercurrent system. In man, the juxtamedullary nephrons deep in the renal cortex have long loops of Henle reaching down into the renal pyramids; the outer cortical nephrons have short loops that do not penetrate deeply into the medulla. Man can elaborate urine at a maximal concentration of 1000 to 1200 mOsm/kg of water. In the desert kangaroo rat, all the nephrons have very long loops of Henle, and the single pyramid projects well into the renal pelvis. Urine concentrations greater than 5000 mOsm/kg of water are attained by this

TABLE 2-1   *Localization of Nephron Functions*

SEGMENT OF NEPHRON	FUNCTIONS
a. Glomerulus	Creates ultrafiltrate of plasma
b. Proximal tubule	Reabsorbs two-thirds of filtered Na^+, Cl^-, H_2O Reabsorbs HCO^-_3, glucose, potassium, phosphate, amino acids, proteins, uric acid Secretes H^+, organic acids and bases, NH^+_4
c. Loop of Henle	Reabsorbs NaCl
d. Distal tubule	Reabsorbs Na^+, Cl^-, H_2O Secretes H^+, K^+, NH^+_4
e. Collecting duct	Reabsorbs Na^+, Cl^-, H_2O Secretes H^+, NH^+_4, K^+

desert rodent. On the other hand, the nephrons of beavers have very few long loops; water is plentiful in their environment.

In addition to its role in the reabsorption of sodium and water, the collecting duct is the site of other secretory processes. Hydrogen ions are added to the urine as sodium ions are reabsorbed. Here also ammonia, produced by deamination of amino acids in the tubular cells, diffuses into the urine, captures a hydrogen ion, and becomes NH^+_4.

Table 2-1 summarizes the major reabsorptive and secretory activities of the nephron. Table 2-2 assigns rough quantitative estimates to the

TABLE 2-2   *Sites of Sodium Chloride and Water Reabsorption in Nephron*[a]

	PERCENT GLOMERULAR FILTRATE REABSORBED		TUBULAR FLUID/PLASMA OSMOLARITY
	SODIUM CHLORIDE	WATER	
Proximal tubules	65	67	1
Loop of Henle	25	5	>1 (descending) <1 (ascending)
Distal tubule	Slight	8	<1
Collecting ducts	9	19	>1 or <1
Totals	99	99	

[a] Data derived from Bennett, C. M., Brenner, B. M., and Berliner, R. W. Micropuncture study of nephron function in the rhesus monkey. J. Clin. Invest. 47:203–216, 1968.

reabsorption of sodium and water in the several segments of the nephron described.

Clearance

Much of current thinking about the function of the kidney is linked to the concept of clearance introduced by van Slyke and associates in 1929 (35) in their description of urea excretion. They defined the renal clearance of urea as the volume of blood that 1 minute's excretion of urine suffices to clear of urea. Since all the blood flowing through the kidney is partially cleared of urea, the calculated value for urea clearance, C_{urea},

$$C_{urea} = \frac{U_{urea}V}{P_{urea}} \qquad (2\text{-}1)$$

(where U_{urea} equals the concentration of urea in mg/ml of urine; V is the urine flow in ml/minute, and P_{urea} equals the plasma urea concentration in mg/ml) is a virtual rather than a real volume. It is the minimal volume of blood required to furnish the quantity of substance excreted in the urine in 1 minute's time. A similar calculation can be made for every solute appearing in the urine. The resulting clearances were found to vary from fractions of a milliliter for substances found only in trace amounts in urine, for example, glucose or amino acids, to several hundred milliliters per minute for the organic anion *para*-aminohippurate (PAH).

It was evident to Rehberg and to Homer Smith that a substance freely filtered through the glomerulus that is not secreted, reabsorbed, or synthesized by the tubule would provide a measure of the absolute volume of glomerular filtrate per minute—the glomerular filtration rate. Rehberg proposed creatinine as such an index substance and Smith suggested inulin. The latter, a polyfructose of some 5000 molecular weight, is today regarded as providing the best measure of glomerular filtration rate. Inulin is freely filtered and neither secreted nor reabsorbed by the tubules. Hence the volume of plasma cleared of inulin equals the volume of filtrate formed:

$$C_{In} = \frac{U_{In}V}{P_{In}} = \sim120 \text{ ml (minute)}^{-1} (1.73 \text{ m}^2 \text{ body surface})^{-1}$$
$$(2\text{-}2)$$

To obtain accurate determinations of inulin clearance, constant plasma levels of inulin, obtained by a prolonged, intravenous infusion of inulin, are required. Urine flow must be copious, and the bladder must be emptied completely and rinsed between collection periods. This limits inulin clearance to a research technique.

Creatinine clearance, by contrast, is more conveniently measured, since the endogenous creatinine, continuously produced by the spontaneous hydrolysis of phosphocreatine from muscle, sustains a constant blood level of creatinine and allows the clearance to be determined without injections or infusions. Creatinine clearance in most normal subjects is essentially identical to the clearance of infused inulin. In disease it may be 50% more than the value of the inulin clearance, but this is still sufficiently representative to be clinically useful in estimating the glomerular filtration rate, especially sequentially during renal disease (36).

Once it had been established that the clearance of inulin measured the glomerular filtration rate, then it could be concluded that substances that were freely filtered through the glomeruli, but had a renal clearance less than that of inulin, must have undergone some reabsorption during passage down the nephron. Most substances of physiological interest undergo reabsorption by either passive diffusion or active transport. Early on it was realized, however, that certain exogenous substances, such as phenol red, diodrast, and hippuran, had clearances higher than that of inulin. These substances must, therefore, be added to the urine in excess of the quantities filtered at the glomerulus. Their transport into the urine by the single layer of renal tubular cells is generally referred to as tubular secretion.

It has been found that the renal clearance of the organic iodine compounds diodrast and hippuran increases and becomes independent of the plasma concentration of these substances when the plasma concentration is below a certain level. Increasing the plasma concentration of these iodinated compounds depresses not only their own clearances, but also the simultaneous clearance of phenol red systematically and reversibly. This indicates that all three substances are secreted by a common tubular mechanism.

In a normal man an average plasma clearance of some 600 ml/ minute is obtained for diodrast or hippuran at low plasma concentrations of these substances. Since these substances reach the kidney only via the blood, their clearances indicate a lower limit for the rate of plasma flow to the kidneys. Knowing the hematocrit, one can estimate the minimal blood flow to the kidneys necessary to account for the hippuran and diodrast clearances as some 1000 ml/minute. Detailed studies have been made with another substance, para-aminohippurate (PAH), which has similar high clearance rates at low plasma concentrations. By applying the Fick principle to the observed clearances of PAH, true values for renal blood flow have been obtained.

$$\frac{U_{PAH}V}{a - v} = \text{True plasma flow} \tag{2-3}$$

where U_{PAH} is urine concentration of PAH (mg/ml), V is urine flow (ml/minute), and a and v are renal arterial and venous plasma concentrations, respectively, of PAH (mg/ml). At concentrations in arterial plasma of up to 1.0 mg/dl, it was found from arterial–venous concentration differences that some 90% of the PAH is cleared from arterial blood on a single passage through the kidneys. The 10% remaining could indicate that extraction of PAH by renal tubules is incomplete or that some blood bypasses the renal tubules as it flows through the kidneys. Whatever the case, it means that the true renal blood flow is about 1200 ml/minute. Since the cardiac output in a resting normal adult is 5 to 6 liters/minute, we can conclude that about 20% of the cardiac output perfuses the kidneys. For two structures whose combined weight in a normal 70-kg adult is about 300 gm, this represents a very high level of perfusion.

Normal functioning of the kidneys requires these high levels of blood flow. The renal arteries supplying the glomeruli are so arranged that some 60% of the aortic arterial pressure is delivered to the afferent glomerular arteriole as the filtration pressure. With a drop in blood pressure or a reduction of cardiac output, perfusion of the kidneys diminishes and the glomerular filtration rate falls. The ratio of glomerular filtration rates to plasma flow (filtration fraction) is normally 0.18 to 0.2 (inulin clearance ~120 ml/minute and PAH clearance ~600 ml/minute). In arterial hypertension, the glomerular filtration rate tends to be sustained, whereas renal plasma flow falls, raising the filtration fraction. In glomerulonephritis, damage to the glomerulus is disproportionate to the blood supply, and the filtration fraction declines. When arterial pressure falls below 60 mm Hg, filtration at the glomerulus ceases. Many disease states affecting the circulatory system and the kidneys reversibly compromise renal function. If the reduction in blood flow is too severe or too protracted, the kidneys are damaged and ischemic renal failure results. The reduced function of the kidney can no longer be reversed simply by correcting the systemic circulatory insufficiency. Glomerular filtration may, however, cease when perfusion of the kidneys is adequate, but when the pressure is too low, as it is during hypotensive anesthesia (high spinal anesthesia). In such circumstances filtration and renal function may resume promptly when the perfusion pressure rises.

THRESHOLD AND Tm

Before the classic micropuncture studies of A. N. Richards and his associates in the 1930s on the composition of glomerular urine, there were two opposing views of kidney function. It was known that some substances, such as glucose, that are present in the blood at significant concentrations are absent or appear only in trace amounts in the urine. One group of physiologists, led by Bowman (1842) and Ludwig (1844) and much later by Cushny (1917), proposed that the initial step in urine formation is the separation in the glomerulus of an ultrafiltrate of plasma. This capsular fluid was thought to contain all the filterable constituents of the plasma (Na, Cl, K, HCO_3, SO_4, urea, amino acids, PO_4, glucose, etc.) in the same concentration per unit volume of water as they exist in plasma except for such inequalities in the distribution of ions as are imposed by the Donnan effect or by binding to serum proteins. Subsequent reabsorption of filtered constituents during passage of the glomerular filtrate down the nephron would lead to the final urine. The opposing view, enunciated by Heidenhain (1874), was that the glomeruli secreted water and salts and that this glomerular secretion was further enriched by the addition of salts, waste products, and foreign substances through specific activity of the tubule cells. It was the meticulous collection and analysis of fluid from individual glomerular capsules by Richards and associates that finally resolved this century-old debate. Richards found that the concentrations of glucose and other small solutes, which he could measure, were the same in glomerular fluid as in plasma water.

Since glucose is filtered freely through the glomerular membranes and appears normally only in traces in the urine, although it may be found in larger quantities in the urine of diabetic subjects with elevated blood sugars, there must be a limit to the rate of glucose reabsorption. This has been studied by titrating the tubular reabsorptive process for glucose (see Fig. 2-11). Glucose is infused intravenously to

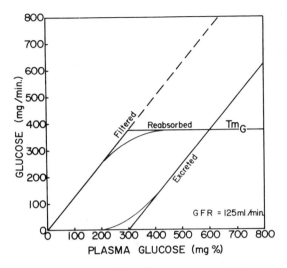

Fig. 2-11 Schematic representation of the classic concept of glucose excretion. It is now recognized that the maximal rate of glucose reabsorption (Tm_G) varies with the functional state of the kidney. From Pitts, Robert F.: *Physiology of the Kidney and Body Fluids.* Copyright © 1974 by Year Book Medical Publishers, Inc., Chicago. Used by permission.

progressively increase plasma concentrations. The rate of glucose filtration, estimated from the simultaneous inulin clearance, and the rate of glucose excretion are then obtained. In most normal individuals elevation of the plasma glucose to 140–190 mg/100 cc produces measurable amounts of glucose in the urine. At these plasma levels the glucose filtration rate is about 144 to 228 mg/minute. Raising the plasma glucose level still further, however, further increases the rate of glucose reabsorption, up to a maximum of about 340 mg/minute.

Glucose reabsorption is an active process that can be inhibited by compounds having an affinity for the glucose transport system. The glucoside phlorizin is such an inhibitor. It completely blocks the reabsorption of glucose, which indicates that the proximal tubule is impermeable to glucose in the absence of its transport system. The plasma glucose concentration at which glucose appears in the urine in significant amounts is referred to as the renal "threshold." The rate of tubular reabsorption is obtained by subtracting the quantity of glucose appearing in the urine per minute from the rate of glucose filtration. The maximal rate of tubular reabsorption (*Tm*) is the rate at which larger amounts presented to the tubules are quantitatively excreted. Thus the Tm_G is some 340 mg/minute for most normally hydrated, healthy individuals, but is not as invariable as was once thought.

The older concept of a maximal tubular rate (Tm) for the reabsorption of various constituents of the body fluids has been reassessed. Instead of a constant glucose reabsorption rate, which is independent of the glomerular filtration rate, tubular absorption of glucose generally varies directly with the filtration rate and also depends on sodium reabsorption, diminishing with decreasing fractional reabsorption of filtered sodium (37, 38, 39, 40). Thus the scheme shown in Figure 2-11 could be obtained only under the unlikely experimental conditions that the glomerular filtration rate and the fractional sodium reabsorption remained constant as the concentration of glucose in plasma varied. Other constituents of body fluids, such as bicarbonate and phosphate, whose reabsorption had also been thought to be governed by a Tm, seem to be similarly variable. But most substances, such as sodium, chloride, water, and urea, that are also reabsorbed by the tubules from the glomerular filtrate do not have a discernible limit to their rate of reabsorption

Within limits, the reabsorption of sodium has been found to be proportional to its rate of filtration. This has given rise to the concept of "glomerular–tubular balance." For a major body constituent such as sodium, severe depletion or retention would rapidly ensue with changes in glomerular filtration rate unless there was some semblance of glomerular–tubular balance. Brenner and associates (41) have pointed out that the glomerular filtration rate, through its effect on the postglomerular colloid osmotic pressure, is a factor in maintaining glomerular–tubular balance. A decrease in filtration pressure in the glomerulus lowers the filtration rate, but also diminishes the rise in colloid osmotic pressure due to concentration of serum proteins in the glomerular capillaries. The lower postglomerular colloid osmotic pressure in turn reduces salt and water reabsorption in the proximal tubule. Increasing the glomerular filtration pressure has the opposite effect (see discussion on p. 29). Changes in reabsorption of salt and water in proximal tubules, accordingly, are directly proportional to changes in the glomerular filtration rate. But there is also much evidence (49, 50, 51) that a feedback system within each nephron adjusts glomerular filtration in response to the rate, apparently, of chloride reabsorption at the macula densa—the distinctive cluster of tall cells in the ascending limb of Henle's loop where the tubule emerges from the medulla and abuts on the vascular pole of its own glomerulus. A high rate of flow at the distal nephron allows increased chloride reabsorption at the macula densa, and this signals either constriction of the adjacent afferent arteriole or dilatation of the efferent glomerular arteriole to reduce the glomerular filtration rate of that nephron. Contrariwise, a low rate of flow at the macula densa increases the single nephron glomerular filtration rate, constricting the efferent or dilating the afferent glomerular arteriole. It remains to be established which arteriolar resistance is affected and whether the juxtaglomerular apparatus, of which the macula densa is a component, participates in the adjustments of arteriolar tone by the release of renin and the formation of angiotensin II locally. However the details are resolved, it is evident that this single nephron feedback mechanism is the major determinant of glomerular-tubular balance.

NATURE OF THE TRANSPORT PROCESSES

The traffic of water and solutes in both directions across the renal tubular epithelium partakes of all modes of membrane transport. Reabsorption of water is entirely, and of urea largely, passive; these substances move down concentration gradients. For many substances of importance—sodium, chloride, calcium, potassium, glucose, and amino acids, to name only a few—specific active transport processes exist; energy from metabolism is used by the renal tubule cells to drive these solutes "uphill" thermodynamically, that is, from states of lower to higher electrochemical potential (or from lower to higher concentrations, in the case of uncharged solutes). In no instance yet reported has the mechanism of active transport in the kidney been elucidated; however, the "carrier" concept has now been proved in bacteria and in the intestine, and seems most likely to account for specific transport processes in the renal tubule cells as well. Mobile molecules, probably proteins, located in the cell membranes are assumed by the carrier hypothesis to bind specific solutes and translocate them across the permeability barriers in the renal tubular cells. The sodium- and potassium-dependent adenosine triphosphatase present in abundance in the membranes of renal tubular cells is thought to provide both the translocating carrier for sodium and the energy transducer.

Most of the energy metabolism of the kidneys, as measured by oxygen consumption, has been found to be directly related to the reabsorption of sodium and chloride from the lumen. This is consistent with the very large quantities of sodium ($\sim$25,000 mEq/day) that must be reabsorbed actively from the glomerular filtrate to maintain sodium balance. But the characteristics of the transport process are not uniform throughout the nephron. In the proximal tubule, the transepithelial electrical potential is close to zero, and large quantities of sodium are transported from lumen to peritubular capillaries by a process incapable of lowering the concentration of sodium in the luminal fluids below 70% of its concentration in plasma. Water normally moves out of the lumen so rapidly, along with the transported sodium, that reabsorption is isotonic in the proximal tubule. The epithelium of the thin descending and ascending limbs of the loop of Henle apparently is not engaged in active sodium transport, but in the thick ascending limb there is a very vigorous active transport process capable of moving sodium and chloride from low luminal concentrations to high concentrations in the medullary interstitium. It is now evident that the vigorous transport system in the thick ascending limb of Henle's loop, at least in the rabbit kidney, primarily transports chloride ions actively; and that sodium moves passively in this segment (27, 28). Unlike the process in the proximal tubule, in the ascending limb and distal nephron, sodium chloride may be reabsorbed without accompanying water, with the result that the tubular fluid may become very dilute. In the distal nephron and collecting tubule sodium reabsorption produces an electrical potential gradient across the nephron with the peritubular surface positive to the lumen. This electrical gradient affects the movement of other charged species across the tubule, as shown in Figure 2-12. When sodium is abundant in the diet, the kidneys may excrete urine having a concentration of sodium of more than 200 mEq/liter, whereas during sodium deprivation the concentration of sodium may fall to less than 1 mEq/liter. This versatility is the result of the reabsorptive activity of the distal nephron and collecting tubule with respect to sodium and water.

Although the cortical portion of the kidneys is abundantly supplied with oxygen, the inner medulla is not. The countercurrent arrangement of the medullary blood vessels and the affinity of their hemoglobin for oxygen produce hypoxia within the renal medulla. Although the cortex has a high rate of oxidative metabolism, the tubules deep in the medulla depend on anaerobic energy sources to supplement the

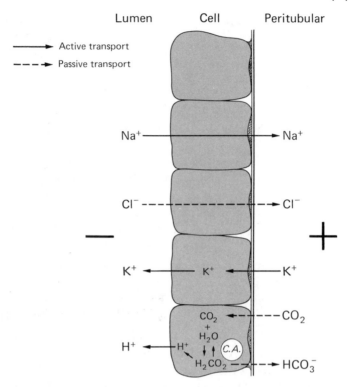

Fig. 2-12 Effect of active sodium transport on movement of Cl^-, K^+, and H^+ in the distal nephron. Active Na^+ reabsorption from lumen to peritubular fluid renders the latter electrically positive to the luminal fluid. This electrical gradient serves as a major driving force to promote Cl^- reabsorption and K^+ secretion. Although H^+ is actively secreted, the electrical gradient produced by Na^+ transport favors secretion of H^+, too.

limited energy available from oxidative metabolism for their active transport processes. Oxygen tension in the urine is low (42), reflecting these hypoxic conditions deep in the medulla through which the collecting ducts must finally pass.

References

1. Handbook of Physiology: Renal Physiology. J. Orloff and R. W. Berliner (eds.), Am. Physiol. Soc., Washington, D.C. 1973.
2. Renkin, E. M. and Gilmore, J. P. Glomerular filtration: *In* Orloff, J. and Berliner, R. W. (eds.): Handbook of Physiology. Section 8, Renal Physiology. Wash., D.C., American Physiology Society, 1973, p. 185.

3. Farquhar, M. G. The primary glomerular filtration barrier—basement membrane of epithelial slits? Kidney Int. 8:197, 1975.

4. Venkatachalam, M. A. and Rennke, H. G. Structural and molecular basis of glomerular filtration. Circ. Res. 43:337, 1978.

5. Karnovsky, M. J. The ultrastructural basis of glomerular permeability. *In* Ching, J. et al. (eds.): Kidney Disease—Recent Studies. Williams & Wilkins, Baltimore, 1979.

6. Rennke, H. G., Cotran, R. S., and Venkatachalam, M. A. Role of molecular charge in glomerular permeability. Tracer studies with cationized ferritins. J. Cell. Biol. 67:638, 1975.

7. Brenner, B. M., Hostetter, T. H., and Humes, H. D. Molecular basis of proteinuria of glomerular origin. New Eng. J. Med. 298:826, 1978.

8. Seiler, M. W., Venkatachalam, M. A., and Cotran, R. S. Glomerular epithelium: Structural alterations induced by polycations. Science 189:390, 1975.

9. Rodewald, R. and Karnovsky, M. J. Porous substructure of the glomerular slit diaphragm in the rat and mouse. J. Cell. Biol. 67:638, 1975.

10. Pappenheimer, J. R. Passage of molecules through capillary walls. Physiol. Rev. 33:387–423, 1953.

11. Brenner, B. M., Troy, J. L., and Daugharty, T. M. The dynamics of glomerular ultrafiltration in the rat. J. Clin. Invest. 50:1776–1780, 1971.

12. Brenner, B. M., Troy, J. L., Daugharty, T. M., Deen, W. M., and Robertson, C. R. Dynamics of glomerular ultrafiltration in the rat. II. Plasma-flow dependence of GFR. Am. J. Physiol. 223:1184, 1972.

13. Robertson, C. R., Deen, W. M., Troy, J. L., and Brenner, B. M. Dynamics of glomerular ultrafiltration in the rat. III. Hemodynamics and autoregulation. Am. J. Physiol. 223:1191, 1972.

14. Deen, W. M., Troy, J. L., Robertson, C. R., and Brenner, B. M. Dynamics of glomerular ultrafiltration in the rat. IV. Determination of the ultrafiltration coefficient. J. Clin. Invest. 52:1500–1508, 1973.

15. Walker, A. M., Hudson, C. L., Findley, T., Jr., and Richards, A. N. The total molecular concentration and the chloride concentration of fluid from different segments of the renal tubule of Amphibia; the site of chloride reabsorption. Am. J. Physiol. 118:121, 1937.

16. Diamond, J. M. and Bossert, W. H. Standing-gradient osmotic flow. J. Gen. Physiol. 50:2061–2083, 1967.

17. Kashgarian, M., Stockle, H., Gottschalk, C. W., and Ullrich, K. J. Transtubular electrochemical potentials of sodium and chloride in proximal and distal renal tubules of rats during antidiuresis and water diuresis. Pflügers Arch. 277:89–106, 1963.

18. Burg, M. B. and Orloff, J. Electrical potential difference across proximal convoluted tubules. Am. J. Physiol. 219:1714–1716, 1970.

19. Barratt, L. J., Rector, F. C., Jr., Kokko, J. P., and Seldin, D. W. Factors governing the transepithelial potential difference across the proximal tubule of the rat kidney. J. Clin. Invest. 53:454–464, 1974.

20. deWardener, H. E., Mills, I. H., Clapham, W. F., and Hayter, C. J. Studies on the efferent mechanism of the sodium diuresis which follows the administration of intravenous saline in the dog. Clin. Sci. 21:249–258, 1961.

21. Daugharty, T. M., Belleau, L. J., Martino, J. A., and Early, L. E. Interrelationship of physical factors affecting sodium reabsorption in the dog. Am. J. Physiol. 215:1442–1447, 1968.

22. Grandchamp, A. and Boulpaep, E. L. Pressure control of sodium reabsorption and intercellular backflux across proximal kidney tubule. J. Clin. Invest. 54: 69–83, 1974.

23. Kashgarian, M., Warren, Y., Mitchell, R. L., and Epstein, F. H. Effect of protein in tubular fluid upon proximal tubular absorption. Proc. Soc. Exp. Biol. and Med. 117:848–850, 1964.

24. Hargitay, B. and Kuhn, W. Das Multiplikationsprinzip als Grundlage der Harnkonzentrierung in der Niere. Zeitschrift fur Elektrochemie und Angewandte Physikalische Chemie 55:539–558, 1951.

25. Wirz, H., Hargitay, B., and Kuhn, W. Lokalisation des Konzentrier-Ungsprozesses in der Niere durch direkte Kryoskopie. Helvetica Physiologica et Pharmacologica Acta 9:196–207, 1951.

26. Scholander, P. F. The wonderful net. Scientific American 196:97–107, April 1957.

27. Pitts, R. J. Physiology of the kidney and body fluids, 2nd ed. Year Book Medical Pub., Inc. Chicago, 1968, p. 266.

28. Gardner, K. D. and Maffly, R. H. An *in vitro* demonstration of increased collecting tubular permeability to urea in the presence of vasopressin. J. Clin. Invest. 43:1968–1975, 1964.

29. Rocha, A. S. and Kokko, J. P. Permeability of medullary nephron segments to urea and water: effect of vasopressin. Kidney Int. 6:379–387, 1974.

30. Burg, M. and Green, N. Function of the thick ascending limb of Henle's loop. Am. J. Physiol. 224:659–668, 1973.

31. Rocha, A. S. and Kokko, J. P. Sodium chloride and water transport in the medullary thick ascending limb of Henle. Evidence for active chloride transport. J. Clin. Invest. 52:612–623, 1973.

32. Imai, M. and Kokko, J. P. Sodium chloride, urea, and water transport in the thin ascending limb of Henle. J. Clin. Invest. 53:393–402, 1974.

33. Kokko, J. P. and Rector, F. C., Jr. Countercurrent multiplication system without active transport in inner medulla. Kidney Int. 2:214–223, 1972.

34. Bennett, C. M., Brenner, B. M., and Berliner, R. W. Micropuncture study of nephron function in the rhesus monkey. J. Clin. Invest. 47:203–216, 1968.

35. Möller, E., McIntosh, J. F., and van Slyke, D. D. Studies of urea excretion. II. Relationship between urine volume and the rate of urea excretion by normal adults. J. Clin. Invest. 6:427–486, 1929.

36. Kim, K. E., Onesti, G., Ramirez, O., Brest, A. N., and Swartz, C. Creatinine clearance in renal disease: A reappraisal. Brit. Med. J. 4:11–14, 1969.

37. Keyes, J. L. and Swanson, R. E. Dependence of glucose Tm on GRF and tubular volume in the dog kidney. Am. J. Physiol. 221:1–7, 1971.

38. Kurtzman, N. H., White, M. G., Rogers, P. W., and Flynn, J. J., III. Relationship of sodium reabsorption and glomerular filtration rate to renal glucose reabsorption. J. Clin. Invest. 51:127–133, 1972.

39. Schultze, R. G. and Berger, H. The influence of GFR and saline expansion on Tm_G of the dog kidney. Kidney Int. 3:291–297, 1973.

40. Kwong, T. –F. and Bennett, C. M. Relationship between glomerular filtration rate and maximum tubular reabsorptive rate of glucose. Kidney Int. 5:23–29, 1974.

41. Brenner, B. M., Troy, J. L., Daugharty, T. M., and MacInnes, R. M. Quantitative importance of changes in postglomerular colloid osmotic pressure in mediating glomerulotubular balance in the rat. J. Clin. Invest. 52:190–197, 1973.

42. Rennie, D. W., Reeves, R. B., and Pappenheimer, J. R. Oxygen pressure in urine and its relation to intrarenal blood flow. Am. J. Physiol. 195:120–132, 1958.

43. Frömter, E. and Diamond, J. Route of passive ion permeation in epithelia. Nature New Biology 235:9–13 (Jan. 5) 1972.

44. Welling, L. W. and Welling, D. J. Shape of epithelial cells and intercellular channels in the rabbit proximal nephron. Kidney Int. 9:385–394, 1976.

45. Hill, A. E. Solute-solvent coupling in epithelia. A critical examination of the standing-gradient osmotic flow theory. Proc. Roy. Soc. Lond. (Biol.) 190:99–114, 1975.

46. DiBona, D. R. and Mills, J. W. Distribution of Na$^+$-pump sites in transporting epithelia. Fed. Proc. 38:134–143, 1979.

47. Andreoli, T. E. and Schafer, J. A. External solution driving forces for isotonic fluid absorption in proximal tubules. Fed. Proc. 38:154–160, 1979.

48. Schmidt-Nielsen, B. Excretion in mammals: role of the renal pelvis in the modification of the urinary concentration and composition. Fed. Proc. 36:2493–2503, 1977.

49. Schnermann, J., Wright, F. S., Davis, J. M., von Stackelberg, W., and Grill, G. Regulation of superficial nephron filtration rate by tubuloglomerular feedback. Pflüger's Arch. 319:147–175, 1970.

50. Thurau, K. Intrarenal action of angiotensin. In Handbook of Experimental Pharmacology. I. H. Page and F. M. Bumpus (eds.), Springer-Verlag, New York 37:475–489, 1974.

51. Arendhorst, W. J., Finn, W. F., and Gottschalk, C. Nephron stop-flow pressure response to obstruction for 24 hours in the rat kidney. J. Clin. Invest. 53:1497–1500, 1974.

3

Regulation of the Volume and Concentration of the Body Fluids

In health both the concentration and volume of the body fluids are jealously guarded within narrow limits, but in disease marked alterations occur. This chapter considers the regulatory processes that normally preserve the concentration and volume of body fluids and the disturbances that may occur in disease states.

ANATOMY OF BODY FLUIDS: BODY FLUID COMPARTMENTS

In the healthy adult male some 60% of body weight is water. In the adult female only about 50% of body weight is water. This percentage is determined mainly by the amount of adipose tissue present; the normal female has more than the male, as anatomical observation indicates. Each gram of body fat is associated with only 0.1 gm of water, in keeping with its function as a compact energy store. On the other hand, approximately 3 gm of water are associated with each gram of protein or glycogen. These are average figures, and within various tissues there are, of course, characteristic differences. Lean muscle contains about 20% dry solids, liver consists of approximately 33% dry solids. The newborn has a higher percentage of water than the adult; aging is associated with progressive desiccation.

Total body water, as well as the water content of each tissue, is generally divided into two main compartments: the fluid actually within cells (intracellular fluid) and the fluid bathing the cells (extracellular fluid). The latter is subdivided into the interstitial and the intravascular fluids. Approximately two-thirds of total body water is intracellular, and the remainder is extracellular. One-third of the extracellular fluid is intravascular, and the remainder interstitial. Thus, in a 70-kg normal adult with about 42 liters of total body water, 28 liters are intracellular and 14 liters extracellular (Fig. 3-1). Of the extracellular fluids some 4 liters are intravascular (plasma), and the rest is extravascular and interstitial.

Since there are no absolute barriers to the movement of water from one compartment to another—in fact, water moves rapidly across most cell membranes—it is the quantity of solute rather than the amount of solvent that defines the size of the compartment. Each body fluid compartment has one solute that, because it is restricted largely to that space, determines the extent of the compartment: serum proteins for the intravascular volume, sodium for the extracellular compartment, and potassium for the intracellular space. In each case it is the osmotic activity of the solute confined largely to the particular compartment that is important.

Fig. 3-1 Body water distribution.

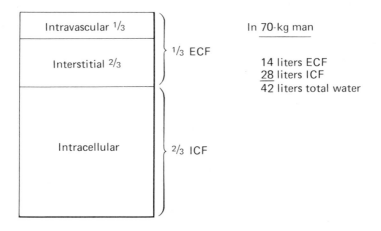

The intravascular volume

The plasma proteins comprise a large number of variegated proteins totaling 7 to 8 gm/dl of plasma. Normally there are about 5 gm of albumin/dl plasma, and the rest are largely globulins. The albumin is homogeneous and has a molecular weight of 69,000, whereas the globulins are diverse and mostly larger. The albumin, present at twice the concentration of other proteins and roughly half their size, provides about 80% of the oncotic pressure (colloid osmotic pressure) of the plasma. Nevertheless, the pressure is small, amounting only to some 0.7 mOsm

$$\frac{5 \times 10 \text{ gm/liter}}{69,000} = 0.7 \text{ millimole or mOsm/liter or kg water}$$

$$(3-1)$$

or an osmotic pressure of approximately 15 mm Hg for the total plasma proteins. From measurements of the freezing point of serum we know that it has a total solute concentration equivalent to about 290 mOsm/kg of water. Small solutes, such as NaCl, glucose, and urea, which pass freely across the vascular endothelium between the intravascular and interstitial fluid, make up nearly all the osmotic pressure of serum. Since only the serum proteins are restricted to the intravascular compartment, it is their small contribution that is responsible for the effective osmotic pressure difference between intravascular and interstitial extracellular fluid.* This small osmotic pressure difference opposes the outward-directed hydrostatic pressure generated by the pumping action of the heart, draws fluid back into the intravascular compartment, and thus maintains its volume. These interrelationships, described by Starling, are depicted in Figure 3-2 (see Chapter 6, Edema, for a more detailed discussion). The net effect of the serum

---

* The reflection coefficient σ is used to express the osmotic effectiveness of a given solute with respect to a given membrane. A reflection coefficient of 1.0 indicates that the membrane is impermeable to the solute. A reflection coefficient of 0 indicates that the membrane does not restrict the solute, so that the concentration of solute in the filtrate is the same as in the initial solution. Expressed more succinctly, $\sigma = \pi_a/\pi_t$ in which π_t is the theoretical osmotic activity of the solute and π_a its apparent osmotic activity relative to the membrane system concerned. Thus, the serum proteins in the intravascular compartment have a $\sigma = 1$ while the small solutes mentioned have a σ approximately 0 in this system.

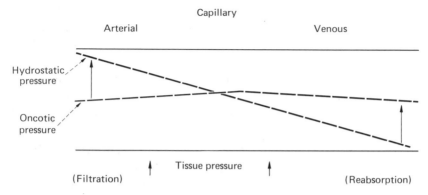

Fig. 3-2 The effects of hydrostatic, oncotic, and tissue pressures on fluid movements across a capillary wall.

proteins is to allow the heart to pump one-third of the extracellular fluid volume around the vascular compartment, which continuously circulates and mixes the entire interstitial fluid (the actual environment of the cells).

The extracellular fluid volume

Physiologists and clinicians have expended much effort to determine the factors that control the extracellular fluid volume. Some mechanisms have been established; others remain controversial and are the subject of active investigation. In this section an attempt is made to present what has been established and to indicate the directions of investigation.

Just as the content of serum proteins within the vascular compartment affects the balance of filtration and reabsorption of interstitial fluid and thus preserves the intravascular volume, so the content of sodium determines the volume of the extracellular fluids. Since the concentration of sodium in the extracellular fluid is kept constant (see the section below, Tonicity of Body Fluids), the content of sodium in the body—the balance between intake and output—determines the extracellular fluid volume.

Valid as this generalization is, considerable amounts of sodium are present in the body outside the diffusable extracellular fluids. Some of this is within cells, some is adsorbed onto the crystalline structure of bone, and some is bound to collagen and connective tissue. Some sodium may be available to support the extracellular fluid volume under conditions of stress, but most is sequestered in forms unavailable to the needs of the extracellular fluid volume—about 750 mEq of the sodium in bone is nonexchangeable (1).

When salt in excess of the body's needs is ingested or administered the extracellular fluid and vascular volumes expand. This leads to an increased perfusion of the kidneys and increased glomerular filtration rate. More sodium is delivered into the lumen of the renal tubules and more sodium is excreted in the urine. Conversely, with depletion of body sodium from any cause, such as sweating, diarrhea, or vomiting, the extracellular fluid volume contracts, glomerular filtration decreases, and less sodium is filtered and less excreted. The reduced amount of sodium that enters the renal tubule is almost entirely reabsorbed and body sodium stores are conserved. Thus, simple changes in the glomerular filtration rate in the direction anticipated for overexpansion or contraction of extracellular volume lead to increased or decreased renal excretion of sodium, respectively, which maintains the extracellular fluid volume.

It has been known since the classic studies of Loeb (2) and of Harrop (3) that removal of the adrenal cortex results in renal sodium wastage and that this sodium loss could be prevented by injections of extracts of the adrenal gland. Not until some 20 years later was the substance responsible for the major sodium-retaining effect of the adrenal gland isolated (4). This is the steroid hormone aldosterone, which stimulates sodium reabsorption by the renal tubular epithelium. Thus, a dual control of sodium excretion by changes in the glomerular filtration rate and in the rate of sodium reabsorption mediated via aldosterone is recognized. It is thought that the glomerular filtration rate remains stable for the most part and that finer adjustments in the sodium content of the body fluids are the result of changes in tubular reabsorption rates. It should be appreciated, however, that the total quantity of sodium filtered through the glomeruli is so large (180 liters $\times$ 150 mEq/liter $=$ 27,000 mEq/day), compared with the urinary excretion of sodium (1–200 mEq/day), that it is difficult to assign changes in urinary excretion to changes either in filtered load or to tubular reabsorption of sodium.

How is the need for increased aldosterone secretion and increased tubular reabsorption of sodium sensed? A number of ingenious experiments indicate that the sodium regulatory mechanism responds to some parameter of intravascular volume, the "effective intravascular volume" (5, 6). This effective intravascular volume, unfortunately, does not lend itself to quantitative measurement. The concept is based on the following sequence of observations.

1. Simple water loss leading to contraction of all body fluid compartments results in increased aldosterone excretion and reduced renal sodium losses. In this situation the intravenous administration of hypertonic sodium chloride sufficient to reexpand the extracellular volume at the expense of further contraction of the intracellular fluid volume reduces aldosterone excretion and increases renal sodium excretion (7).

2. In a sodium-depleted subject whose intracellular volume is presumably normal, aldosterone secretory rates are high and extracellular fluid volume is contracted. Again, intravenous administration of hypertonic sodium chloride may correct the extracellular volume deficit by drawing water from cells so that no change in total body water occurs. The redistribution of water in the body with expansion of extracellular fluid volume shuts off aldosterone excretion and increases renal sodium excretion (see Fig. 3-3) (7).

3. In certain clinical conditions the concentration and content of serum proteins within the intravascular compartment decrease. As a result the intravascular volume is contracted. Patients with such disorders have high rates of aldosterone excretion, but excrete very little sodium, so that ingested sodium is nearly quantitatively retained. This sodium retention leads to gross over-expansion of the interstitial extracellular fluid, that is, to massive edema. Administering hyperoncotic serum albumin in such instances draws interstitial fluid back into the intravascular compartment and thus reduces aldosterone excretion and enhances sodium excretion (see Fig. 3-4) (6).

4. Finally, it has been shown that the readjustments in intravascular volume associated with a simple change from the upright to the recumbent position are accompanied by a decrease in aldosterone excretion and an increase in sodium excretion (8).

These observations all indicate that some parameter of the intravascular volume is sensed by the volume-regulating mechanism. Changes

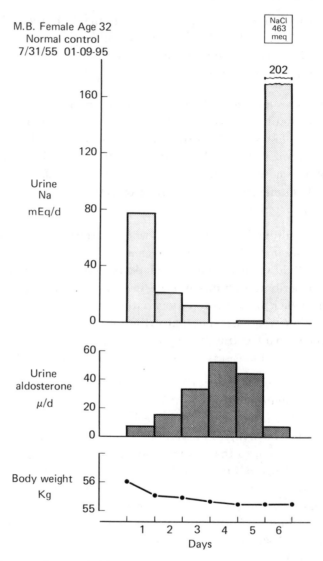

Fig. 3-3 Urinary sodium and aldosterone and body weight in a normal subject, who received hypertonic saline intravenously, on restricted water and sodium intake (7). Reprinted from (7) with permission of the *Journal of Clinical Investigation*.

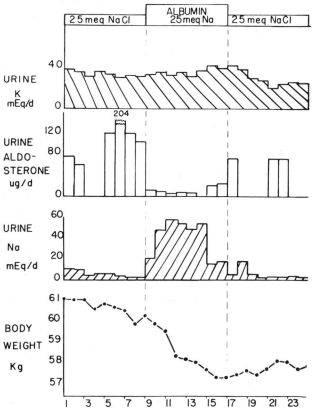

N.W. ♀ AGE 26

01-05-57

1/22/56
IDIOPATHIC HYPOPROTEINEMIA

Fig. 3-4 The effect of intravenous albumin on urinary sodium, potassium, and aldosterone, and on body weight in a woman with idiopathic hypoproteinemia on constant regimen. Destruction of albumin proceeded at a greatly increased rate in this subject. The dose of albumin was 50 gm/day. Reprinted from (6) with permission from *Metabolism*.

in serum sodium concentration, by contrast, bear no definite relationship to sodium excretion or conservation. Simple water lack leads to hypernatremia, with contracted body fluid volumes and decreased sodium excretion, whereas infusion of 5% sodium chloride solutions also produces hypernatremia, but with greatly increased sodium excretion. Sodium depletion contracts extracellular fluid volume, and hyponatremia in this state is associated with virtual disappearance of sodium from the urine. Administering water together with vasopressin (antidiuretic hormone), which inhibits excretion of the administered water, dilutes the body fluids and also produces hyponatremia, but with an associated large diuresis of sodium (9). Although sodium concentration can be dissociated from renal sodium excretion, in each instance the renal response is appropriate for correcting the disturbance in extracellular or intravascular volume.

Having determined that some change in intravascular volume is monitored, we next ask how and where such monitoring occurs. Although we have no real answers, there is increasing evidence that stretch receptors in the walls of the large low-pressure capacitance vessels near the heart serve as the first-line monitors of intravascular volume (38, 40, 41). These vessels are 100 to 200 times more distensible than arteries and are capable of holding a large fraction of the total blood volume, estimated to be as high as 80%. The moderate, day-to-day fluctuations in extracellular fluid and intravascular volumes mainly affect the filling of these capacitance vessels and thereby the amount of sensory information from this part of the circulation. As long as sufficient blood is flowing through the capacitance vessels to sustain left ventricular filling, cardiac output and arterial blood pressure need not be measurably compromised, while the volume of blood in the capacitance vessels may vary greatly. These low-pressure vessels thus serve as buffers to sustain cardiac output and arterial blood pressure, but in so doing, their stretch or cardiopulmonary "mechanoreceptors" provide continuous afferent stimuli regarding the adequacy of the intravascular volume. The afferent pathway from the mechanoreceptors to the brain apparently is via the vagus nerves.

In extreme extracellular and/or intravascular volume deficiency, sufficient to compromise cardiac filling, the arterial baroreceptors are affected. When this happens the arterial baroreceptors also contribute to volume regulation, but this probably represents a back-up emergency response, with the low-pressure capacitance vessels through mechanoreceptors serving the usual monitoring function.

Physiological and clinical studies by Davis (5), Bartter (7), Denton (10), Genest (11), and others have implicated the renin–angiotensin mechanism in this volume regulation. Morphologic studies by Hartroft (12) and Tobian (13) of the renal juxtaglomerular apparatus have supported this view. Thus, renin is thought to be secreted in response to stimulation of cardiopulmonary mechanoreceptors (38). A decrease of right atrial pressure, cardiopulmonary blood volume, and cardiac output, which follows pooling of blood in the legs of normal human volunteers caused by inflation of cuffs about the thighs, was associated with increased plasma renin activity. There were no detectable changes in the intra-arterial systolic and diastolic pressures or in the pressure amplitude during this maneuver. The increase in plasma renin activity is most likely a reflex, as it was prevented by the beta-adrenergic antagonist propranolol and did not occur in patients who had functioning, but denervated, transplanted kidneys. Systemic injections of small amounts of isoproterenol, a potent beta-adrenergic agonist, will also elevate plasma renin activity, but this effect is abolished by nephrectomy. It is likely that, at least in some species, reduction in blood flow or perfusion pressure within the kidney will also cause release of renin by a direct, local effect.

Renin has long been known to be a specific proteolytic enzyme whose substrate is an α-globulin of plasma. It splits off a decapeptide chain from this α-globulin (see Fig. 3-5). This peptide fragment, an-

Fig. 3-5 Renin-angiotensin system.

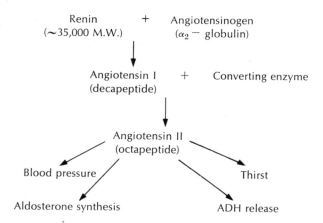

giotensin I, is inactive until another enzyme (converting enzyme) cleaves off two amino acids, leaving the octapeptide angiotensin II.

This octapeptide, one of the most potent pressor agents known, acts on arterial smooth muscle to directly maintain blood pressure despite fluid volume deficits. But it has other actions that set into motion long-range, slower adjustments to correct deficits of intravascular and extracellular volume. It initiates biosynthesis of aldosterone by the adrenal cortex, to decrease renal sodium losses. It also acts via receptors within the circumventricular organs (primarily the subfornical organ), the specialized tissues of the third and fourth ventricles, which are outside the blood-brain barrier, to induce thirst and to effect the release of antidiuretic hormone (39). Thus it both increases water intake and conserves body sodium and water. In some species it stimulates salt appetite as well, but this effect is not known to occur in man. Angiotensin II thus has a central role in the regulation of extracellular and vascular volume.

Recently it has been found that the C-terminal heptapeptide fragment of angiotensin II [(des-Aspartyl)-angiotensin II] is also an agonist. It occurs naturally and elicits qualitatively similar, though quantitatively different, effects as angiotensin II on steroidogenesis and blood pressure (43). For these reasons it has been termed "angiotensin III."

Figure 3-6 summarizes the self-correcting feedback system just described. In addition to indicating how excesses or deficits in extracellular or intravascular volume are corrected, this scheme also suggests the aberrations in volume regulation that may occur in disease. Thus, a failing cardiac output due to heart disease might be indistinguishable in this system from an actual reduction in intravascular volume and could set off the same mechanisms for sodium retention. But in heart disease the retained sodium does not correct the primary disturbance; it produces an increase in extracellular fluid volume, and edema, while the stimulus to sodium retention persists. Similarly, diseases of kidney and liver leading to excessive loss or deficient synthesis of serum proteins, respectively, are associated with a contracted intravascular volume. This sets off the mechanisms for sodium and water retention shown in Figure 3-6. But the deficiency of serum proteins diminishes the proportion of the retained sodium and water held in the intravascular compartment to correct the insufficiency of its volume, the stimulus for sodium and water retention persists and large

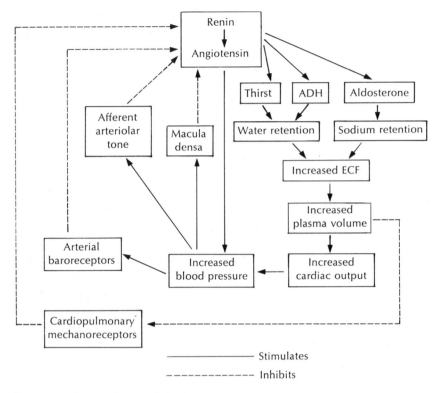

Fig. 3-6 Regulation of extracellular fluid volume (ECF).

volumes of extracellular fluid accumulate in the interstitial spaces, and edema ensues. The retained sodium and water are partitioned mostly into the interstitial space, so that correction of intravascular volume is relatively or absolutely retarded.

The very simplicity of this regulatory system should by now have aroused the reader's suspicion that the story is still incomplete. Other factors undoubtedly are involved. Experiments by de Wardener and Mills in 1961 (14, 15) focused on the inadequacy of this formulation. These workers, and their associates administered saline intravenously to dogs that had received large amounts of mineralocorticoids, which excluded the possibility that decreased adrenocortical secretion might be responsible for the resulting large sodium excretion. Furthermore, they reduced glomerular filtration during the saline infusion by inflating a balloon in the aorta above the renal arteries. Nevertheless, increased sodium excretion persisted. The search continues for the factor or factors responsible for increased sodium excretion in these experiments (16, 17). The noncommital term "third factor" has been applied to the determinants of sodium excretion that operate independently of changes in glomerular filtration rate and adrenocorticoid effects. Third factor may well represent several distinct influences on renal sodium excretion. At present, hemodynamic factors and the oncotic pressure of the proteins in the peritubular capillaries are the best characterized additional factors. Dilution of plasma proteins in the peritubular capillaries secondary to expansion of the volume of extracellular fluids reduces the proportion of filtered sodium and water reabsorbed in the proximal tubules, whereas increases in the concentration of plasma proteins in these vessels have the opposite effect on sodium reabsorption in the proximal tubule (18, 19). This effect promotes sodium excretion when extracellular volume expands and sodium retention when it contracts and thus tends to stabilize the volume of extracellular fluid. An active search continues for other humoral and hemodynamic factors that may be involved in this important regulatory process (16–20).

The intracellular volume

Much less attention has been paid to changes in the volume of the intracellular fluid compartment in health and disease, but a very dynamic regulation of its water content must occur. The difficulty in sampling the intracellular fluids and our almost total ignorance of what activity or osmotic coefficients to apply to the estimated chemical concentrations of intracellular solutes have retarded understanding in this important area. In this section we attempt a plausible hypothesis to further our understanding.

The first fact emerging from a consideration of the regulation of the intracellular fluid volume is that it is a highly individual process solved independently by each cell in the body. Since about two-thirds of total body water exists within cells but body weight normally fluctuates by only 1 to 2% from day to day, each cell must accomplish this regulation on the average with remarkable precision. Studies by Loewenstein (21) have emphasized the electrical coupling that occurs between adjacent cells in some tissues. His evidence that solutes may move much more readily between certain adjacent cells that are in contact than between the intracellular compartment of a cell and its extracellular environment suggests cooperative cellular activity in volume regulation within certain tissues, but basically this regulation must depend on the function of each individual cell.

Isotope techniques show that cell membranes are quite permeable to water and, to varying degrees, permeable to nearly all the small solute molecules and ions in their environment. It is also known that cells contain many poorly diffusible macromolecules that are both fixed and soluble in cytoplasm and organelles. These soluble macromolecules enveloped within the plasma membranes must exert an osmotic pressure, tending to draw extracellular fluid into the cell, with resultant swelling of the cell. There are only two ways in which this catastrophic occurrence can be avoided, as it obviously is.

1. Each cell could be surrounded by a tough membrane that would withstand the high osmotic pressures involved and prevent cell swelling. Although this solution to the problem has been adopted by plant cells, each encased in a cellulose wall, what information we have about animal cells indicates that their plasma membranes have very low tensile strength (22).

2. Some solute could be retained in an extracellular position to balance the osmotic effects of intracellular, nondiffusible molecules. The sodium ion appears to fulfill this requirement.

All determinations of the sodium content of tissues indicate that some sodium is present outside the diffusible extracellular space of the tissue as estimated with extracellular markers such as inulin, chloride, and sulfate. This sodium, generally allocated to an intracellular position, may be only ~10 mEq/kg of intracellular water in muscle or ~30 mEq/kg of intracellular water in cells isolated from a transporting epithelium (23). The intracellular concentration, however, must be considerably lower than that of the surrounding extracellular fluid. Studies with isotopic sodium have shown that this predominantly extracellular position of sodium does not result from impermeability of cell membranes to sodium. Rather, sodium is continuously diffusing into cells from the extracellular fluid and is continuously being pumped out to maintain its low intracellular concentration.

When micropipets are inserted into individual cells so that the electrical potential within the cell can be compared with that of a reference electrode in the extracellular fluid, most cells prove to be electrically negative to their environment with a potential difference of some 30 to 90 mV established across the thin plasma membrane. This membrane potential may be regarded as arising from the slight separation of charge that occurs when the positive sodium ions Na^+ are pumped out of the cell and the negatively charged nondiffusible anions A^{n-} are left behind. Alternatively, if the active removal of Na^+ is obligatorily coupled to the uptake of the potassium ions K^+ so that no separation of charge occurs, the membrane potential may be regarded as a diffusion potential due to the outward diffusion of K^+ from its high intracellular to low extracellular concentration. Thus, for muscle

$$E = RT \ln \frac{(K_i)}{(K_e)} = RT \ln \frac{164}{4} = 94 \, \text{mV} \qquad (3\text{-}2)$$

The measured membrane potential of skeletal muscle ($\sim$90 mV) is slightly less than the calculated diffusion potential. This indicates that, although potassium distribution between the cell and its extracellular fluid is close to its equilibrium electrochemical potential, the plasma membrane is significantly permeable to other ions besides K^+, the activity coefficient for intracellular potassium is low, or potassium is actively accumulated by the cell. All three factors are generally thought to be involved.

For the present discussion it is assumed that the outward movement of sodium ions is the major transport activity of cells. Since sodium is being transported out of the cell against both an electrical and a chemical concentration gradient, work must be performed in maintaining the external position of sodium. The energy for this process derives from the metabolism of the cell.

Figure 3-7 schematically represents the distribution of ions in a normally metabolizing cell and in a cell with impaired metabolism. The steady state is maintained by a continuous supply of metabolic energy that is used to "pump out" the sodium that is constantly streaming down its electrochemical potential gradient into the cell. The result is a predominantly extracellular position of sodium that counterbalances osmotically the effect of nondiffusible, intracellular molecules and thus stabilizes the normal intracellular volume. Because of the electronegativity of the intracellular fluid, chloride and other diffusible anions are largely kept out of the cell.

The steady-state nature of this regulation can be demonstrated by

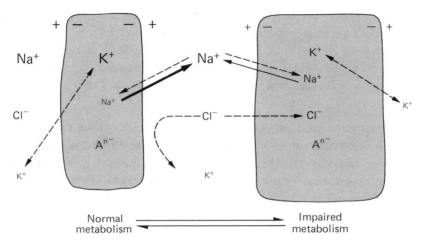

Fig. 3-7 Regulation of cell volume. Reprinted by permission from the *American Journal of Medicine,* 49:293, 1970.

inhibiting tissue metabolism. This may be accomplished simply and reversibly by cooling the tissue. Without sufficient energy, sodium can no longer be pumped out of the cell and it accumulates there. This leads to depolarization of the cell membranes potential so that chloride also accumulates in the cell. Potassium is lost, but it has been shown that the gain of sodium and chloride must exceed the loss of potassium (24). A net gain of intracellular solute occurs, and swelling of the cell ensues. If metabolism is restored before cell death occurs, sodium is again pumped out of the cell, chloride follows, potassium reaccumulates, and the steady-state conditions, including a normal intracellular volume, are reestablished.

This method of preserving cell volume has several advantages for the animal cell. Our very mobility, as compared to sessile members of the vegetable kingdom, derives from this method of preserving cell volume, which obviates the necessity for the rigid wall that surrounds every plant cell. A low cell membrane tension is a prerequisite for motility. Furthermore, the potential energy stored within the ion gradients across cell membranes is adapted in specialized tissues, such as nerves and muscles, for conduction of electrical impulses.

One may wonder why primary disturbances in the regulation of intracellular fluid volume are not more commonly encountered in clinical medicine. Several answers to this question are probably relevant.

1. Our ability to recognize changes in cell volume is very limited. If our histologic preparatory techniques preserved an increase in cross-sectional area of cells by 50%, which might or might not be detected by microscopy, an increase in intracellular volume of 72% would have had to occur. But it is dubious that an increase of only 50% in area would be detectable.

2. Depolarization of the cell membrane potential can be expressed as the logarithm of the intracellular-to-extracellular concentration ratio of potassium, or the extracellular-to-intracellular concentration ratio of chloride. Thus, large changes in ion gradients are necessary before large changes in volume can occur. In many cells such changes may not be compatible with life.

Despite our ignorance in these matters, disturbances in the regulation of cell volume may play an important part in two of the major causes of death, heart attacks and strokes. An initial ischemia in heart muscle (25) or brain tissue (26) may interfere with the supply of energy necessary for the sodium pump and lead to swelling of the affected cells. Prevention or reversal of this swelling by the infusion of hypertonic, poorly penetrating solutes reduces the amount of subsequent cell necrosis in the heart (25) and kidneys (44).

TONICITY OF BODY FLUIDS

The normal serum sodium concentration
In health the serum sodium concentration ranges between 136 and 143 mEq/liter of serum, despite large individual variations in the intake of salt and water. Since serum normally has a water content of 93%, the sodium concentration expressed more rigorously per liter or kilogram of serum water is about 7% higher than these values. The serum sodium concentration is maintained at constant levels because the salts of sodium comprise the major osmotically active solutes in the serum and the body zealously preserves the total solute concentration of the serum in health within narrow limits of some 275 to 290 mOsm/kg of water.

Maintenance of the constancy of total solute activity of serum is the function of the thirst–neurohypophyseal–renal axis, about which there is now considerable understanding. Figure 3-8 shows the operation of

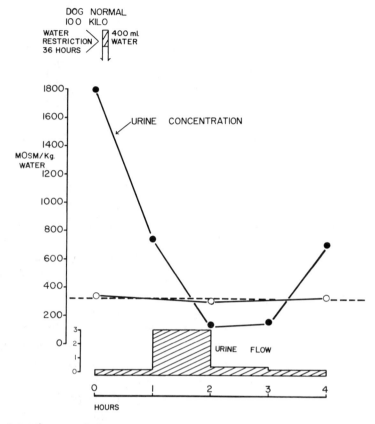

Fig. 3-8 The normal diuretic response. Reprinted from (27) with permission of the *Journal of Clinical Investigation.*

the neurohypophyseal–renal portion of this axis in a dog; similar results have been obtained in man (27). After 36 hours of fluid restriction, the serum total solute concentration was found to be very slightly elevated above the normal level for the dog (indicated by the horizontal broken line in Fig. 3-8). The urine, however, was maximally concentrated. (In man urinary concentrations of 900 to 1200 mOsm/kg of water are maximal.) After water was administered by stomach tube, there was a slight fall in serum total solute concentration, along with a marked reduction in urinary concentration, and a water diuresis. As the administered water was excreted, the serum solute concentration rose and urinary concentration again increased.

Antidiuretic hormone

In terms of the classic studies of Verney (28), these simple observations can be interpreted as follows. The continuous obligatory losses of water during the period of restricted fluid intake resulted in an increased concentration of the body fluids. But a rise of only 1 or 2% in the effective total solute concentration of serum is sufficient to stimulate maximal release of antidiuretic hormone from the neurohypophysis. The antidiuretic hormone then acts on the renal tubules to increase reabsorption of water. Water is maximally conserved by the production of a small volume of concentrated urine. When water is ingested, the resulting dilution of the body fluids inhibits secretion of antidiuretic hormone, tubular reabsorption of water is reduced, and a diuresis of dilute urine rids the body of the excess water load. Thus, with water deficit or excess, this sensitive feedback mechanism acts to preserve the total solute concentration of serum within the narrow normal limits.

The antidiuretic hormone, arginine vasopressin in man, is an octapeptide. It is synthesized in nuclei of the hypothalamus, chiefly in the supraoptic nuclei, from which it passes down the supraopticohypophyseal tract within the axons as identifiable granules to be stored and subsequently released from the posterior pituitary gland. The latter is thus the site of storage, but not of biosynthesis of the hormone. The eight amino acids comprising the hormone are arranged with a five-member ring containing an S–S bond and a tail composed of three amino acids:

glycinamide
|
arginine
|
proline
cys————aspartamide
S   glutamide
S   phenylalanine
cys————tyrosine

The ring structure, but not the disulfide bond, is essential for hormonal activity. The hormone exerts its action on the target cells in the kidney by activating the appropriate adenylate cyclase to produce 3′,5′-cyclic adenosine monophosphate, which mediates the permeability changes attributed to the hormone in the luminal plasma membrane of the cells lining the collecting ducts.

Thirst

Regardless of how effective the above mechanism is in reducing renal water loss, the continuous obligatory extrarenal dissipation of water would result in a progressive increase in total solute concentration of body fluids if there were no means to alert the individual to the need for more water. The sensation of thirst obviously provides for this need. As a result largely of the studies of Bengt Andersson (29), we now appreciate the close anatomic and physiologic relations of the thirst and antidiuretic systems. Andersson found that instillation of small amounts of hypertonic saline solution into the anterior hypothalamus of goats through capillary pipettes, or direct electric stimulation of the same area, results in thirst. The sensation is apparently so pronounced that, if the stimulus is prolonged, the animals drink themselves into a state of water intoxication with intravascular hemolysis from hypotonicity. It is particularly pertinent to this discussion that the stimulation of the anterior hypothalamus in Andersson's experiments, which was effective in producing thirst, would often elicit antidiuresis.

There are two distinct and separable stimuli for thirst, and in all probability, for secretion of antidiuretic hormone as well. These are cellular dehydration and extracellular fluid volume depletion.

Reductions in cell volume by hypertonic solutions of solutes that penetrate cell membranes poorly elicit drinking behavior in animals. Thus intravenous injections of hypertonic solutions of sodium chloride, sodium sulfate, sodium acetate, or sucrose in nephrectomized rats provoke an intake of an amount of water that fairly precisely is that needed to dilute the injected solution to isotonicity (40). The threshold for drinking has been estimated for man to be a reduction of cellular water content by $1.23 \pm 0.48\%$ (42) which is consistent with the estimated 1 to 2% rise in serum osmolality that will stimulate thirst and release antidiuretic hormone. Verney (28) had localized the receptors responsive to osmotic stimuli to the circulation of the internal carotid artery. Careful ablation experiments in the rat and rabbit localize thirst receptors to the lateral preoptic areas, but it is likely that

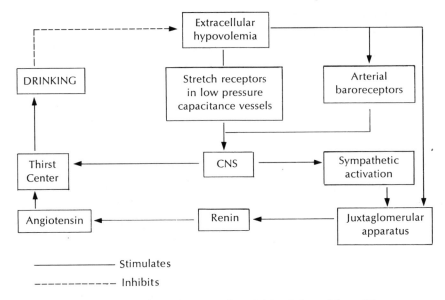

Fig. 3-9 Extracellular hypovolemia as a stimulus of thirst (adapted from 40).

these are anatomically separate from the osmoreceptors that are concerned with the release of antidiuretic hormone, which lie more caudally in the supraoptic area (40).

Reductions in extracellular fluid volume also stimulate thirst (Fig. 3-9). It seems likely that extracellular volume reduction or hypovolemic thirst depends on sensory information from stretch receptors in the low-pressure capacitance vessels near the heart and in the atria; these, the receptors that comprise the afferent side of the reflex arcs, influence secretion of vasopressin and aldosterone and thus control excretion of water and sodium in response to extracellular volume changes (Fig. 3-9). The vagi carry afferent impulses to the central nervous system where the thirst center is stimulated directly. Sympathetic pathways to the kidney are also activated, resulting in the release of renin. The angiotensin II produced acts via receptors within the circumventricular organs, the specialized tissues of the third and fourth ventricles outside the blood-brain barrier, to stimulate the thirst center. Thus a dual mechanism provokes thirst when extracellular fluid volume is compromised.

The thirst induced by cell dehydration and by extracellular fluid volume reduction is simply additive. This absence of interaction between the components is evidence for the functional independence of the mechanism mediating cellular and extracellular thirst. There is evidence also that the neural systems mediating the thirst resulting from these two stimuli are anatomically separate. The osmosensitive neurons responding to cellular dehydration seem to be in the lateral preoptic area; they can be selectively destroyed without affecting the drinking response to depletion of extracellular fluid volume. The neurons that mediate the latter are more diffusely spread. Both neural systems converge posteriorly so that they become inseparable in the lateral hypothalamus (40).

In man, loss of body weight of some 0.8% from water lack will stimulate thirst. The stimulus in this situation is a combination of cellular and extracellular dehydration acting additively.

The renal concentrating and diluting mechanism

The function of the renal countercurrent systems, and their role in the elaboration of dilute and concentrated urine (30–33), was described in Chapter 2. To review briefly:

1. Isotonic tubular fluid, consisting of about 25% of the glomerular filtrate, enters the descending limb of the loop of Henle.

2. This fluid becomes progressively more concentrated as it enters the hypertonic inner medulla, where water is extracted from it.

3. After rounding the hairpin turn deep in the medulla, the concentrated fluid enters the thick ascending limb of the loop of Henle, where sodium chloride is pumped out.

4. This creates a medullary interstitium that is progressively more hypertonic toward the papillary tips, leaving a dilute fluid of some 150 mOsm/liter to enter the distal convoluted tubule in the cortex.

5. In the absence of antidiuretic hormone, this dilute fluid passes through the distal tubule and collecting duct. A further reabsorption of salt without water may occur, leaving a dilute, copious urine to be excreted.

6. In the presence of antidiuretic hormone, the tubular fluid still proceeds through the distal convoluted tubule without changing

significantly in concentration. The hormone, however, has rendered the cells lining the collecting duct permeable to water. A large reduction in the volume of tubular fluid occurs in the cortical portions of the collecting duct as the dilute contents equilibrate with the isotonic cortical interstitium. The remaining small volume of tubular urine passes down the collecting duct through the progressively more concentrated medullary interstitium, to which it loses water. A small volume of concentrated urine thus emerges from the papillary tip. In normal man maximal urinary concentrations of 900 to 1200 mOsm/kg of water can be achieved.

The bookkeeping for the process of concentrating and diluting the urine is credible. As urine is concentrated, an isotonic filtrate is formed and a hypotonic reabsorbate is returned to the circulation from the collecting ducts, leaving a hypertonic, scanty urine to be excreted. During water diuresis an isotonic fluid is again delivered to the kidney, but a hypertonic fluid is returned to the circulation from the medullary interstitium, leaving a hypotonic, copious urine to be excreted.

It should be clear from these requirements that any condition that prevents the delivery of a sufficient volume of fluid containing sodium chloride to the ascending limb of the loop of Henle interferes with both the maximal concentrating and diluting abilities of the kidney. If too little salt and water are delivered to this segment during antidiuresis, there is insufficient sodium chloride to achieve maximal solute concentrations in the hypertonic medullary interstitial zone. Even in the presence of antidiuretic hormone, urinary concentrations fall, therefore, short of the maximum by the amount that the hypertonic medullary interstitial zone achieves less than its highest tonicity. On the other hand, water diuresis is also diminished by a reduced volume of fluid reaching the ascending limb. In this situation reabsorption of sodium chloride, no matter how nearly complete, leaves a lesser volume of dilute urine to be excreted. Furthermore, it seems that the collecting tubules are somewhat permeable to water, even in the absence of antidiuretic hormone. As the small volume of dilute urine passes down the collecting duct through the zone of high interstitial fluid osmolality, there is a net loss of water, with a subsequent increase in concentration (34). Thus, it is apparent whenever there is a decrease in glomerular filtration per nephron, the concentrating and diluting capabilities of the kidney are both impaired.

Conversely, whenever there is an increase in glomerular filtration per nephron, a condition associated with over-expansion of the extracellular volume or high cardiac output, the concentrating and diluting capabilities of the kidney are also impaired. This is the case during osmotic diuresis, when the concentration of the urine tends toward isotonicity with that of serum, irrespective of the presence or absence of antidiuretic hormone. Superimposing a large osmotic load (i.e., by intravenous infusion of mannitol, glucose, or urea) on a water diuresis brings such a large volume of fluid to the thick ascending limb of the loop of Henle that reabsorption of sodium and chloride at this site does not appreciably dilute the fluid entering the distal nephron, and urine concentration rises toward that of plasma. And during antidiuresis, the increased blood flow through the medulla, associated with the osmotic load, "washes out" the high concentrations of solute in the interstitium, preventing formation of maximal urinary concentrations.

Largely from studies on amphibian tissues—skin (35) and urinary bladder (36)—we know that vasopressin exerts its antidiuretic action by making the responsive epithelium more permeable to water and urea. In the presence of this hormone and an osmotic gradient, the tubular epithelium of the cortical segments of collecting ducts permits passage of large quantities of water with very little solute; in the medulla the permeability of collecting ducts, to both water and urea, is increased. The hormone acts on the responsive plasma membrane at the luminal surface of the tubular cells to accommodate the large reabsorption of water.

The integrated functions of the thirst–neurohypophseal–renal system that regulate normal tonicity of body fluids are summarized in Figure 3-10.

Tonicity of intracellular fluids

Thus far our discussion has focused on regulation of the extracellular fluid tonicity. It is well established that the intracellular fluids are isotonic with the extracellular fluids (37). Although the solute composition within cells differs considerably from that of extracellular fluids, cell membranes do not constitute a barrier to water, which attains a uniform activity inside and outside cells. Only in the renal medulla, where concentrated or dilute urine is formed, and in glands with anisosmolar secretions, does tonicity differ from that of serum. Hence the same mechanism that stabilizes the total solute or sodium concentration of the serum also regulates the tonicity of the larger

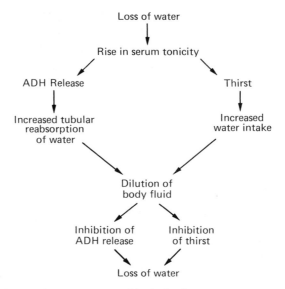

Fig. 3-10 Regulation of concentration of body fluids.

volume of intracellular fluids. The serum sodium concentration consequently serves as an index of the concentration, or activity, of water throughout the body fluids.

References

1. Moore, F. D. Metabolic care of the surgical patient. W. B. Saunders, Philadelphia, 1959, 1011, 10.
2. Loeb, R. The adrenal cortex and electrolyte behavior. The Harvey Lectures, Series 37, Lancaster, Pa., Science Press Printing Co., 1942.
3. Harrop, G. A., Soffer, L. J., Ellsworth R., and Trescher, J. H. Studies on the suprarenal cortex. III. Plasma electrolytes and electrolyte excretion during suprarenal insufficiency in the dog. J. Exper. Med. 58:17–38, 1933.
4. Simpson, S. A., Tait, J. F., Wettstein, A., Neher, R., vonEuw, J., and Reichstein, T. Isolierung eines neuen kristallisierten Hormons aus Nebennieren mit besonders hober Wirksamkeit auf den Mineral Stoffwechsel. Experientia 9:333–335, 1953.
5. Davis, J. O. The control of aldosterone secretion. The Physiologist 5:65–86, 1962.
6. Bartter, F. C. Role of aldosterone in normal homeostatis and in certain disease states. Metabolism 5:369–383, 1956.
7. Bartter, F. C., Liddle, G. W., Duncan, L. E., Jr., Barber, J. K., and Delea, C. The regulation of aldosterone secretion in man: The role of fluid volume. J. Clin. Invest. 35:1306–1315, 1956.

8. Müller, A. F., Riondel, A. M., and Manning, E. L. Mechanismes regulateurs de l'aldosterone chez l'homme. Helv. Med. Acta 23:610, 1956.

9. Leaf, A., Bartter, F. C., Santos, R. F., and Wrong, O. Evidence in man that urinary electrolyte loss induced by pitressin is a function of water retention. J. Clin. Invest. 32:868–878, 1953.

10. Denton, D. A., Goding, J. R., and Wright, R. D. Control of adrenal secretion of electrolyte-active steroids. Brit. Med. J. 2:447–456, 522–530, 1959.

11. Genest, J., Biron, P., Koiw, E., Nowaczynski, W., Chretien, M., and Boucher, K. Adrenocortical hormones in human hypertension and their relation to angiotensin. Circ. Res. 9:775–791, 1961.

12. Pitcock, J. A. and Hartroft, P. M. The juxtaglomerular cells in man and their relationship to the level of plasma sodium and to the zona glomerulosa of the adrenal cortex. Am. J. Path. 34:863–883, 1958.

13. Tobian, L. Physiology of the juxtaglomerular cells. Ann. Int. Med. 52:395–410, 1960.

14. deWardener, H. E., Mills, I. H., Clapham, W. F., and Hayter, C. J. Studies on the efferent mechanism of the sodium diuresis which follows the administration of intravenous saline in the dog. Clin. Sci. 21:249–258, 1961.

15. Mills, I. H., deWardener, H. E., Hayter, C. J., and Clapham, W. F. Studies on the afferent mechanism of the sodium chloride diuresis which follows intravenous saline in the dog. Clin. Sci. 21:259–264, 1961.

16. Berliner, R. W. Intrarenal mechanisms in the control of sodium excretion. Fed. Proc. 27:1127–1131, 1968.

17. Pearce, J. W. Renal nervous and spinal pathways and the reflex regulation of extracellular fluid volume. Fed. Proc. 27:1132–1148, 1968.

18. Earley, L. E. Influence of hemodynamic factors on sodium reabsorption. Ann. N.Y. Acad. Sci. 139:312–327, 1966.

19. Lewy, J. E. and Windhager, E. E. Peritubular control of proximal tubular fluid reabsorption in the rat kidney. Am. J. Physiol. 214:943, 1968.

20. Levinsky, N. G. Nonaldosterone influences on renal sodium transport. Ann. N.Y. Acad. Sci. 139:295–303, 1966.

21. Loewenstein, W. R., Socolar, S. J., Higashino, S., Kanno, Y., and Davidson, N. Intercellular communication: renal, urinary bladder, sensory, and salivary gland cells. Science 149:295–298, 1965.

22. Harvey, E. N. Tension at the cell surface. Protoplasmatologia 2:E5, 1954.

23. Gatzy, J. T. and Berndt, W. O. Isolated epithelial cells of the toad bladder. Their preparation, oxygen consumption and electrolyte content. J. Gen. Physiol. 51:770–784, 1968.

24. Leaf, A. On the mechanism of fluid exchange of tissues *in vitro*. Biochem. J. 62:241–248, 1956.

25. Powell, W. J., Jr., DiBona, D. R., Flores, J., and Leaf, A. The role of cell swelling in myocardial ischemia and the protective effect of hypertonic mannitol. J. Clin. Invest. 52:66a, 1973.

26. Ames, A., Wright, R. L., Kowada, M., Thurston, J. M., and Majno, G. Cerebral ischemia II. The no-reflow phenomenon. Am. J. Path. 52:437–453, 1968.

27. Leaf, A. and Mamby, A. R. The normal antidiuretic mechanism in man and dog; its regulation by extracellular fluid tonicity. J. Clin. Invest. 31:54–59, 1952.

28. Verney, E. B. The absorption and excretion of water: the antidiuretic hormone. Lancet 2:781–783, 739–744, 1946.

29. Andersson, B. Polydipsia, antidiuresis and milk ejection caused by hypothalamic stimulation. The neurohypophysis, H. Heller, ed., Butterworths, London, pp. 131–140, 1957.

30. Hargitay, B. and Kuhn, W. Das Multiplikationsprinzip als Grundlage der Harnkonzentrierung in der Niere. Zeitschrift für Elektrochemie und Angewandte Physikalische Chemie 55:539–558, 1951.

31. Wirz, H., Hargitay, B., and Kuhn, W. Lokalisation des Konzentrierungsprozesses in der Niere durch direkte Kryoskopie. Helvetica Physiologica et Pharmacologica Acta 9:196–207, 1951.

32. Berliner, R. W., Levinsky, N. G., Davidson, D. G., and Eden, M. Dilution and concentration of the urine and the action of antidiuretic hormone. Am. J. Med. 24:730–744, 1958.

33. Gottschalk, C. W. Osmotic concentration and dilution of the urine. Am. J. Med. 36:670–685, 1964.

34. Berliner, R. W. and Davidson, D. G. Production of hypertonic urine in absence of pituitary antidiuretic hormone. J. Clin. Invest. 36:1416–1427, 1957.

35. Koefoed-Johnsen, V., Ussing, H. H., and Zehran, K. The contributions of diffusion and flow to the passage of D_2O through living membranes. Acta Physiologica Scandinavica 28:60–76, 1953.

36. Leaf, A. Action of neurohypophyseal hormones on the toad bladder. Gen. and Comparative Endocrinol. 2:148–160, 1962.

37. Maffly, L. H., and Leaf, A. The potential of water in mammalian tissues. J. Gen. Physiol. 42:1257–1275, 1959.

38. Kiowski, W. and Julius, S. Renin response to stimulation of cardiopulmonary mechanoreceptors in man. J. Clin. Invest. 62:656–663, 1978.

39. Fitzsimmons, J. T. Angiotensin, thirst and sodium appetite: retrospect and prospect. Fed. Proc. 37:2669–2675, 1978.

40. Fitzsimmons, J. T. Thirst. Physiol. Rev. 52:468–560, 1972.

41. Gauer, O. H. and Henry, J. P. Neurohormonal control of plasma volume. Int. Rev. Physiol. 9:145–190, 1976.

42. Wolf, A. V. Thirst: Physiology of the Urge to Drink and Problems of Water Lack. Charles C. Thomas, Springfield, Ill. 1958.

43. Carey, R. M., Vaughan, Jr., E. D., Peach, M. J., and Ayers, C. R. Activity of (des-Aspartyl)-angiotensin II and angiotensin II in man. J. Clin. Invest. 61:20–31, 1978.

44. Frega, N. S., DiBona, D. R., and Leaf, A. The protection of renal function from ischemic injury in the rat. Pflugers Archiv. 381:159–164, 1979.

4

Acid–Base Regulation

The hydrogen ion activity of the extracellular fluids is a jealously guarded parameter of body composition. Its quantitative statement is the pH, the negative logarithm to the base 10 of the hydrogen ion concentration. Ideally, pure water dissociates

$$H_2O = [H^+] [OH^-]$$

so that the concentration of both $[H^+]$ and $[OH^-]$ is equal to 10^{-7} molar; the pH of such neutral water is thus 7.00. The reaction of extracellular fluid is normally slightly alkaline, with a pH of 7.40; hydrogen ion activity $[H^+]$ equals 40 nM (nanamolar). The range of pH compatible with life is approximately 7.0 to 7.6, which defines a four-fold change in hydrogen ion activity or concentration* (100 to 25 nM). Thus, though we regard regulation of hydrogen ion as precise, the body tolerates considerable percent change in the concentration of this

---

* The glass electrodes conventionally used measure hydrogen activity directly, but custom permits use of the term *concentration* interchangeably with *activity* in referring to hydrogen ions, terminology not permitted in referring to other ions in aqueous solution.

ion as compared with other important ions, such as calcium and potassium.

It is not understood why reactions of the extracellular fluid outside these limits are not tolerated. Presumably, some essential biochemical process is affected. Whatever the explanation, serious impairment of function intervenes whenever the upper or lower limit is approached.

The pH of the body fluids is protected by three lines of defense: (1) the body buffers, (2) pulmonary regulation of the concentration of carbon dioxide in the body, and (3) renal excretion of acid or alkali. They act in complementary fashion, first to minimize changes in reaction of the body fluids and then to correct any disturbance in acid–base balance by the appropriate retention or excretion of hydrogen ions.

BUFFERS

A buffer is a substance that can give or accept protons in a way that tends to minimize changes in pH. An acid is a proton donor and a base is a proton acceptor. We generally speak of buffer pairs:

$$H_2CO_3-NaHCO_3$$
$$\text{H protein–Na protein}$$
$$NaH_2PO_4-Na_2HPO_4$$

All buffer pairs of physiologic interest (with the exception of urinary $NH_3-NH^+_4$) are weak acids and the salt of a strong alkali with the weak acid.

The reaction of the buffer pair to a strong acid, e.g., hydrochloric acid, is

$$NaHCO_3 + HCl \rightarrow H_2CO_3 + NaCl$$

In reacting with this strong acid, sodium bicarbonate ($NaHCO_3$) produces a neutral salt, sodium chloride ($NaCl$) and a weak acid, carbonic acid (H_2CO_3). The latter undergoes further degradation to yield CO_2 and H_2O and the CO_2 is removed via the lungs. In reacting with a strong alkali, such as sodium hydroxide,

$$H_2CO_3 + NaOH \rightarrow NaHCO_3 + H_2O$$

the products are a weakly alkaline salt, sodium bicarbonate, and water. In both instances the effect of the strong acid or alkali on the pH has been minimized, *but not abolished* by interaction with the buffer pair.

The effect of buffers is to mitigate, but not abolish changes in pH. This can be understood by examining the dissociation constant K for a weak acid $[HA] = [H^+] + [A^-]$

$$K = \frac{[H^+][A^-]}{[HA]} \qquad (4\text{-}1)$$

This can be rearranged

$$[H^+] = K\frac{[HA]}{[A^-]}$$

and the logarithm taken

$$\log[H^+] = \log K + \log\frac{[HA]}{[A^-]}$$

Since $pH = -\log[H^+]$, the familiar Henderson–Hasselbalch equation is obtained

$$pH = pK + \log\frac{[A^-]}{[HA]}$$

From this it is evident that pH is determined by the ratio of free buffer anion to undissociated acid. For the major buffer system of the extracellular fluids (H_2CO_3–$NaHCO_3$), this equation is

$$pH = 6.1 + \log\frac{[HCO^-_3]}{[H_2CO_3]}$$

The pK value defines the pH at which the ratio $[A^-]/[HA]$ equals 1.0; it is the pH at which buffering capacity is maximal. The physiologic pH of the extracellular fluid (7.4) is, however, remote from the pK value of this buffer system and in fact represents an $[HCO^-_3$ to $[H_2CO_3]^*$ ratio of 20/1. The peculiar effectiveness of this buffer derives from the fact that one component, $[H_2CO_3]$, is directly regulated by pulmonary ventilation.

In the normal person, with a plasma pH of 7.40, the total carbon

---

* $[H_2CO_3]$ is taken as the sum of dissolved CO_2 and H_2CO_3 in practice. Some 99.9% of this quantity is, in fact, the concentration of dissolved CO_2 rather than of free acid, Thus, the pK of 6.1 is an apparent value.

dioxide released by addition of strong acid to a volume of plasma is approximately 27 millimolar. Thus

$$pH = 6.1 + \log\frac{26}{1.3} = 7.4$$

and the ratio $[HCO^-_3]/[H_2CO_3]$ necessary to yield a pH of 7.4 is 20/1. The absolute values of bicarbonate or carbonic acid are unimportant in this regard; only the ratio of their concentrations is pertinent to establishing the pH of the blood or body fluids.

Measurement of any two of the three variables in the Henderson–Hasselbalch equation suffices to define the system completely. Classically, the pH, together with the total CO_2 content of a sample of blood, carefully collected under oil, were measured (the quantity of CO_2 liberated from a given volume of plasma by a strong acid, which included, therefore, all HCO^-_3 *and* H_2CO_3). Technical advances now permit accurate, simple measurement of pH and pCO_2 ([H_2CO_3] directly with appropriate electrodes.

Two further facts should be appreciated:

1. Since the dissociation of water yields $[H^+]$ and $[OH^-]$, the dissociation constant for water is

$$K_{HOH} = [H^+]\,[OH^-] = 10^{-14}$$

    Thus, any change in $[OH^-]$ must be represented by a reciprocal change in $[H^+]$, so that their product remain 10^{-14}.

2. With excess CO_2 in body fluids, the reaction $CO_2 + [OH^-] = [HCO^-_3]$ occurs, catalyzed by the enzyme carbonic anhydrase, and the HCO^-_3 in the extracellular fluid is the physiologic expression of the strong base OH^-. Gain or loss of HCO^-_3, if H_2CO_3 remains constant, is equivalent, therefore, to loss or gain of H^+ in the extracellular fluids.

Body buffers

It would be erroneous to leave the impression that bicarbonate is the only base participating in the buffering of acids added to the body or that all buffering occurs within the extracellular fluid. Indeed, all buffers exposed to the same ambient hydrogen ion activity of the extracellular fluids contribute to the total buffering capacity of the body. The extent of this contribution, for a given deviation of pH from normal, is quantitatively determined by the amount of the buffer in the system and its pK. Phosphate and proteins are the two other major contributors but are of less quantitative importance than bicarbonate in the extracellular fluids. Other organic acids contribute only negligibly because of their low concentrations.

The intracellular compartment, or more correctly the "extraextra-cellular fluid" compartment, contributes very significantly to the body's buffering capacity. When strong acid is added to the extracellular fluid, hydrogen ion from the extracellular fluid may exchange with intracellular sodium and potassium of muscle or with Na^+ and Ca^{++} of bone. The result is buffering of the extracellular fluids at the expense of an increased hydrogen ion concentration in structures outside the diffusible extracellular fluids (see Fig. 4-1).

Pitts and associates (1–3) have estimated the quantitative aspects of such buffering in nephrectomized dogs in which the amount of H^+ buffered outside the volume of distribution of $^{35}SO^=_4$ was measured ($^{35}SO^=_4$ is generally thought not to enter cells, or to enter them only very slowly, and thus serves as a marker for the extracellular fluid volume). The steady-state concentration of $^{35}SO^=_4$ in the plasma divided into the quantity of $^{35}SO^=_4$ injected into the animal served as the measure of diffusible extracellular space. Since the amount of an administered load of H^+ or OH^- buffered in this compartment was determined, the remainder must have been buffered outside this "space." Figure 4-2 shows the distribution of buffering of an acid load in Pitts' experiments, and Figure 4-3, the distribution of the buffering of strong alkali (3). There is some evidence to suggest that the distribution of buffering is not very dissimilar in man and that the proportion of buffering accomplished by extracellular fluid and by fluids outside the

Fig. 4-1 Buffering of acid by tissues.

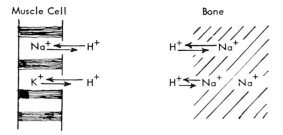

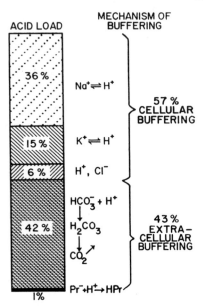

METABOLIC ACIDOSIS

Fig. 4-2 Distribution in body fluids of the buffering of acid. From Pitts, Robert F.: *Physiology of the Kidney and Body Fluids.* Copyright © 1974 by Year Book Medical Publishers, Inc., Chicago. Used by permission. (Adapted from Swan, R. C., and Pitts, R. F.: *J. Clin. Invest.* 34:205, 1955.)

extracellular compartment does not change greatly except in association with very low plasma bicarbonate levels, in which case a disproportionately large share of the buffering seems to occur outside the extracellular fluid compartment (4).

This information is pertinent to correcting systemic acidosis and alkalosis clinically. The magnitude of the disturbance is greatly underestimated if this nonextracellular fluid buffering is ignored. Thus, in dealing with an acidotic patient, one determines the decrement in serum bicarbonate concentration from the ideal normal of 26 mM and multiplies this decrement by the estimated volume of the patient's extracellular fluid volume (normally about 20% of lean body weight). But the resulting value must be doubled to account for the H^+ buffered outside the extracellular fluid. Only in this manner can the total excess of hydrogen ion be calculated and the amount of base estimated that would be necessary to correct the deficit in buffering capacity that occurred. In practice one does not replace the total amount abruptly, but may administer half the total within 24 hours, depending on the severity of the acidosis and the patient's condition.

In alkalosis the bicarbonate excess in the extracellular fluid volume is calculated and then multipled by 3/2 to obtain the total excess sustained. Because intracellular buffers differ from those in extracellular fluids, their pK values also differ. Thus, there is no reason to expect buffering capacity outside the extracellular fluids to be symmetrical around pH 7.40. In fact, these buffers are more effective in buffering an acidic than an alkaline load.

PULMONARY REGULATION OF CARBONIC ACID
In mitigating the effect of adding strong acid to the buffer system, HCO^-_3–H_2CO_3, $[HCO^-_3]$ decreases and $[H_2CO_3]$ increases; adding

Fig. 4-3 Distribution in body fluids of the buffering of alkali. From Pitts, Robert F.: *Physiology of the Kidney and Body Fluids.* Copyright © 1974 by Year Book Medical Publishers, Inc., Chicago. Used by permission. (Adapted from Swan, R. C., et al.: *J. Clin. Invest.* 34:1795, 1955.)

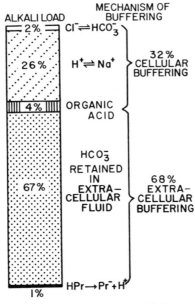

alkali has the opposite effect. In both situations changes in pulmonary excretion of carbon dioxide will shift the pH toward normal values.

The response of the bicarbonate buffer system to acidosis may be illustrated as follows. Consider a liter of fluid containing 26 mM of bicarbonate in a closed system with a gaseous environment that contains sufficient carbon dioxide to maintain a concentration of $[H_2CO_3]$ equal to 1.3 mM. With plasma a pCO_2 of 40 mm Hg suffices. This situation is depicted in column A of Figure 4-4. Here we see that our conditions $[HCO^-_3]/[H_2CO_3] = 26/1.3 = 20/1$ define a pH of 7.4. Addition of 13 mEq of a strong acid, such as HCl, to this system promptly converts HCO^-_3 to H_2CO_3, and the ratio $[HCO^-_3]/[H_2CO_3]$ falls to 10/11 and the pH to 6.0 if the extra H_2CO_3 formed cannot be "blown off." If the pCO_2 of the gaseous phase were kept at 40 mm Hg, then the ratio would rise to 10/1. This would yield a pH of 7.1, which would represent a severe, but not fatal acidosis in a patient. A patient with a normal respiratory system could do even better in compensat-

Fig. 4-4 The effect of strong acid on pH of a bicarbonate solution. In *A*, 26 mEq of bicarbonate in a liter of fluid is in equilibrium with a gas phase with carbon dioxide at a pressure of 40 mm Hg. *B* represents the effect of adding 13 mEq of strong acid to this system. In *C* the carbon dioxide partial pressure is reduced again to 40 mm Hg. In *D* carbon dioxide tension is even lower.

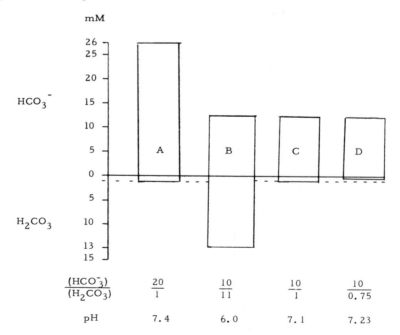

ing for the acidosis. By hyperventilating he could actually lower the pCO_2 of the alveolar air below 40 mm Hg and the concentration of H_2CO_3 in the body fluids correspondingly. The consequences of such a respiratory effort may be similar to the situation depicted in Column *D* of Figure 4-4. The final pH of the system is brought back up to 7.23, which is equivalent only to a moderate acidosis. If the H_2CO_3 concentration had actually been reduced to 0.65 mM, the ratio would have been $13/0.65 = 20/1$, and the pH would have again been 7.40. Such compensation is thus possible through pulmonary excretion of CO_2 with nothing being done to correct the loss of buffer, HCO^-_3, suffered as the initial and inescapable effect of adding strong acid to the system.

Clinically, the increased ventilation in the acidotic patient should be discernible to the physician as a deep, unhastened breathing, referred to as Kussmaul respiration. By this type of breathing the acidotic patient increases his tidal volume so as to dilute the concentration of CO_2 in alveolar air. It is the alveolar CO_2 tension that, of course, establishes the tension of CO_2 in body fluids and the concentration of H_2CO_3. The slow, deep breathing characteristic of acidosis should be distinguished from the shallow, rapid breathing that characterizes pulmonary congestion from pulmonary edema, infarction, or infection.

In the past, acidosis was deliberately induced in patients by feeding them ammonium chloride in large amounts as a diuretic or an adjunct to mercurial diuretics. The ammonium of this neutral salt is converted quantitatively in the liver to urea, leaving in effect hydrochloric acid. But today this practice has been abandoned so that acidosis does not usually arise from the clinical administration or ingestion of strong acid. More commonly it results from metabolic disturbances in which large amounts of endogenous organic acids accumulate, that is, diabetic ketoacidosis, in which acetoacetate and β-hydroxybutyric acids accumulate, or tissue anoxia, in which lactic acid may accumulate. Severe acidosis can develop rapidly, especially in infants, from loss of alkaline intestinal fluids in diarrhea. One of the most common causes of acidosis is renal failure. This may take two forms: (1) simple inability of a diseased kidney to rid the body of hydrogen ions at the rate of their production during metabolism or (2) wasting of bicarbonate in the urine. These aspects of renal function will be considered in more detail shortly.

In these kinds of acidosis a drop in the serum bicarbonate level results either from accumulation of acids in the body that are stronger than carbonic acid or directly from loss of bicarbonate via urine or stool. Acidoses from these causes are generally grouped together as "metabolic acidoses."

Alkalosis may arise clinically from the ingestion or administration of excessive amounts of alkali, generally sodium bicarbonate, or from the loss of acid from the body. Vomiting secondary to pyloric obstruction or other cause may produce large losses of gastric hydrochloric acid that result in systemic alkalosis. Potent diuretics may so enhance the renal excretion of acid as to cause alkalosis. In such alkalosis the serum bicarbonate levels, or CO_2 content, may be markedly elevated and serum chloride concomitantly reduced. These states are commonly referred to as "metabolic alkaloses." Excessive and prolonged exposure to adrenocortical hormones may also be associated with metabolic alkalosis resulting from increased renal excretion of hydrogen ions, an effect of mineralocorticoids that is augmented in dogs by potassium deprivation (28).

In contrast to the respiratory response to metabolic acidosis, hypoventilation occurs in "metabolic alkalosis." This permits an increase in the concentration of alveolar CO_2 and, hence, an increase in its partial pressure in the body fluids. The increase in the concentration of H_2CO_3 in the body fluids tends to compensate for the alkalosis. Thus, a patient with pyloric obstruction secondary to a peptic ulcer may vomit sufficiently to increase his serum CO_2 content to 53 mM. With normal values of pCO_2 this would yield a ratio of $[HCO^-_3]/[H_2CO_3] = 52/1.3 = 40/1$, which in turn defines a pH of 7.70. If sufficient CO_2 is retained to increase $[H_2CO_3]$ to 2.0, the ratio becomes $52/2 = 26/1$, and the pH falls to 7.52. Retention of CO_2 to levels of 2.6 mM would clearly result in complete compensation of pH to a normal value of 7.4, but in reality alveolar hypoventilation does not produce such complete compensation. This failure of complete respiratory compensation for metabolic acidosis or alkalosis is probably important, as we shall see, in allowing the kidneys to sense the disturbed acid–base balance and to take appropriate action to secrete the excess acid or alkali so as finally to correct the disturbance.

PRIMARY RESPIRATORY DISTURBANCES

Since the Henderson–Hasselbalch equation indicates that the pH is determined by the ratio of $[HCO^-_3]/[H_2CO_3]$, it is evident not only that gains or losses of strong acids affecting [HCO$^-$$_3$] can produce metabolic acidosis or alkalosis, respectively, but also that primary changes in [H$_2$CO$_3$] may disturb the normal pH. Carbon dioxide retention from lung disease, common with pulmonary emphysema, or central nervous system depression, or injury to the respiratory center, causes a decrease in the bicarbonate/carbonic acid ratio with concomitant acidosis. Hyperventilation, which may result in hypocapnia, may increase this ratio and cause alkalosis. Hysterical hyperventilation, rare postencephalitic disturbances of the respiratory center, and the hyperventilation that accompanies pulmonary congestion may all result in excessive CO$_2$ loss. Certain medicines, such as salicylates, may directly stimulate the respiratory center and thus cause hyperventilation. Since salicylic acid itself is stronger than carbonic acid, salicylates may produce a mixed metabolic and respiratory disturbance of acid–base balance (5). These conditions of primary CO$_2$ retention or loss result in "respiratory acidosis" and "respiratory alkalosis," respectively.

Any compensation that the body can make to respiratory acidosis or alkalosis must clearly be through alterations in the concentration of bicarbonate: increasing it in respiratory acidosis and decreasing it in response to respiratory alkalosis. The kidney responds appropriately by excreting bicarbonate ions in response to a reduction in pCO$_2$ of the body fluids and by excreting hydrogen ions in response to an elevated pCO$_2$. The result of these responses is that plasma changes in metabolic acid–base disturbances are quite distinct from those in respiratory acid–base disturbances:

| | PLASMA | | |
	CO$_2$ CONTENT	pH	pCO$_2$
Metabolic acidosis	↓	↓	↓
Metabolic alkalosis	↑	↑	↑
Respiratory acidosis	↑	↓	↑
Respiratory alkalosis	↓	↑	↓

ROLE OF THE KIDNEYS

Although the body buffers and pulmonary control of CO$_2$ excretion are the first line of defense in protecting the pH of the extracellular fluids, it is the action of the kidneys that ultimately corrects the disorder. The kidneys excrete the excess acid or alkali responsible for the disturbance.

Response to alkalosis

The mechanism used by the kidneys to correct metabolic alkalosis is, at least descriptively, simple. The kidneys excrete an alkaline urine containing the excess bicarbonate. A urine of the same pH as that of plasma should contain at least the same concentration of bicarbonate as the plasma. But the kidneys can do better than this. They can elaborate a urine of pH greater than that of plasma, approximately as high as 7.8. This defines a ratio $[HCO^-_3]/[H_2CO_3]$ of about $50/1$ and allows bicarbonate to be excreted at concentrations in excess of its concentration in plasma. But, in addition, careful measurements have shown that the $[H_2CO_3]$ or pCO_2 of alkaline urine may be double that of plasma. This also contributes to the capacity for excretion of bicarbonate within the limits of urinary pH.

With such efficient mechanisms for correcting metabolic alkalosis, how then does severe alkalosis ever occur? It is difficult to induce alkalosis in a normal individual even by administering very large quantities of alkali because of the efficiency of renal excretion of bicarbonate. Severe alkalosis is associated with sodium deficiency. Only when the quantity of sodium in the extracellular fluids is inadequate to maintain optimal volume of this compartment can severe metabolic alkalosis develop. Bicarbonate can be excreted in the urine only with a fixed cation, which, for practical purposes, means Na^+ or K^+. When no sodium is excreted in the urine because this ion is needed to maintain extracellular fluid volume, then little bicarbonate is excreted. It is true that some bicarbonate is excreted as its potassium salt under such conditions, but this mechanism is limited quantitatively and is more significant clinically as the cause of potassium depletion with alkalosis than it is physiologically as a means of correcting metabolic alkalosis. In addition to an adequate supply of sodium ions with which to excrete the excess bicarbonate, chloride ions must be available to replace the bicarbonate in the extracellular fluid as the latter is excreted (6). Administration of sodium chloride satisfies both of these needs, and in patients with intrinsically normal kidney function this is generally all that is necessary to correct metabolic alkalosis. Because potassium depletion so commonly accompanies alkalosis, supplements of this ion, preferably as potassium chloride, should also be provided.

In the renal compensation for respiratory alkalosis, the same considerations apply, but here the excretion of the "excess" bicarbonate reduces the plasma levels below normal as the ratio $[HCO^-_3]/[H_2CO_3]$ falls toward 20/1.

Response to acidosis

The renal mechanisms for excretion of acid are more complex. Three distinguishable but interrelated processes have been described: (1) the reabsorption of filtered bicarbonate, (2) the excretion of "titrable acids," and (3) the production of ammonia. Even in the absence of disease or iatrogenic stress on these mechanisms, there is a continuous requirement for excretion of the excess acid produced by the daily metabolism of ingested foodstuff. The average American diet yields, on catabolism, an excess of some 50 to 100 mEq of hydrogen ion daily, which must be excreted to preserve normal acid–base balance. This acid is derived largely from metabolism of the sulfur-containing amino acids to sulfuric acid, so that the magnitude of the acid load is mainly a function of the quantity of dietary protein.

The process of reabsorbing the filtered bicarbonate is an essential "housekeeping" function of the kidney and one of considerable magnitude. Because of the seemingly inefficient design and operation of this organ, a normal adult with 26 mM bicarbonate in his plasma and a volume of glomerular filtrate of about 180 liters/24 hours filters about 4700 millimoles of bicarbonate each day. Just to maintain the status quo, all of this huge quantity of bicarbonate (equivalent to nearly 395 gm of sodium bicarbonate) must be reabsorbed. Loss of bicarbonate is the physiological equivalent of loss of hydroxyl ions or retention of hydrogen ions in the body, since, in the presence of the large amounts of carbon dioxide generated during metabolism, hydroxyl ions are promptly buffered by interaction with CO_2:

$$OH^- + CO_2 \rightarrow HCO^-_3$$

The mechanism by which the renal tubules reabsorb filtered bicarbonate (Fig. 4-5) is clearly a devious process. $NaHCO_3$ is filtered through the glomerulus, CO_2 produced in the renal tubular epithelium or brought to the kidney from other tissues by the blood, reacts with water in the presence of carbonic anhydrase to form carbonic acid,

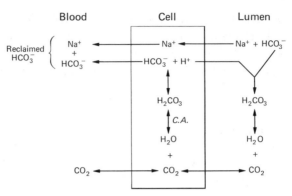

Fig. 4-5 Reabsorption of filtered bicarbonate by H^+ secretion.

which in turn dissociates to produce hydrogen and bicarbonate ions. Alternatively, water dissociates, providing OH^-, which reacts directly with CO_2 in the presence of carbonic anhydrase to yield bicarbonate ions. The hydrogen ions produced by either process are then available to exchange for the sodium in the glomerular filtrate. The secreted proton interacts with tubular fluid bicarbonate to form urinary H_2CO_3. This in turn dissociates to H_2O and CO_2, and the diffusible CO_2 equilibrates across the renal tubular epithelium; some is excreted via the lungs. Meanwhile the urinary sodium ion reabsorbed by exchange with tubular cell hydrogen ions is transported across the tubular epithelium into the blood accompanied by bicarbonate as counterion. In the process of reabsorption, the original bicarbonate ion has been destroyed, and sodium is returned to the body fluids accompanied by a new partner, the bicarbonate generated within the tubule. The net effect for acid–base economy is, however, that one bicarbonate ion has been filtered and one has been reabsorbed. This "housekeeping" subsistence function of the kidney has been accomplished; no acid or alkali has been gained by or lost from the body.

Formation of titratable acid is a variant of this same process. This is illustrated in Figure 4-6. Hydrogen ions formed in the renal tubular epithelial cells are again exchanged for filtered sodium in the luminal fluid. The hydrogen ion this time encounters a phosphate ion, $HPO_4^=$ (bicarbonate ions having become scarce) and converts this to $H_2PO_4^-$. Thus

$$Na_2HPO_4 + H^+ \rightarrow NaH_2PO_4 + Na^+$$

Again, a sodium ion has been reabsorbed from the glomerular filtrate and returned to the body fluids accompanied by the bicarbonate ion generated in the renal tubular cell. In this instance a hydrogen ion is excreted from the body and a new bicarbonate ion added, so that there is a net loss of acid and the body buffers are reconstituted. At the pH of the body fluids, four-fifths of the phosphate is present as the mono-hydrogen anion $HPO_4^=$ and one-fifth as the dihydrogen phosphate $H_2PO_4^-$. This is, of course, defined by the Henderson–Hasselbalch equation:

$$7.4 = 6.8 + \log \frac{[HPO_4^=]}{[H_2PO_4^-]}$$

In the urine, titration of $HPO_4^=$ by secreted hydrogen ions changes the ratio $[HPO_4^=]/[H_2PO_4^-]$ downward from $4/1$, and the urine becomes more acid. At the lower limits of urinary pH, about 4.5, virtually all the $HPO_4^=$ has been converted to the acid form, $H_2PO_4^-$. Other weak acids in the urine are similarly titrated to their undissociated free-acid form by this addition of hydrogen ions. Although phosphate usually comprises the major urinary buffer, other weak acids, such as creatinine, become increasingly important quantitatively as the urinary pH falls.

The amount of buffer anions in the urine and the lower limit of urinary pH set the limit on the quantity of hydrogen ion that can be excreted as titratable acids. But the kidney has a highly efficient means of overcoming this limitation: it produces ammonia within the renal tubular cells, largely by enzymatic deamination of amino acids, primarily glutamine. As seen in Figure 4-7, the NH_3 diffuses into the acid urine, where it buffers H^+ and is trapped as NH_4^+,

$$NH_3 + H^+ = NH_4^+$$

Fig. 4-6 Urinary acidification; the excretion of titratable acid.

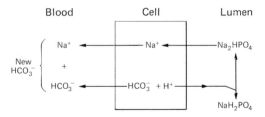

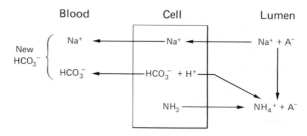

Fig. 4-7 Urinary acidification; the secretion of ammonium.

since the uncharged NH_3 freely crosses cell membranes, which are highly impermeable to charged species (see Fig. 4-7). The conversion of a hydrogen ion to the neutral cation, NH^+_4, decreases the hydrogen ion concentration of the urine and thus permits increased excretion of protons from the body within the limits of urinary pH. At a urine pH of 4.5 the concentration of free H^+ is under 0.1 mEq/liter. By the devices of titrable-acid excretion and ammonium formation the net removal of hydrogen ions per liter of urine can greatly exceed the urine's content of free hydrogen ions.

"Titratable acids" received their name because they have long been measured in terms of the milliequivalents of sodium hydroxide that must be added to a liter of urine to return its pH to 7.4. This value, plus the NH^+_4 content and minus the bicarbonate content of the urine, is the quantitative measure of net acid excretion from the body. Since any bicarbonate in the urine represents a loss of alkali or a gain of acid, any excretion of bicarbonate must be subtracted from the sum of titratable acids plus ammonium to obtain the net excretion of acid in the urine. Of course, at pH 4.5 the amount of bicarbonate present in the urine is neglible as defined by the Henderson–Hasselbalch equation when urinary pCO_2 equals that of the extracellular fluids.

With an average American diet yielding some 70 mEq of hydrogen ions per day, the titrable-acid excretion may be expected to account for about 30 mEq of acid, while ammonium excretion makes up the remainder. Under conditions of chronic acidosis, as in diabetic keto-acidosis or prolonged administration of the acidifying salt, ammonium chloride, several hundred milliequivalents of hydrogen may require excretion daily. This is accomplished largely by an increase in the excretion of ammonium, which may attain levels of 200 to 300 mEq daily. During chronic acidosis an adaptation occurs in the renal tubular mechanisms for forming NH_3 so that the very high rates of ammonium excretion can be attained. A period of 4 to 6 days is required for this adaptation to reach its maximum.

The site of acidification in the renal tubule has long been a subject of speculation and, more recently, of attempts at direct localization. Knowledge that bicarbonate reabsorption was largely accomplished in the proximal tubule and appreciation that this "reabsorption" occurred by a process of hydrogen ion excretion, as described above, led to the inescapable conclusion that most of the hydrogen ion added to the urine was secreted in the proximal tubule. The argument that bicarbonate is "reabsorbed" by a process of hydrogen ion secretion rather than directly is based largely on the proportion of filtered bicarbonate that can be excreted when renal carbonic anhydrase is inhibited by progressively increasing amounts of acetazolamide (7); micropuncture techniques have also been used to show this (8). It is possible, however, that some bicarbonate is absorbed directly as the anion (9). Whatever the actual situation, the secretion of hydrogen ions into urine containing bicarbonate buffers the hydrogen ion with little change in pH. Whereas in the distal nephron, after absorption of bicarbonate, a relatively small further secretion of hydrogen ions drives the urinary pH down to its final levels.

REGULATION OF RENAL BICARBONATE REABSORPTION BY pCO_2

The elegance of the carbonic acid–bicarbonate buffer system lies in the complementary, but independent control of carbonic acid concentrations by the lungs and of bicarbonate concentrations by the kidneys. How and where the pCO_2 of body fluids influences respiration is unresolved, despite a great deal of research and speculation. It is apparent that renal reabsorption or generation of bicarbonate is a direct function of the plasma pCO_2 (10), as shown in Figure 4-8. Whether the pCO_2 measures the availability of CO_2, which, in the presence of carbonic anhydrase, is the substrate for the reaction that yields H^+ for secretion and HCO^-_3 for "reabsorption" by renal tubular cells, or whether some more subtle influence exists is not known. The consequences of this relationship are happy indeed. A decrease in pCO_2 from hyperventilation reduces bicarbonate reabsorption or hydrogen ion secretion.

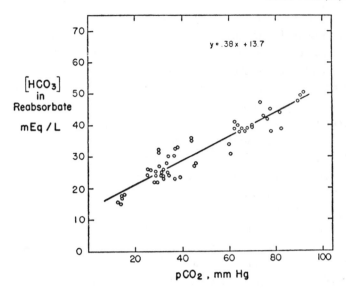

Fig. 4-8 The relation of reabsorbate bicarbonate concentration to plasma pCO_2. The plasma pH was never less than 7.45. Reprinted from (10) with permission of the *Journal of Clinical Investigation*.

The resulting alkaline urine lowers the serum bicarbonate, and the ratio $[HCO^-_3]/[H_2CO_3]$ falls toward normal to compensate for a respiratory alkalosis. In response to hypercapnia the kidneys increase hydrogen ion secretion and add a significant quantity of bicarbonate to the body fluids and thus compensate for a respiratory acidosis. In this manner the kidneys adjust appropriately to primary respiratory disorders of acid–base regulation even as the lungs help out when metabolic disturbances affect primarily the bicarbonate concentration. But whereas the pulmonary response is prompt, the renal response requires a day or more before excretion or generation of bicarbonate takes place in quantities sufficient to affect its concentration in the body fluids significantly. Furthermore, whether it is respiratory compensation for a metabolic disturbance or renal compensation for a respiratory disorder, the adjustment always falls short of being complete. Perhaps it is necessary to have some slight residue of the primary disorder reflected in the pH so that the feedback mechanisms can sense persistence of the disturbance and, when possible, correct the primary defect. But then perhaps we are indulging in teleology when what is really needed is a better understanding of the mechanisms under discussion.

Other factors that may modulate the acid–base status have been studied. A reduction in extracellular fluid volume in itself seems to increase the plasma bicarbonate through increased secretion of hydrogen ions in the proximal tubule (11). The frequent occurrence of a moderate elevation of plasma bicarbonate in patients receiving diuretic therapy on a chronic basis is probably one clinical manifestation of this phenomenon.

It is also apparent that the parathyroid hormone has some effect on the acid–base balance. An increase in this hormone reduces proximal reabsorption of bicarbonate, sodium, and phosphate. This causes a mild metabolic acidosis. In contrast, patients who lack this hormone as a consequence of idiopathic hypoparathyroidism or of surgical ablation have a mild metabolic alkalosis. Excessive amounts of mineralocorticoids also cause increased acid excretion and mild metabolic alkalosis, as seen in Cushing's syndrome or hyperaldosteronism.

The factors currently known to cause increased renal bicarbonate absorption include:

increased pCO_2
decreased serum chloride
decreased serum potassium
increased adrenal steroids
decreased parathyroid hormone
decreased extracellular fluid volume

CLINICAL ACID–BASE DISORDERS

Simply to recognize and treat acidosis or alkalosis is not sufficient. It is important to recognize specific causes and to manage the underlying disorders as well. Fortunately, the simple plasma analyses necessary to establish the presence of the acid–base disturbance often yield important clues that, when combined with the patient's clinical history, usually reveal the underlying disorder.

Metabolic acidosis

Metabolic acidosis may be classified according to the presence or absence of an "anion gap." If the sum of serum chloride and bicarbonate concentrations is subtracted from the serum sodium concentration, the resulting difference is referred to as the "anion gap":

$$[Na^+] - ([Cl^-] + [CO_2]) = 142 - (103 + 27)$$
$$= 12 \ mEq/liter \ anion \ gap$$

Thus, the usual anion gap is some 10 to 16 mEq/liter. When values greater than 16 are encountered with metabolic acidosis, they signify the addition of acid stronger than carbonic acid to the body at rates that exceed the rate of disposal of the anion from the body. Examples of such anion gap acidoses are diabetic ketoacidosis and lactic acidosis. In the former acetoacetic and β-hydroxybutyric acids are produced at rates that exceed the rate of their metabolism by tissues and excretion by the kidneys. Severe tissue hypoxia may enhance glycolysis and liberate lactic acid more rapidly than it can be oxidized or reconverted by the liver to glucose or glycogen. In the acidosis of renal failure, the rate of production of strong acid in the body may not be excessive, but the decreased renal function, especially the low glomerular filtration rate, prevents excretion of the anions of the strong acids produced during metabolism, and sulfate, phosphates, and other anions accumulate at the expense of a lowered plasma bicarbonate concentration. In every case, however, it is the retained hydrogen ion, not the retained anion, that is responsible for the systemic acidosis!

A number of intoxicants are associated with metabolic acidosis and a large anion gap. Methanol poisoning causes acidosis from formic acid. Ethylene glycol ingestion yields oxalic acid, and the oxalate in turn may profoundly lower the serum calcium concentration because of the insolubility of calcium oxalate. An elevated anion gap occurs in salicylate intoxication and is probably due to lactic acid, salicylate, and other organic anions. Thus, with an anion gap greater than 16 mEq/liter and metabolic acidosis one suspects

1. Diabetic ketoacidosis
2. Lactic acidosis
3. Renal failure
4. Poisoning

When the anion gap is less than 12 mEq/liter in metabolic acidosis, different etiologic factors must be considered. A low anion gap metabolic acidosis is a hyperchloremic acidosis with serum chloride levels

generally in excess of 107 mEq/liter, but in the presence of hyponatremia, estimation of the anion gap is more informative than the
absolute concentration of chloride. Hyperchloremic acidosis occurs in
severe diarrhea because of losses in the stool of alkaline intestinal and
pancreatic secretions. It may occur with ingestion of NH_4Cl, an acidifying salt, or acetazolamide (Diamox), a carbonic anhydrase inhibitor
that prevents tubular reabsorption of bicarbonate and, hence, loss of
this ion in the urine. Ureterosigmoid transplant, or more rarely today,
ileal loops, for diversion of urine from bladder to bowel when the
former must be removed has often been associated with hyperchloremic
acidosis. Reabsorption of urinary chloride by the bowel in exchange
for bicarbonate, which is then lost in the stool, is the main cause of
the acidosis and can be prevented by emptying the colon or the ileal
loop frequently so that such ionic exchanges cannot occur.

There has been great interest in a group of acidotic hyperchloremic
patients with a nonazotemic renal acidification defect—the so-called
renal tubular acidosis or RTA (12). Actually, all patients with renal
disease and acidosis suffer from an inability of the renal tubules to
secrete hydrogen ions (or reabsorb bicarbonate), and this is the cause
of their acidosis. Patients with RTA, however, have a urinary pH that
is generally too high for their degree of systemic acidosis.

Two forms of RTA are recognized, the proximal and the distal (13,
14). The distal constitutes the classic RTA that is characterized by an
inability of the distal nephron to establish or maintain a normal hydrogen ion gradient. The normal kidney can excrete an acid urine of
pH 4.7, which represents a urine/plasma concentration ratio for hydrogen ions of approximately 800/1. By contrast, the patient with
distal RTA cannot excrete a urine more acidic than pH ~6.0, irrespective of the severity of his systemic acidosis. A lower limit of urine
pH of 6.0 in turn, limits the amount of H^+ that can be excreted as
NH^+_4. Since the amount of buffers in the urine is limited, the pH of
6.0 also limits the excretion of titrable acid. The inability to excrete
hydrogen ions at their rate of formation in the body produces systemic
acidosis. If urinary buffer is increased, more hydrogen ions can be excreted within the limitation of urine pH. This indicates that the defect is in the formation of an adequate hydrogen ion gradient between
the urine and the plasma rather than in the quantity of hydrogen ion
that may be excreted. Although the rate of ammonium excretion in
patients with distal RTA is high for the relatively alkaline urine, it is

insufficient to provide the cation for such fixed anions as $SO_4^=$ and $HPO_4^=$ in the urine. Hence, these anions obligate fixed cations Na^+, K^+, and Ca^{++} for their excretion. This results in depletion of these cations with reduction of extracellular fluid volume, potassium depletion, and rickets or osteomalacia. The increased calcium and phosphate excreted into the alkaline urine often cause kidney stones or nephrocalcinosis.

Since proximal reabsorption of the major moiety of filtered bicarbonate is intact in distal RTA, the amount of sodium bicarbonate needed to correct the hyperchloremic acidosis is relatively small and equals the acid load of approximately 70 mEq produced each day in metabolism. Furthermore, this modest amount of sodium bicarbonate prevents the potassium depletion and demineralization of bone.

Distal or gradient RTA is seen in
   Primary (idiopathic) form
      sporadic
      familial
   Drug- or toxin-induced damage by
      amphotericin B
      vitamin D excess
      lithium
   Miscellaneous conditions
      certain hypergammaglobulinemic states
      Sjogren's syndrome
      hepatic cirrhosis
      renal transplant rejection
      pyelonephritis
      nephrocalcinosis
      medullary sponge kidney

In proximal RTA there may be a very large wasting of bicarbonate in the urine. The disorder of bicarbonate reabsorption in the proximal tubule may deliver quantities of bicarbonate into the distal nephron that overwhelm the limited bicarbonate reabsorptive capacity in this portion of the tubule. An alkaline urine is excreted, and a hyperchloremic, systemic acidosis ensues. When plasma bicarbonate falls to very low levels, however, the distal tubule may be able to reabsorb the small amount of bicarbonate that is filtered. The urine may then again become maximally acidified to pH 4.7, which indicates that the distal tubular hydrogen ion secretory mechanism is intact. The proximal nature of the reabsorptive defect of bicarbonate is usually indicated by concomitant defects in proximal reabsorptive activity, so that aminoaciduria, glycosuria, and phosphaturia may be present as well.

In proximal RTA, attempts to bring the serum bicarbonate up to normal levels by administering sodium bicarbonate are generally doomed to failure. The higher the plasma bicarbonate level, the larger the quantity of bicarbonate that escapes proximal reabsorption and is excreted in the urine. The loss of sodium in the alkaline urine results in contraction of the extracellular fluid volume, which in turn, enhances aldosterone secretion. In the presence of increased aldosterone, the large quantities of sodium delivered to the distal tubule enhance potassium secretion into the urine, and potassium depletion ensues. Demineralization of the skeleton occurs as the result of phosphate loss, systemic acidosis, and secondary hyperparathyroidism, so that the condition in these respects resembles distal RTA. The inability to correct the hyperchloremic acidosis completely, except with huge amounts of sodium bicarbonate, the failure of such therapy to prevent the potassium loss, the reduction of urinary pH at low levels of plasma bicarbonate, and the frequent association with other proximal tubular reabsorptive defects all distinguish the proximal from the distal types of RTA.

Proximal or bicarbonate-wasting RTA is seen

1. Associated with multiple proximal tubular defects
    a. Fanconi syndrome as a result of genetically transmitted systemic diseases, for example, cystinosis, Wilson's disease, hereditary fructose intolerance, tyrosinosis, and Lowe's syndrome or intoxications from heavy metals and drugs, for example, outdated tetracyclines
    b. Disorders of protein excretion, for example, nephrotic syndrome and multiple myeloma
    c. Vitamin D deficiency

2. Without other defects of proximal tubular function
    a. Primary form, either familial or sporadic
    b. Drug induced, for example, sulfonamides (including acetazolamide)

Metabolic alkalosis

At a urine pH of 7.8 the bicarbonate concentration would be 66 mM if urine pCO_2 equaled the normal value for extracellular fluid. Since the pCO_2 of alkaline urine may exceed that of plasma by a factor of two or more, the bicarbonate concentration in alkaline urine may be considerably higher than 65 mM. The kidneys are able to excrete a great excess of bicarbonate during metabolic alkalosis. In practical terms this means that metabolic alkalosis is essentially limited to situations in which the kidneys are either damaged or constrained to conserve sodium ions, that is, depletion of extracellular fluid volume or excessive levels of adrenal mineralocorticoids.

ALKALI INGESTION

Alkalosis caused by administration of such alkaline salts as sodium bicarbonate is rarely encountered today. Not long ago sodium bicarbonate was prescribed in the treatment of peptic ulcer. With the then popular Sippy powders, patients might receive 40 to 60 gm of sodium bicarbonate daily, and it is a tribute either to the capacity of the kidneys to excrete alkali or to the unreliability of patients in taking prescribed medications that more cases of severe alkalosis did not occur. In addition to a daily intake of 500 mEq or more of sodium bicarbonate, milk or calcium carbonate was administered on alternate hours during the day. Potassium depletion from the alkali was common, and the high calcium intake, in the presence of alkaline body fluids and urine, resulted in kidney stones, nephrocalcinosis, renal damages, and hypercalcemia—the so-called milk–alkali syndrome. It is now known that hypercalcemia stimulates gastric acid secretion; thus the regimen was self-defeating in its therapeutic goals as well as harmful. But even during the decades when Sippy powders constituted the accepted therapy for peptic ulcer and dyspepsia, severe alkalosis was uncommon.

LOSS OF GASTRIC SECRETIONS

Loss of gastric secretions due to vomiting or suction is a more common cause of metabolic alkalosis. The primary secretion of the parietal cells is 150 mM hydrochloric acid. Loss of this acid obviously leaves the body fluids alkaline. The concentration of acid in vomitus or aspirate need not reach this limit to produce significant H^+ losses and metabolic alkalosis. Vomiting also causes loss of some sodium and may restrict further sodium intake. Thus, depletion of extracellular volume accompanies the alkalosis and prevents its renal correction. The stimulus to retain sodium prevents the kidneys from excreting the sodium bicarbonate which is necessary to correct the alkalosis. Not until sodium or potassium chloride is administered to alleviate the depletion of extracellular volume can the kidneys excrete the sodium or potassium bicarbonate and correct the alkalosis. This situation, termed *chloride depletion alkalosis,* is in fact due to a deficit of both chloride and sodium, and both are required for its correction. However, hydrochloric acid or ammonium chloride will temporarily correct the alkalosis, without, of course, correcting the sodium depletion. Sodium chloride reexpands extracellular fluid volume, allowing sodium to be excreted with bicarbonate in an alkaline urine and the alkalosis thereby to be corrected. Without sufficient sodium chloride to correct the volume deficit during metabolic alkalosis, there may be a paradoxical aciduria, a lowering of urinary pH to 6.0 to 6.5 despite severe systemic alkalosis. In the process of conserving sodium, potassium and hydrogen ions are secreted by the renal tubules. The potassium depletion that ensues augments the production of ammonium, and this enhances the renal hydrogen ion loss, thereby preventing correction of the metabolic alkalosis by the kidneys. Volume depletion in itself may impair renal function with prerenal azotemia from reduced renal perfusion and a low glomerular filtration rate.

DIURETICS

Metabolic alkalosis of varying degrees regularly accompanied the use of organic mercurials in the treatment of edematous states. The stimulus to sodium reabsorption by the distal nephron in the edematous patient is great, so that sodium that escapes reabsorption proximally is avidly taken up in the distal nephron. This enhances potassium, hydronium, and ammonium secretion, producing metabolic alkalosis with potassium depletion.

Modern oral diuretics may have a similar effect. Both furosemide and ethacrynic acid have their major inhibitory effect on reabsorption in the ascending limb of the loop of Henle. There is evidence that chloride reabsorption may be the primary transport activity in this segment of the nephron, since the lumen is electrically positive to the peritubular fluid (15, 16). Direct inhibition of this active chloride transport with loss of chloride, and more distal reabsorption of sodium, accompanied by hydronium and ammonium secretion may be responsible for the alkalosis these diuretics can produce.

The thiazide diuretics are widely used in the management of hypertension. The modest reduction in extracellular fluid they provoke is an important feature of their antihypertensive action. But a reduced extracellular fluid volume is itself a stimulus for increased bicarbonate reabsorption with resulting aciduria and metabolic alkalosis. A rigorous maximum rate of tubular reabsorption of bicarbonate (Tm_{HCO-_3}) can be demonstrated only at constant extracellular fluid volume, and with reduction in that volume, bicarbonate reabsorption/dl of glomerular filtrate increases (11). When cannulated isolated segments of proximal tubule are perfused with a solution containing 25 mM bicarbonate, the slower the rate of delivery of the perfusate through the tubule segment, the more of the bicarbonate in the luminal fluid is reabsorbed (28). This may be analagous to the situation that occurs when extracellular fluid volume is reduced secondary to diuretic or other cause so that the filtration rate per nephron diminishes. Elevated plasma bicarbonate and hypokalemia are commonly seen in chronic antihypertensive regimens that include thiazide diuretics.

HORMONALLY INDUCED ALKALOSIS

Metabolic alkalosis is seen in hyperaldosteronism and also in Cushing's syndrome due to excess glucocorticoids. Alkalosis and potassium depletion may be pronounced in the Cushing's disease associated with lung or other cancer in which no aldosterone excretion may be detected. The mechanism of the alkalosis accompanying adrenocortical steroid excess is not clear, since aldosterone administration for as long as 3 months in normal subjects fails to produce significant alkalosis (17). In the dog, however, potassium depletion together with large doses of a mineralocorticoid will produce alkalosis, whereas either alone will not (29). Potassium depletion stimulates renal ammonium excretion. In the rat it also causes renal chloride wasting by depressing chloride reabsorption in the proximal tubule, in the loop of Henle, and in the collecting duct (30). Chloride thus becomes a poorly reabsorbable anion. In the presence of the increased distal sodium reabsorption induced by the excessive adrenal corticosteroids, the poorly reabsorbable chloride enhances the electronegativity of the luminal fluid of the distal nephron and net acid excretion is increased (see Fig. 2-12).

Parathyroid hormone increases urinary bicarbonate excretion, and the absence of this hormone is associated with an increased reabsorption of bicarbonate and consequent mild metabolic alkalosis (18).

INTRACELLULAR pH

Another area of intensive investigation is the intracellular pH and its relation to the pH of the extracellular fluids we have been discussing. Here, unfortunately, the experimental evidence is contradictory. Depending on the technique of measurement, highly divergent results have been obtained. If hydrogen ions distribute between intracellular and extracellular fluids simply passively, then the pH should be lower in skeletal muscle than in plasma. With a membrane potential of 90 mV (intracellular fluids negative), the intracellular pH might be as low as 5.9.

Techniques used to estimate intracellular pH include (1) dyes as pH indicators (9); (2) application of the Henderson–Hasselbalch equation to estimates of intracellular concentrations of bicarbonate and plasma pCO_2 (20); (3) measurement of the distribution of weak organic acids, particularly DMO (5,5-dimethyl-2,4-oxazolidinedione), between extracellular and intracellular fluids (21, 22); and (4) direct measurements with sensitive glass electrodes inserted into individual muscle cells (23). All reports agree that intracellular pH is lower than plasma pH, but sharp controversy rages over whether the value is near 6.0 or 7.0. The DMO method yields results averaging 7.1, though readings with glass electrodes from different laboratories vary from 6 to 7 (23, 24). In view of the complexity of membrane-bounded subcellular organelles, it is highly probable that no single, uniform pH prevails through the intracellular compartment; compartmentation of hydrogen ions is likely, and activities vary with the state of metabolism.

Perhaps of even more importance to the present discussion than the level of intracellular pH is how it reflects changes in the extracellular fluid. From what has been said about the contribution of the intracellular fluids to extracellular acidosis and alkalosis, it can be predicted that changes in the intracellular compartment generally reflect those in the extracellular fluids. But because of the permeability barrier afforded by the plasma membrane that separates the two compartments, significant, if transient, discrepancies may occur.

Small undissociated molecules generally penetrate cells much more readily than ions do. Thus, carbon dioxide and undissociated carbonic acid penetrate cell membranes rapidly compared with the bicarbonate ion. Rapid introduction of sodium bicarbonate into the extracellular fluids produces alkalosis, leading to diminished respiration with retention of carbon dioxide. The increased pCO_2 equilibrates across the cell membrane before the bicarbonate equilibrates. This may produce intracellular acidosis, even when the extracellular fluids are alkalotic. Episodes similar to this, in which cerebrospinal fluid (CSF) rather than intracellular fluid was sampled, have been documented (25). The CSF became more acid as the extracellular fluid pH was increased by alkali therapy. It may take 6 to 12 hours before plasma and CSF bicarbonate attain equilibrium after a change in the former, whereas carbon dioxide equilibrates more rapidly.

These paradoxical pH shifts may also be clinically significant in their effect on the distribution of weak acids or bases between intracellular and extracellular fluids. In severe liver disease ammonia intoxication may result from the failure of the liver to convert blood ammonia arising in the kidneys or gut to urea. Here sudden alkalinization of the extracellular fluids increases the pNH_3, and ammonia readily penetrates cells, while the relatively low intracellular pH increases the concentration of NH^+_4 within cells. Hepatic coma may develop or worsen to the extent that the central nervous system absorbs some of this shift (26).

Phenobarbital is a weak organic acid, and its distribution is also influenced by the pH of body fluids. Extracellular fluid acidosis increases the proportion present as the undissociated free acid, driving more into cells, including those of the brain, and thus increasing the degree of central nervous system depression; alkali administration has the opposite effect (27).

We should never be made so complacent by the ease of sampling changes in the plasma and extracellular fluid that we fail to consider that deleterious, even opposite, changes may be occurring in the critical intracellular compartment out of reach of our sampling needle. Ignorance limits our thinking in this area, but it does not take great imagination to sense the importance of increasing our understanding.

References

1. Swan, R. C. and Pitts, R. F. Neutralization of infused acid by nephrectomized dogs. J. Clin. Invest. 34:205–212, 1955.
2. Swan, R. C., Axelrod, D. R., Seip, M., and Pitts, R. F. Distribution of sodium

bicarbonate infused into nephrectomized dogs. J. Clin. Invest. 34:1795–1801, 1955.

3. Pitts, R. F. Physiology of the kidney and body fluids. Year Book Medical Publishers, Inc., Chicago, 1974, Chapters 10 and 11.

4. Garella, S., Dana, C. L., and Chazan, J. A. Severity of metabolic acidosis as a determinant of bicarbonate requirements. N. Eng. J. Med. 289:121–126, 1973.

5. Singer, R. B. The acid–base disturbance in salicylate intoxication. Medicine 33:1–13, 1954.

6. Kassirer, J. P., Berkman, P. M., Lawrenz, D. R., and Schwartz, W. B. The critical role of chloride in the correction of hypokalemic alkalosis in man. Am. J. Med. 38:172–189, 1965.

7. Schwartz, W. B., Falbriard, A., and Relman, A. S. An analysis of bicarbonate reabsorption during partial inhibition of carbonic anhydrase. J. Clin. Invest. 37:744–751, 1958.

8. Rector, F. C., Jr., Carter, N. W., and Seldin, D. W. The mechanism of bicarbonate reabsorption in the proximal and distal tubules of the kidney. J. Clin. Invest. 44:278–290, 1965.

9. Maren, T. H. Carbonic anhydrase: chemistry, physiology, and inhibition. Physiol. Rev. 47:595–781, 1967.

10. Relman, A. S., Etsten, B., and Schwartz, W. B. The regulation of renal bicarbonate reabsorption by plasma carbon dioxide tension. J. Clin. Invest. 32:972–978, 1953.

11. Kurtzman, N. A. Regulation of renal bicarbonate reabsorption by extracellular volume. J. Clin. Invest. 49:586–595, 1970.

12. Morris, R. C. Renal tubular acidosis. N. Eng. J. Med. 281:1405–1413, 1969.

13. Soriano, J. R., Boichis, H., Start, H., and Edelmann, C. M., Jr. Proximal renal tubular acidosis: a defect in bicarbonate reabsorption with normal urinary acidification. Pediat. Res. 1:81–98, 1967.

14. Soriano, J. R., Boichis, H., and Edelman, C. M., Jr. Bicarbonate reabsorption and hydrogen ion excretion in children with renal tubular acidosis. J. Pediat. 71:802–813, 1967.

15. Burg, M. and Green, N. Function of the thick ascending limb of Henle's loop. Am. J. Physiol. 224:659–668, 1973.

16. Rocha, A. S. and Kokko, J. P. Sodium chloride and water transport in the medullary thick ascending limb of Henle. J. Clin. Invest. 52:612–623, 1973.

17. Kassirer, J. P., London, A. M., Goldman, D. M., and Schwartz, W. B. On the pathogenesis of metabolic alkalosis in hyperaldosteronism. Am. J. Med., 49:306–315, 1970.

18. Hellman, D. E., Au, W. Y. W., and Bartter, F. C. Evidence for a direct effect of parathyroid hormone on urinary acidification. Am. J. Physiol. 209:643–650, 1965.

19. Rous, P. The relative reaction within living mammalian tissues. J. Exper. Med. 41:739–759, 1925.

20. Conway, E. J. and Fearon, P. J. The acid-labile CO_2 in mammalian muscle and the pH of the muscle fibre. J. Physiol. (Lond.) 103:274–289, 1944.

21. Waddell, W. J. and Butler, T. C. Calculation of intracellular pH from the distribution of 5,5-dimethyl-2,4-oxazolidinedione (DMO): Application to skeletal muscle of the dog. J. Clin. Invest. 38:720–729, 1959.

22. Adler, S. The simultaneous determination of muscle cell pH using a weak acid and weak base. J. Clin. Invest. 51:256–265, 1972.

23. Caldwell, P. C. Intracellular pH. Int. Rev. Cytology 5:229–277, 1956.

24. Carter, N. W., Rector, F. C., Jr., Campion, D. S., and Seldin, D. W. Measurement of intracellular pH of skeletal muscle with pH-sensitive glass microelectrodes. J. Clin. Invest. 46:920–933, 1967.

25. Posner, J. B. and Plum, F. Spinal-fluid pH and neurologic symptoms in systemic acidosis. N. Eng. J. Med. 227:605–613, 1967.

26. Stabenau, J. R., Warren, K. S., and Rall, D. P. The role of pH gradients in the distribution of ammonia between blood and cerebrospinal fluid, brain and muscle. J. Clin. Invest. 38:373–383, 1959.

27. Waddell, W. J. and Butler, T. C. The distribution and excretion of phenobarbital. J. Clin. Invest. 36:1217–1226, 1957.

28. Hulter, H. N., Sigala, J. F., and Sebastian, A. Potassium deprivation potentiates the renal alkalosis-producing effect of mineralocorticoid. Am. J. Physiol. 235:F298–F309, 1978.

29. Warnock, D. G. and Burg, M. G. Urinary acidification: CO_2 transport by the rabbit proximal straight tubule. Am. J. Physiol. 232:F20–F25, 1977.

5
Pathophysiology of Potassium Excess and Deficiency

Although the older medical literature contains sporadic references to the importance of potassium in certain clinical conditions, as was pointed out in the historical review by Gamble (1), our current understanding of its importance began with the study of experimental potassium depletion by Heppel (2). With the studies of Darrow and his associates (3) further progress followed rapidly. After extensive experimental characterization of potassium depletion in rats, Darrow (4) demonstrated by repletion studies the importance of potassium deficits in the mortality of infantile diarrhea. Since these early studies many important contributions have been made to an understanding of both the basic physiology of potassium metabolism and its role in clinical medicine.

DISTRIBUTION IN TISSUES
Potassium has long been known to be quantitatively the major cation within animal cells. The ability to accumulate potassium and extrude sodium in the presence of large amounts of sodium and small amounts of potassium in the surrounding fluid is a fundamental characteristic of living cells (5–11). With death of the cell these ionic gradients

are rapidly dissipated. Tracer techniques with radioactive isotopes have demonstrated that these gradients are maintained by living cells despite readily measurable permeabilities of cell membranes to both ions. Hence, this ionic distribution derives from steady-state conditions maintained at the expense of energy from cellular metabolism and is not simply an equilibrium state resulting from absolute impermeabilities of the cell membranes to one or more ions, as thought earlier.

The importance of these ionic gradients to the regulation of cell volume is well known (6)—see the section "The Intracellular Volume," Chapter 3. In this section we indicated that the high intracellular concentration of potassium is probably the result of two factors: (1) the active outward extrusion of sodium from cells, which leaves the cell's interior electrically negative to the exterior and thereby favors the intracellular accumulation of the positive potassium ion and (2) an active uptake of potassium by cells. In either case the ionic gradient is maintained in a steady state by energy supplied by cellular metabolism. Our understanding of how metabolic energy is coupled to the movements of ions by cell membranes is still incomplete, despite many studies. Descriptive explanations for most clinical observations must serve us, for the most part.

MEASUREMENT OF INTRACELLULAR COMPOSITION

The reason our understanding of the changes that occur in tissue composition has lagged so far behind our understanding of extracellular fluid composition is, of course, the difficulty of measuring tissue constituents during life and the rapid changes that occur after death. Techniques for determining intracellular composition quantitatively are still cumbersome and largely indirect. If a normal constituent of extracellular fluid is completely or very nearly excluded from the intracellular compartment, or if one injects into the extracellular fluid some substance with this limited distribution, then a basis is established for estimating the amount of any other substance present within cells (or, more accurately, outside the volume of distribution of the extracellular marker). For such measurements it has been useful to assume for muscle—the major tissue mass—that chloride ions are almost entirely extracellular. Alternatively inulin, radioactive sulfate, and many other exogenous substances have been assumed to distribute solely in the extracellular fluids after intravenous infusion or addition to media in which isolated tissues are incubated. If we know the steady-state concentration of the marker in the plasma or medium and the total amount of marker in the tissue, we can calculate the volume of "extracellular fluid." Subtracting this from total tissue water gives us the intracellular fluid volume. Any constituent of extracellular fluid or medium can similarly be partitioned between extracellular and intracellular fluids. This principle can readily be applied, in conjunction with balance studies, to partition the losses or gains between the extracellular and intracellular compartments.

Isotopic methods can be used to determine tissue composition both *in vivo* and *in vitro*. After ^{24}Na, or ^{42}K, has been injected intravenously and the constant specific activity of the ion determined in any body fluid (usually urine is examined), the quantity of "exchangeable" sodium or potassium can be readily calculated. Values for normal adults are 40 mEq of sodium and 45 mEq of potassium per kilogram (12). Clearly, these techniques must be used with an extracellular marker to partition the ions between intracellular and extracellular fluids, but the total extracellular fluid potassium is such a small fraction of total body potassium that changes in "exchangeable" potassium reflect changes in the intracellular content of this ion.

There are many limitations to the use of extracellular markers. No marker is likely to measure the true extracellular fluid volume. Adsorption, exclusion from collagenous tissues or bone, and secretion into the gastrointestinal tract are only a few of the processes that affect the validity of such methods. Furthermore, it should be obvious from a glance at an electron micrograph of the interior of most cells that many organelles and vesicles subdivide the intracellular compartment. Rather than any prevailing uniform intracellular composition, there is undoubtedly compartmentation of intracellular solutes, and these methods can yield only average values. Nevertheless, a considerable amount has been learned through the use of such methods.

Figure 5-1 compares the ionic composition of the intracellular compartment of muscle with that of the extracellular fluids—plasma and interstitial fluid. Intracellular ionic composition is known to vary from one cell type to another, but the general pattern is similar.

RENAL TRANSPORT OF POTASSIUM

As with most other ionic constituents of the body, the ultimate amount of potassium in the body is determined by the balance between its

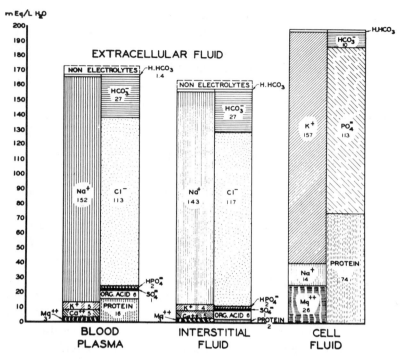

Fig. 5-1 Comparison of approximate normal ionic concentrations in plasma, interstitial fluid, and intracellular fluid of muscle. For comparison, concentrations are all expressed as millequivalents per liter of water (mEq/liter H₂O).

intake and excretion. Since dietary intake is largely unplanned, and for potassium ranges between 40 and about 140 mEq/day, the brunt of regulating body content of this ion falls on the kidneys. Renal handling of potassium involves both reabsorption and secretion.

Berliner (13) suggested that the potassium filtered at the glomerulus is largely reabsorbed proximally and what appears in the urine is largely secreted distally. This has been confirmed by micropuncture studies in rats (14). From recent studies it can be calculated that 80–95% of the filtered potassium is reabsorbed by the time the fluid has reached the beginning of the distal tubule. This proximal reabsorption of potassium seems to be an obligatory process. Thus the wide range of potassium content of the urine reflects the wide range of secretory activity in the terminal parts of the nephron. Normally, at least 75% of urinary potassium can be accounted for by distal tubular secretion, and under such conditions as potassium loading or administration of diuretics, even higher fractions obtain.

In the distal nephron, distal convoluted tubule, and collecting duct, potassium is both reabsorbed and secreted. Paradoxically, reabsorption is an active process, whereas secretion is largely passive. Potassium moves up an electrochemical gradient from luminal to peritubular fluids, whereas the electrical driving force (lumen electronegative to peritubular fluid) more than suffices to account for the potassium concentrations in the urine. The electrical gradients are determined largely by the reabsorption of sodium from the urine. The membrane potentials arising from active sodium transport, rather than any rigid obligatory coupling of sodium and potassium ions, appear to account for the dependence of potassium excretion on the presence of sodium. Thus, Giebisch (15) has found that any factor that increases the electronegativity of the luminal fluid increases potassium secretion. High intraluminal sodium concentrations and unreabsorbable anions such as sulfate or bicarbonate increase the membrane potentials and also the urinary losses of potassium. However, there is evidence for an active secretion of potassium in the distal nephron of isolated, perfused rabbit renal tubules (16, 17).

Other factors modulate the effect of the transepithelial membrane potential on secretion of potassium (18):

1. Changes in intracellular potassium concentration of the distal tubular epithelial cells would affect the quantity of potassium secreted in response to a given electrical driving force. Suppression of cellular potassium uptake from peritubular fluid by cardiac gycosides reduces intracellular potassium in tubular cells as well as distal tubular secretion of potassium. The very high rates of distal tubular secretion of potassium by animals who have been adapted to large intakes of potassium is also, in part at least, the result of the high levels of intracellular potassium that occur under such conditions. Renal Na–K-ATPase levels are increased significantly in potassium adaptation (59).

2. Adrenal hormones, primarily aldosterone, are necessary for normal rates of potassium secretion and for the adaptation of the secretory mechanisms that occur in response to a prolonged high intake of potassium. How the adrenal hormones lubricate the

pathways for passive secretion, or more likely, how they increase sodium transport and thereby increase the electrical driving force for potassium secretion, is not yet fully understood. Adrenal corticoids also increase Na–K-ATPase levels which increase potassium levels within tubular cells and thus favor potassium secretion.

3. Potassium secretion by the distal tubule appears to be flow limited. That is, the concentration in luminal fluid remains nearly constant irrespective of the rate of flow through this portion of the nephron. Hence, factors promoting high rates of flow increase excretion of potassium in the urine, whereas low flow rates decrease potassium excretion. It seems that for passive secretion of potassium to occur, the membrane potential across the luminal plasma membrane sets the ratio of intracellular to urinary (luminal) potassium concentrations. As the luminal fluid flows through this portion of the nephron its potassium concentration is maintained; the more rapid the flow, therefore, the more potassium will be secreted. Although this occurs in the distal tubule, it is proximal to the sites of action of antidiuretic hormone. Thus, water diuresis has little effect on the rate of potassium secretion, though it may profoundly affect the rates of final urine flow. Osmotic and other diuretics and a high salt intake that increase the rate of flow through the distal nephron, on the other hand, may enhance potassium excretion by this means as well as by presenting more sodium for reabsorption to this portion of the nephron. The higher sodium concentrations will increase transtubular electrical potential differences and enhance potassium secretion.

4. The acid–base balance of the body is another factor that affects potassium secretion. The pH of the extracellular fluids probably affects the potassium concentrations in the distal tubular cells. During extracellular alkalosis hydrogen ions leave and potassium ions move into the cells. Administration of sodium bicarbonate will produce alkalosis, increasing plasma pH, with a fall in plasma potassium as potassium moves into muscle cells, primarily; simultaneously an enhanced uptake of potassium across the peritubular cell membrane into the distal tubule cells occurs. This stimulates potassium secretion. Alkalosis may be a potent stimulus to potassium secretion and, if prolonged, may result in severe potassium depletion. Thus factors other than the extracellular to intracellular shifts of potassium that accompany a rise in plasma pH

must be involved. Though these shifts of potassium into or out of cells with alkalosis or acidosis, respectively, significantly affect plasma potassium concentrations, they are quantitatively much too small to account for the magnitude of renal potassium wasting in alkalosis. The total amount of potassium in extracellular fluids is simply too small.

Acidosis of the extracellular fluids has the opposite effects, causing transfer of hydrogen ions into cells in exchange for intracellular potassium. Thus, plasma potassium concentrations are elevated. Initially the loss of potassium from distal tubular cells produces a transient decrease in potassium secretion. But, prolonged acidosis increases potassium secretion, and severe depletion of body potassium stores may ensue. This results from the presence of poorly reabsorbable anions in the urine and loss of extracellular volume stimulating aldosterone secretion, both of which increase the electrical potential across the distal tubular cells and thus enhance potassium secretion.

The micropuncture studies of Giebisch and associates (18) have dispelled the notion that the limited ability of the kidneys to excrete potassium under conditions of very low sodium excretion, that is, salt deprivation or acute reductions in glomerular filtration rate, is a direct result of an inadequate supply of luminal sodium for a one-to-one exchange with cellular potassium. Not only is there no evidence for such a direct exchange process but also the amount of sodium reabsorbed along the distal tubule greatly exceeds the amount of potassium secreted. Thus, the supply of sodium could not be limiting for such an exchange with potassium if this, in fact, were the means by which potassium secretion took place. Furthermore, the distal tubule is the site of most potassium secretion, whereas the activity of the collecting ducts accounts for the very low urinary sodium excretion in these states. It is more likely that low luminal sodium limits potassium secretion indirectly, by causing a lower transepithelial electrical potential. This would both reduce the passive secretion of potassium into the urine and favor its active reabsorption.

POTASSIUM EXCESS
The very efficient renal tubular secretory process makes it difficult to overload a normal subject with potassium. Particularly if subjects are

adapted gradually to increasing amounts of potassium, secretion rates of several hundred milliequivalents daily can be attained. Under such conditions in animal experiments it was found that the quantity of potassium in the urine considerably exceeded the amount filtered. This provided the first definite proof of tubular secretion of potassium. Only with a diminished capacity to excrete potassium can overloading and intoxication occur. Decreased perfusion of the kidneys from any cause—low cardiac output, salt depletion, adrenal cortical insufficiency, and renal disease, both acute and chronic, associated with reduced glomerular filtration rate—is the usual condition for limiting tubular secretion of potassium. In acute tubular necrosis the suppression of renal function, and the increased release of potassium into the extracellular fluid from traumatized, infected, or ischemic tissues, often present in the clinical setting in which acute tubular necrosis occurs, create situations in which hyperkalemia develops quickly and may be life threatening.

Normal serum concentrations of potassium range from 3.5 to 5.0 mEq/liter. Concentrations greater than 7 mEq/liter are considered dangerous, and concentrations of 10 to 12 mEq/liter are likely to be fatal. The cause of death is cardiac arrhythmia or cardiac arrest.

Excitability of nerves and muscles depends on the difference between the resting membrane potential and the threshold potential; for muscle this may be -90 and -65 mV, respectively (with the cell interior electrically negative to the extracellular fluid). During excitation the release of acetylcholine at synaptic junctures and muscle end plates depolarizes the membrane, raising the membrane potential toward the threshold potential. When the threshold is reached, excitation occurs. Any factor that alters the resting membrane potential or the threshold potential affects the responsiveness of excitable tissues (see Fig. 5-2).

The membrane potential depends on many factors, including the concentration of ions in the extracellular fluids. These may change sufficiently in a variety of clinical conditions to affect neuromuscular irritability significantly. An increase in potassium concentration (hyperkalemia) depolarizes the cell membranes of nerve and muscle, resulting in hyperexcitability of these tissues. When resting potentials rise to the level of the threshold potential, repolarization cannot occur, and after a single response the tissue is no longer excitable. Conversely, a decrease in serum potassium (hypokalemia) lowers the resting

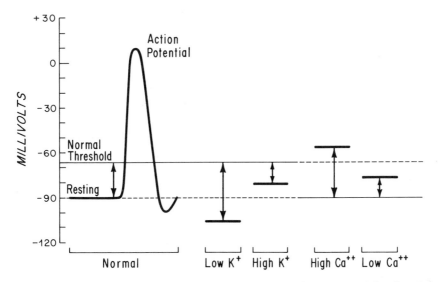

Fig. 5-2 Effects of serum calcium and potassium on membrane potentials of excitable tissues. The concentration of potassium in extracellular fluids affects the resting potential, whereas calcium concentrations alter the threshold potentials.

membrane potential, producing hyperpolarization. This stabilizes the membrane so that it is less influenced by stimuli, and excitability is again lost. The end result of both hypokalemia and hyperkalemia is, therefore, similar, and flaccid paralysis may be seen with both. With hyperkalemia, however, fatal cardiac arrhythmias or arrest usually supervenes before paralysis is fully developed.

The dependence of neuromuscular excitability on the concentration of potassium in the extracellular fluid varies greatly because of the effects of other ions, tissue metabolism, drugs, etc., on the resting membrane and threshold potentials. Calcium and hydronium ions also modify this system significantly. Extracellular acidosis generally decreases irritability, and alkalosis increases it. An increase in ionized calcium (hypercalcemia) decreases irritability, whereas a decrease (hypocalcemia) increases irritability. The concentration of ionized calcium affects the threshold potential (19); low values decrease (make more negative—see Fig. 5-2) and high values raise the threshold potential. Low values thus reduce the difference between resting and threshold potentials, making the neuromuscular system vulnerable to stimuli, and irritability is increased. A high serum concentration of ionized

120   Renal Pathophysiology

calcium increases the threshold potential, reducing excitability. Undoubtedly, other ionic and metabolic factors further affect the functioning of this system, so that fatal cardiac arrest may occur with hyperkalemia at serum potassium concentrations of 8 mEq/liter in one patient but not until 12 mEq/liter in another. With hypokalemia, total flaccid paralysis, including the muscles of respiration, may occur in some patients at serum potassium concentrations of 1.5 mEq/liter, whereas others may be virtually symptomless with the same potassium concentration. The electrocardiogram, which reflects the functional consequences of potassium excess or depletion rather than of the serum potassium concentration alone, is an excellent means of warning of impending disaster.

It is difficult to overload a normal subject with potassium because of its rapid renal excretion and its rapid uptake by tissues. Potassium equilibrates so rapidly with muscle, liver, and other tissues that a single circulation through a limb may reequilibrate intracellular and extracellular potassium. If potassium is given intravenously, however, toxic concentrations may bathe the heart before peripheral concentrations rise. Since the heart is the first organ to encounter the infused potassium and thus may be exposed to lethal concentrations very soon after it is given, fluids containing potassium in concentrations in excess of 40 mEq/liter must be administered slowly and with careful supervision. When given by mouth potassium salts are quite safe in almost any amount that can be tolerated without causing gastrointestinal upset, provided excretory mechanisms are functioning normally. During a period of sodium depletion or deprivation, however, even a normal individual has a low tolerance to potassium, since potassium secretion depends on sufficient amounts of sodium in the urine of the distal nephron.

No tissue changes characterize potassium excess. If it were not for the peculiar vulnerability of excitable tissues to hyperkalemia, the condition might be well tolerated.

Physiologic and pharmacologic methods may be used to reduce the concentration of serum potassium when it rises to dangerous levels. Since potassium moves with glucose across cell membranes, glucose administered with insulin reduces potassium in the serum by transferring it into cells, probably chiefly in the liver. Alkalosis also lowers extracellular concentrations of potassium by causing the ion to move into cells. Thus, administering sodium bicarbonate reduces the danger of hyperkalemia. Administering calcium intravenously may also protect excitable tissues. These are temporary measures, but they can buy valuable time until the usual excretory pathways, cation exchange resins administered orally or by enema, or dialysis can remove the excessive, life-threatening amounts of potassium from the body.

POTASSIUM DEFICIENCY

Potassium deficiency alone, or more commonly in association with other electrolyte and fluid disturbances, is of clinical importance.

Experimental Potassium Depletion

The work of Heppel (2), Darrow (3), and Ferrebee and his associates (20) called attention to the increase in cellular sodium that accompanies loss of cellular potassium. Figure 5-3 shows the alterations in the electrolyte composition of muscle, observed by Heppel (2), of rats maintained for a considerable period on potassium-deficient diets. The loss of muscle potassium and the gain in muscle sodium are contrasted with the normal values in control animals. It is generally accepted that nearly all the chloride in muscle is extracellular. Hence, the similar chloride content in the tissue obtained from the control

Fig. 5-3 Effect of low K diet for 45 days on Na and K of a rat muscle. Adapted from data of Heppel (2) with permission of the American Physiological Society.

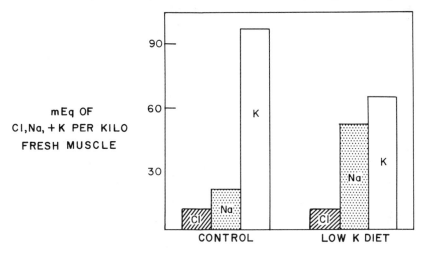

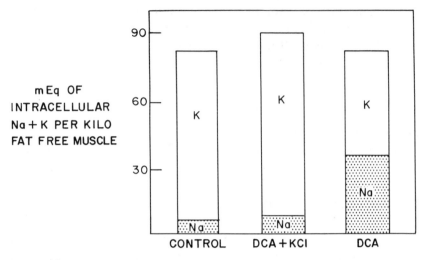

Fig. 5-4 Effect of deoxycorticosterone on concentration of intracellular Na and K in dog muscle. Adapted from data of Ferrebee et al. (20) with permission of the American Physiological Society.

animals and from those on potassium-free diets is interpreted as indicating that the potassium loss and sodium gain in the muscle of the potassium-depleted animals represent a change in intracellular ionic composition.

It is of clinical interest that administering adrenal steroids can produce the same changes in tissue composition that are encountered in simple deficiency of potassium intake. This is shown in Fig. 5-4, which was constructed from data taken from the work of Ferrebee and his associates (20). These investigators produced potassium depletion in dogs by repeated injection of deoxycorticosterone acetate. This compound has an effect on the kidneys similar to that of the physiologic adrenal hormone aldosterone, causing a diuresis of potassium. If the urinary loss of potassium exceeds its dietary intake, body potassium is depleted. Figure 5-4 contrasts the intracellular sodium and potassium concentrations in the muscle of dogs receiving deoxycorticosterone acetate injections, control animals on the same diet, but without injections, and animals receiving deoxycorticosterone acetate in addition to liberal dietary supplements of potassium chloride. Here, again, it is demonstrated that body potassium can be depleted experimentally and that cellular potassium is replaced by approximately equivalent quantities of sodium. This point has been established in many other types of animal and human studies.

From the clinical point of view we are interested in what, if any, disturbances in cellular functions accompany such alterations in intracellular ionic composition. The protocols of experiments such as the one described above reveal that the animals become ill and fail to gain weight and develop in contrast with control littermates. Their fur is less thick; they become anorectic. A gradual paralysis develops, and the dogs die if the potassium depletion is prolonged.

The functional disturbances have a morphologic counterpart. Postmortem examination of tissues from potassium-depleted animals shows characteristic degenerative changes in the myocardium, with patchy fibrosis and round-cell infiltration (21). The immediate cause of death from potassium depletion is usually cardiac arrest. Electrocardiographic changes occur commonly in potassium depletion and are of considerable diagnostic importance.

Muscular weakness, postural hypotension, and paralysis may be prominent features of the clinical picture in advanced potassium depletion. In experimental potassium deficiency, the refractory period of muscle increases, indicating diminished muscular excitability, as well as degenerative histologic changes (22). Skeletal muscles of the extremities are involved primarily, but when the disturbance is profound, paralysis of the muscles of respiration may occur, creating an urgent need for prompt medical attention to forestall death from asphyxia. A similar paralysis often affects the smooth muscle of the gastrointestinal tract, causing ileus. The kidneys show extensive, clear, vacuolar changes in the tubular epithelium (21) that are known to be associated with impaired renal function (23). Failure of the renal concentrating mechanism in potassium depletion explains the polyuria that is occasionally prominent in the clinical picture. This polyuria does not diminish on administration of antidiuretic hormone (23) and, hence, can be attributed directly to tubular dysfunction, not to any deficiency of neurohypophyseal hormones. Figure 5-5 shows the time-course and magnitude of the concentrating defect induced by experimental potassium deficiency in man (24). The renal effects of potassium depletion seem to be largely reversible, both morphologically and functionally upon potassium repletion and do not *per se* cause renal failure.

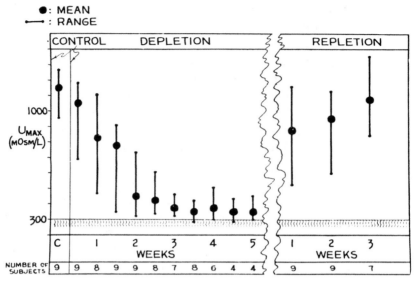

Fig. 5-5 Urine concentration during hydropenia in potassium depletion. Reprinted from (24) with permission of the *Journal of Clinical Investigation*.

Effects of potassium depletion on cellular function

Whether the deleterious effects on tissue function are attributable to the loss of potassium from the cells or to the secondary gain of intracellular sodium, so far as the two changes are separable, has been investigated by Cannon and associates (25). Growing rats were subjected to a low sodium and potassium diet. Though the effect of this diet was to retard and arrest the normal growth rate, the animals did not die until their sodium intake was increased. This suggests that, only with an abundant sodium intake, do sodium ions replace the intracellular potassium and give rise to serious functional disturbances. The role of sodium, discussed below, in increasing urinary excretion of potassium and thus aggravating potassium depletion may also be important.

There is a growing list of enzymes whose functions are known to be influenced by the concentrations of sodium and potassium ions in their immediate environment (26, 27). Since many of the vital enzymatic processes of cells occur in the intracellular fluid, it is not surprising that changes in the composition of this fluid result in disturbances in vital processes and functions of the cells. That such disturbances occur was demonstrated *in vitro* in an interesting way

Table 5-1 Effect of ionic composition of incubating medium on glycogen synthesis from glucose by liver slices *in vitro.*

	Glycogen mg/100 gm liver	
Solution	Without glucose	With glucose
Extracellular, mEq/l Na—150 K—5 Ca—2 Mg—1	10	39
Intracellular, mEq/l Na—0 K—130 Ca—0 Mg—40	40	161
Control (Zero time)	33	

some years ago by Hastings (28). Table 5-1 presents the results of his experiments in which rat liver slices were made to synthesize glycogen from glucose *in vitro.* When liver slices containing 38 mg of glycogen/ 100 gm of tissue were placed in a medium high in sodium, as is extracellular fluid, there was no synthesis of glycogen, although glucose was present in the medium. But in rat liver slices incubated with glucose for an hour in a medium containing no sodium, but high in potassium and magnesium as is intracellular fluid, definite *in vitro* synthesis of glycogen occurred. This demonstrates that a certain electrolyte pattern within the cell is necessary to maintain the cell's normal enzymatic activity and function.

Clinical Potassium Deficiency

Deficiencies of tissue potassium are common because many factors may affect potassium balance. The general clinical states most often associated with potassium depletion are alkalosis, acidosis, abnormal gastrointestinal losses, excessive adrenal corticosteroids, and diuretic therapy. Each will be considered separately.

Alkalosis

Potassium deficiency is frequently associated with metabolic alkalosis, and primary alkalosis may produce potassium depletion. Both administration of alkali and chronic vomiting with alkalosis produce loss of potassium in the urine and clinical potassium deficiency. Gastric secretions generally do not contain potassium at concentrations greater than about 12 mEq/liter, and it is the renal losses secondary to the alkalosis of vomiting rather than the potassium lost in the vomitus that cause significant depletion. The increased urinary potassium excretion following administration of alkali has been repeatedly demonstrated experimentally (29). As mentioned above, research on the process of distal tubular secretion of potassium has disproved the earlier assumption that sodium in the distal convoluted tubule is reabsorbed via an obligatory exchange with potassium or hydrogen ions. The notion that there is a direct competition for secretion between hydrogen and potassium ions in the distal nephron with potassium secretion favored when hydrogen ions are rendered scarce by alkalosis is also undoubtedly incorrect. Perhaps the presence of bicarbonate in the distal nephron during alkalosis serves as a non-reabsorbable anion that augments the transepithelial potential and thus enhances passive potassium secretion. An increased concentration of potassium in tubular cells may also contribute (18). It has been demonstrated that alkalosis directly stimulates secretion of potassium in the distal tubule (15). Further research is needed to explain the renal mechanism of potassium wasting with alkalosis. In chronic vomiting, as in pyloric obstruction, the additional factors of potassium loss in the vomitus and reduced dietary intake of potassium are present, contributing to the effect of alkalosis. Surgery in such cases, with resultant stimulation of adrenocortical activity, intubation, and administration of sodium-containing solutions, further complicates the picture.

Since metabolic alkalosis is usually associated with hypochloremia, hypokalemia, and a contracted extracellular fluid volume (or some other stimulus for sodium retention, as in the edematous states), the role of each ion deficiency (H^+, Na^+, Cl^-, and K^+) has been considered in the etiology of the acid–base disturbance. The importance of the concomitant chloride depletion in sustaining the metabolic alkalosis has been emphasized (30). Patients who lose gastric secretions become alkalotic and hypochloremic because of the loss of hydrochloric acid; they also lose potassium via the kidneys. But the vomiting and reduced intake of sodium, in addition, compromise extracellular fluid volume so that the kidneys avidly conserve sodium. Although in theory the kidneys could correct the alkalosis in this situation simply by excreting sodium bicarbonate, this does not occur. Conservation of sodium and, hence, of extracellular fluid volume seems to take priority over correction of the acid–base disturbance. The result is that the hypochloremia causes a disparity between the availability of chloride to be reabsorbed and the requirement to conserve sodium; this promotes an exchange of sodium ions for hydrogen and potassium ions in the renal tubules. The hydrogen ion loss sustains the alkalosis, and the potassium loss, the depletion of that ion. Providing sufficient chloride as the sodium salt generally corrects the alkalosis, and the potassium deficit is then repaired, even without supplementing the potassium intake of the diet. This type of "saline responsive" alkalosis is associated with deficiencies of potassium of less than 500 mEq, and patients generally have less than 10 mEq of chloride/liter in their urine. It has been conveniently labeled *chloride depletion alkalosis,* but its genesis, as indicated, is multifactorial.

With more severe potassium depletion, that is, total body potassium deficits of 1000 mEq, a "saline-resistant" alkalosis may develop. Potassium as well as chloride replacement may be required to relieve this type of alkalosis (31). Serum potassium is usually under 2.0 mEq/liter. A modest chloride wasting is part of the associated nephropathy, so that urinary chloride concentrations are usually greater than 10 mEq/liter. This situation may be seen with hyperadrenocorticism or other causes of severe potassium depletion.

Acidosis

Whenever acidosis appears clinically in the absence of severe glomerular insufficiency, potassium depletion should be anticipated. Diabetic acidosis and renal tubular acidosis are the most commonly encountered types. In diabetic acidosis the rate of hydrogen ion secretion fails to keep pace with the rate of formation of acids in the body. Acidosis ensues, and the obligatory anion excretion preempts the excretion of fixed cations, including potassium. In renal acidosis the acid loads requiring excretion are no more than normal, but the diseased kidney's reduced ability to secrete hydrogen ions calls for an increased excretion of fixed cation to accompany non-reabsorbed anions.

In recognizing and treating potassium depletion in the presence of acidosis one must bear in mind the distinction between the ion's serum and intracellular levels. As first shown *in vitro* by Fenn and Cobb (32), acidosis tends to make potassium ions leave the cells, whereas alkalosis has the opposite effect. In intact and nephrectomized animals it has similarly been shown that acidosis causes a slight rise and alkalosis a slight reduction in serum potassium concentrations (33, 34). In alkalosis, however, the large renal losses of potassium result in potassium depletion despite the general tendency in alkalosis for potassium to move from the extracellular to the intracellular fluid. In acidosis the shift of potassium from intracellular to extracellular fluids may maintain normal or occasionally elevated serum potassium levels, even in the presence of severe intracellular deficits. Diabetic acidosis, in which potassium depletion may be associated with severe dehydration and prerenal azotemia, is the classic example of this situation. If therapy fails to include potassium, correction of the dehydration, acidosis, and disturbed carbohydrate metabolism may subsequently decrease serum potassium concentrations to lethal levels (35).

In renal tubular acidosis large potassium deficits secondary to the impaired renal acidifying mechanism may occur (36). In chronic renal failure with azotemia the kidneys are excreting potassium at a rate usually sufficient to preserve potassium balance and normal serum potassium levels. The quantities of potassium in the urine may considerably exceed the small amounts of potassium delivered to the nephrons by the markedly reduced filtration rate (37). This suffices to enable most patients in terminal renal failure to preserve potassium balance (38). The rate of potassium secretion, however, is fixed in these patients. Excess potassium in the diet easily overloads the fixed rate of secretion, causing an elevated serum potassium level to toxic concentrations. On the other hand, a low intake of potassium, as may occur with anorexia, nausea, and vomiting, together with the fixed renal losses of potassium, may lower serum potassium concentration and result in potassium depletion.

Gastrointestinal losses

Loss of gastric secretions, either by vomiting or through gastric suction, has already been mentioned as a cause of potassium depletion. Loss of small bowel and large bowel contents may also produce severe potassium depletion. Diarrhea from infection or malabsorption syndrome and prolonged aspiration of intestinal contents cause the loss of the alkaline intestinal and pancreatic secretions, together with considerable quantities of potassium, and produce acidosis, dehydration, and potassium depletion. When potassium depletion occurs from such causes, the disturbance in bowel function usually is clinically obvious. But the studies by Schwartz and Relman (39) of patients with severe potassium depletion induced by chronic self-administration of laxatives for "constipation," have shown that even mildly increased gastrointestinal motility persisting over long periods can produce severe potassium deficiency despite apparently normal dietary intakes of potassium.

Often a patient presents with hypokalemia without any apparent cause for potassium depletion. The question then must be answered, "Was the loss of potassium via the kidneys or the gastrointestinal tract?" The kidneys cannot conserve potassium in the presence of potassium depletion as efficiently as they do sodium when there is a deficiency of that ion. However, urinary losses of potassium are reduced to some 10 to 20 mEq daily if potassium intake is curtailed or if the potassium depletion is the result of gastrointestinal losses. If excessive renal losses have caused the depletion, higher rates of urinary excretion may be anticipated. Because the kidney conserves this ion poorly, deficiency can result from low intake. Potassium is, however, so ubiquitous in nearly all foodstuffs that low intake is almost never a factor in potassium depletion, except when patients are maintained entirely on parenteral fluids from which potassium has been excluded.

Adrenocortical overactivity
Whether endogenous or iatrogenic, excesses of adrenocortical hormones have long been known to be associated with potassium deficiency. This has been recognized in Cushing's syndrome (40, 41), with excessive production of 17-hydroxycorticosteroids, and also in hyperaldosteronism (42), with excessive production of the specific sodium-retaining steroid. Although the remarkably potent action of aldosterone on renal sodium and potassium excretion is appreciated, potassium depletion may result from excessive amounts of the 17-hydroxycorticosteroids alone, in the absence of increased aldosterone. This situation has been encountered clinically in Cushing's syndrome and with administration of cortisone and other 17-hydroxycorticosteroids. When potassium depletion results from excessive adrenocortical activity, alkalosis is almost always seen. The action of adrenal steroids to increase renal hydrogen ion and ammonium excretion (43), is most likely responsible for the alkalosis, and this action is enhanced by the associated potassium depletion (44).

Recent studies have shown that normal subjects are surprisingly resistant to the development of alkalosis and potassium depletion when given excessive amounts of adrenal hormones. Thus, large doses of aldosterone administered for periods up to 3 months produced only a modest elevation in plasma bicarbonate and a modest reduction in serum potassium levels (45). Other factors beside the excessive amounts of adrenal steroid may be essential in producing the degree of alkalosis and potassium depletion seen clinically in hyperadrenocorticism. Whether or not they are causally related, there is some correlation between the elevation of plasma bicarbonate and the reduction of serum potassium in patients with primary hyperaldosteronism (45).

A characteristic of the potassium depletion associated with excessive adrenocortical activity is its resistance to therapy. So long as excessive corticosteroid activity persists, the administration of large amounts of potassium only transiently corrects the potassium depletion. On the other hand, the renal potassium losses that result in potassium depletion depend on a normal or high intake of sodium. When sodium intake is restricted, administering adrenal hormones fail to produce potassium diuresis and depletion (46). Even the potassium depletion of hyperaldosteronism is reversed by potassium administration if sodium intake is reduced. Apparently one action of adrenal steroids is to stimulate tubular reabsorption of sodium ions at some distal site in the renal tubule, which increases the transepithelial potential. This, in turn, facilitates passive movement of potassium into the urine. When sodium intake is restricted, so that little sodium reaches this distal tubular site, membrane potentials are lowered and less potassium is secreted despite continued adrenal hormone activity. This dependence of potassium loss on the presence of sodium in the tubular urine probably explains part of the deleterious effect of the administration of saline solution to patients with potassium deficiency. The administered sodium facilitates further renal losses of potassium, aggravating potassium depletion as well as making more sodium available to replace the potassium lost from the intracellular fluid.

Diuretics
Alkalosis with potassium depletion and hypokalemia is a relatively common occurrence during treatment of edematous states with potent diuretics. It is now recognized that the edema of congestive heart failure, nephrosis, and cirrhosis is generally associated with an increased output of aldosterone (47, 48). This hormone, perhaps in conjunction with the reduced filtration rate common to these states, increases the renal tubular reabsorption of sodium, causing sodium retention and

edema. As sodium disappears from the urine, insufficient quantities are available to sustain high transepithelial potentials in the distal nephron, and excessive losses of potassium are not ordinarily encountered (49). But when a potent diuretic inhibits the reabsorption of sodium more proximally (50), more of that ion arrives at the distal tubular site, where it can undergo reabsorption; high potentials are sustained, and potassium (and hydrogen) ion secretion is favored. This secretion is heightened by the excessive adrenal hormone levels; an acid urine high in potassium content is excreted. This produces the alkalosis and potassium depletion so commonly encountered during prolonged therapy with diuretics. The reduced extracellular fluid volume resulting from the action of the diuretics may further enhance tubular reabsorption of bicarbonate, which adds to the alkalosis (51, 52). Hence, potassium depletion is appearing with greatly increasing frequency as use of these potent diuretics (thiazides, furosemide and ethacrynic acid) increases. In the digitalized patient the occurrence of even mild potassium depletion entails the added hazard of inducing digitalis intoxication.

REGULATION OF HORMONES BY POTASSIUM

The state of potassium repletion, probably through the serum concentration of potassium, directly affects the secretion of three hormones: (1) renin, (2) aldosterone, and (3) insulin.

High serum potassium depresses renin secretion and low serum potassium stimulates its output. Thus, potassium depletion in dogs was found to raise plasma renin activity; this effect was unrelated to changes in sodium balance (53). Potassium infused directly into the renal artery of normal or salt-depleted dogs at rates sufficient to raise the arterial potassium concentration by 1.65 to 2.85 mM reduced renal vein renin immediately in the ipsilateral kidney, and renin levels returned to control values when the infusion of potassium was stopped (54). In man as well, potassium administration depresses renin activity and potassium depletion increases it (55).

Potassium excess stimulates aldosterone biosynthesis (increasing the conversion of corticosterone to aldosterone) and secretion (56, 57). Potassium depletion has the opposite effect. Again, these direct effects of potassium are not mediated by concomitant changes in sodium balance. In fact, sodium depletion stimulates aldosterone through the renin–angiotensin system, whereas potassium retention inhibits renin secretion. Since sodium depletion is so often associated with potassium retention, it is likely that the potassium effect augments the effect of sodium depletion in enhancing aldosterone secretion.

Potassium chloride infusions in dogs also increase insulin secretion and decreases plasma glucose levels (58). Potassium depletion has the opposite effect, impairing glucose tolerance by inhibiting insulin release. Since insulin lowers serum potassium by sequestering potassium in liver and muscle in association with glucose, this constitutes a feedback loop. Therefore, elevated serum potassium levels activate insulin, which moves potassium into liver and muscle, and aldosterone, which enhances excretion of potassium from the body. Both effects help to protect the body from the disastrous consequences of hyperkalemia on sensitive and critical conduction systems.

With these basic principles in mind, together with an awareness of the diversity of clinical conditions in which factors operate to induce potassium depletion or excess, the wary internist and surgeon will be constantly on the lookout for their occurrence and quick and persistent in their prevention and treatment.

References

1. Gamble, J. L. Early history of fluid replacement therapy. Pediatrics 11:554–567, 1953.
2. Heppel, L. A. Electrolytes of muscle and liver in potassium-depleted rats. Am. J. Physiol. 127:385–392, 1939.
3. Darrow, D. C. Tissue water and electrolyte. Ann. Rev. Physiol. 6:95–122, 1944.
4. Darrow, D. C. Retention of electrolyte during recovery from severe dehydration due to diarrhea. J. Pediat. 28:515–540, 1946.
5. Krogh, A. Active and passive exchanges of inorganic ions through surfaces of living cells and through living membranes generally: Croonian Lecture. Proc. Roy. Soc., London, s. B. 133:140–200, 1946.
6. Leaf, A. Maintenance of concentration gradients and regulation of cell volume. Ann. New York Acad. Sci. 72:396–404, 1959.
7. Steinbach, H. B. Sodium and potassium balance of muscle and nerve. In Modern trends in physiology and biochemistry: Woods Hole lectures dedicated to memory of Leonor Michaelis, E. S. G. Barron, ed. 538 pp. Academic Press, New York, 1952, pp. 173–192.
8. Hodgkin, A. L., Ionic basis of electrical activity in nerve and muscle. Biol. Rev. 26:339–409, 1951.
9. Glynn, I. M. Sodium and potassium movements in human red cells. J. Physiol. 134:278–310, 1956.

10. Adrian, R. H. Effect of internal and external potassium concentration on membrane potential of frog muscle. J. Physiol. 133:631–658, 1956.

11. Koefoed-Johnsen, V. and Ussing, H. H. Nature of frog skin potential. Acta Physiol. Scand. 42:298–308, 1958.

12. McMurrey, J. D., Boling, E. A., Davis, J. M., Parker, H. V., Magnus, I. C., Ball, M. R., and Moore, F. D. Body composition: Simultaneous determination of several aspects by dilution principle metabolism. 7:651–667, 1958.

13. Berliner, R. W. Renal mechanisms for potassium excretion. Harvey Lect., Series 55:141–171, 1961.

14. Giebisch, G. and Windhager, E. E. Renal tubular transfer of sodium, chloride and potassium. Am. J. Med. 36:643–669, 1964.

15. Giebisch, G. Functional organization of proximal and distal tubular electrolyte transport. Nephron 6:260–281, 1969.

16. Grantham, J., Burg, L. B., and Orloff, J. The nature of transtubular Na and K transport in isolated rabbit renal collecting tubules. J. Clin. Invest. 49:1815–1826, 1970.

17. Stoner, I. C., Burg, M. B., and Orloff, J. Ion transport in cortical collecting tubule; effect of amiloride. Am. J. Physiol. 227:453–459, 1974.

18. Giebisch, G., Klose, R. M., and Malnic, G. Renal tubular potassium transport. Proc. 3rd Int. Congress Nephrol., Washington 1:62–75, 1966.

19. Shanes, A. M. Electrochemical aspects of physiological and pharmacological action in excitable cells. Pharmacol. Rev. 10:165–273, 1958.

20. Ferrebee, J. W., et al. Certain effects of desoxycorticosterone: Development of "diabetes insipidus" and replacement of muscle potassium by sodium in normal dogs. Am. J. Physiol. 135:230–237, 1941.

21. Follis, R. H., Jr., Orent-Keiles, E., and McCollum, E. V. Production or cardiac and renal lesions in rats by diet extremely deficient in potassium. Am. J. Path. 18:29–39, 1942.

22. Glaser, G. H. and Stark, L. Excitability in experimental myopathy. II. Potassium deficiency: Initial study. Neurology 8:708–711, 1958.

23. Relman, A. S. and Schwartz, W. B. Nephropathy of potassium depletion: Clinical and pathological entity. New Eng. J. Med. 255:195–203, 1956.

24. Rubini, M. E. Water excretion in potassium-deficient man. J. Clin. Invest. 40:2215–2224, 1961.

25. Cannon, P. R., Frazier, L. E., and Hughes, R. H. Sodium as toxic ion in potassium deficiency. Metabolism 2:297–312, 1953.

26. Muntz, J. A. Effect of ions on activity of enzymes derived from cardiac tissue. Ann. New York Acad. Sci. 72:415–426, 1959.

27. Lubin, M. Intracellular potassium and control of protein synthesis. Fed. Proc. 23:994–1001, 1964.

28. Hastings, A. B. Electrolytes of tissue and body fluids. Harvey Lect. (1940–1941) 36:91–125, 1941.

29. Leaf, A., Couter, W. T., and Newburgh, L. H. Some effects of variations in sodium intake and of different sodium salts in normal subjects. J. Clin. Invest. 28:1082–1090, 1949.

30. Schwartz, W. B., Van Ypersele de Strihou, C., Kassirer, J. P. Role of anions in metabolic alkalosis and potassium deficiency. New Eng. J. Med. 279:630–639, 1968.

31. Garella, S., Chazan, J. A., and Cohen, J. J. Saline-resistant metabolic alkalosis or "chloride-wasting nephropathy." Ann. Int. Med. 73:31–38, 1970.

32. Fenn, W. O. and Cobb, D. M. Potassium equilibrium in muscle. J. Gen. Physiol. 17:629–656, 1934.

33. Abrams, W. B., Lewis, D. W., and Bellet, S. Effect of acidosis and alkalosis on plasma potassium concentration and electrocardiograms of normal and potassium depleted dogs. Am. J. Med. Sci. 222:606–515, 1951.

34. Keating, R. E., Weichselbaum, T. E., Alanis, M., Magraf, H. W., and Elman, R. Movement of potassium during experimental acidosis and alkalosis in nephrectomized dog. Surg., Gynec. & Obst. 96:323–330, 1953.

35. Holler, J. W. Potassium deficiency occurring during treatment of diabetic acidosis. JAMA. 131:1186–1189, 1946.

36. Albright, F., Burnett, C. H., Parsons, W., Reifenstein, E. C., Jr., and Roos, A. Osteomalacia and late rickets: Various etiologies met in United States with emphasis on that resulting from specific form of renal acidosis, therapeutic indications for each etiological subgroup, and relationship between osteomalacia and milkman's syndrome. Medicine 25:399–479, 1946.

37. Leaf, A. and Camara, A. A. Renal tubular secretion of potassium in man. J. Clin. Invest. 28:1526–1533, 1949.

38. Elkinton, J. R., Tarail, R., and Peters, J. P. Transfers of potassium in renal insufficiency. J. Clin. Invest. 28:378–388, 1949.

39. Schwartz, W. B. and Relman, A. S. Metabolic and renal studies in chronic potassium depletion resulting from overuse of laxatives. J. Clin. Invest. 32:258–271, 1953.

40. MacQuarrie, I., Johnson, R. M., and Ziegler, M. R. Plasma electrolyte disturbance in patient with hypercorticoadrenal syndrome contrasted with that found in Addison's disease. Endocrinology 21:762–772, 1937.

41. Willson, D. M., Power, M. H., and Kepler, E. J. Alkalosis and low plasma potassium in case of Cushing's syndrome: Metabolic study. J. Clin. Invest. 19:701–707, 1940.

42. Conn, J. W. Presidential address: painting background: Primary aldosteronism, new clinical syndrome. J. Lab. & Clin. Med. 45:3–17, 1955.

43. Sartorius, O. W., Calhoon, D., and Pitts, R. F. Studies on interrelationships of adrenal cortex and renal ammonia excretion by rat. Endocrinology 52:256–265, 1953.

44. Hulter, H. N., Sigala, J. F., and Sebastian, A. K^+ deprivation potentiates the renal alkalosis-producing effect of mineralocorticoid. Am. J. Physiol. 235:F298–F309, 1978.

45. Kassirer, J. P., London, A. M., Goldman, D. M., and Schwartz, W. B. On the pathogenesis of metabolic alkalosis in hyperaldosteronism. Am. J. Med. 49:306–315, 1970.

46. Relman, A. S. and Schwartz, W. B. Effect of DOAC on electrolyte balance in normal man and its relation to sodium chloride intake. Yale J. Biol. Med. 24:540–558, 1952.

47. Luetscher, J. A., Jr., and Johnson, B. B. Observations on sodium-retaining corticoid (aldosterone) in urine of children and adults in relation to sodium balance and edema. J. Clin. Invest. 33:1441–1446, 1954.

48. Liddle, G. W., Duncan, L. E., Jr., and Bartter, F. C. Dual mechanism regulating adrenocortical function in man. Am. J. Med. 21:380–386, 1956.

49. Bartter, F. C. Symposium: Water and electrolytes: Role of adolsterone in normal homeostasis and in certain disease states. Metabolism 5:369–383, 1956.

50. Pitts, R. F. Some reflections on mechanisms of action of diuretics. Am. J. Med. 24:745–763, 1958.

51. Purkerson, M. L., Lubowitz, H., White, R. W., and Bricker, N. S. On the influence of extracellular fluid volume expansion on bicarbonate reabsorption in the rat. J. Clin. Invest. 48:1754–1760, 1969.

52. Kurtzman, N. A. Regulation of renal bicarbonate reabsorption by extracellular volume. J. Clin. Invest. 49:586–595, 1970.

53. Abbrecht, P. N. and Vander, A. J. Effect of chronic potassium deficiency on plasma renin activity. J. Clin. Invest. 49:1510–1516, 1970.

54. Vander, A. J. Direct effects of potassium on renin secretion and renal function. Am. J. Physiol. 219:455–459, 1970.

55. Brunner, H. R., Baer, L., Sealey, J. E., Ledingham, J. G. G., and Laragh, J. H. The influence of potassium administration and of potassium deprivation on plasma renin in normal and hypertensive subjects. J. Clin. Invest. 49:2128–2138, 1970.

56. Boyd, J. E., Palmore, W. P., and Mulrow, P. J. Role of potassium in the control of aldosterone secretion in the rat. Endocrinology 88:556–565, 1971.

57. Boyd, J. E. and Mulrow, P. J. Further studies of the influence of potassium upon aldosterone production in the rat. Endocrinology 90:299–301, 1972.

58. Hiatt, N., Davidson, M. D., and Bonorris, G. The effect of potassium chloride infusion on insulin secretion *in vivo*. Horm. Metab. Res. 4:64–68, 1972.

59. Schon, D. A., Silva, P., and Hayslett, J. P. Mechanism of potassium excretion in renal insufficiency. Am. J. Physiol. 227:1332–1330, 1974.

6

Edema

Edema is the accumulation of excessive interstitial fluid—that portion of extracellular fluid outside the vascular compartment and outside the cells. Edema may be either localized, as in inflammation, or generalized, as in the anasarca that may accompany the nephrotic syndrome, cirrhosis of the liver, or congestive heart failure. It may represent the accumulation of a few milliliters of fluid at the site of a bee sting, for example, or more than 100 lb of fluid when generalized. It is often stated that such fluid excess may not be apparent clinically in the adult until some 5 liters or more of excess extracellular fluid are retained. This is highly variable, however, and many healthy individuals with normal extracellular fluid volumes have noted puffiness of their feet after sitting long hours, in a bus or airplane, especially in warm weather.

LOCALIZED EDEMA

In Chapter 3, the forces that determine the distribution of fluid between capillaries and interstitial fluids were discussed. The balance between the hydrostatic pressure in the vessels favoring filtration and the oncotic pressure of the serum proteins plus the interstitial hydro-static fluid pressure favoring reabsorption, determine the direction of net transfer of fluid between capillary and interstitium. At the arterial end of the capillary these forces generally favor filtration, whereas at the venous end of the capillary the force vector favors reabsorption from interstitium back to capillary. The drop in intravascular hydro-static pressure, as resistance is overcome in the movement of blood through the capillaries, and the increased concentration and osmotic pressure of plasma proteins, which remain intravascular as the filtra-tion process proceeds, reverse the fluid movement. On the average, a perfect balance pertains such that the volume of interstitial fluid re-mains surprisingly constant, as does its distribution in any one part of the body.

Expressed in more quantitative terms, the pressure promoting ultra-filtration through the capillary is

$$P_u = \Delta P - \Delta \pi \\ = (P_c - P_t) - (\pi_c - \pi_t) \tag{6-1}$$

in which ΔP is the difference of hydrostatic pressure in the capillary, P_c, and interstitium, P_t; $\Delta \pi$ is the difference between the oncotic pres-sure of the intravascular proteins, π_c, and the opposing oncotic pres-sure of proteins in the interstitial fluids, π_t. The net rate of fluid ex-change across the capillary, J_v, is thus

$$J_v = L_p A \left[(P_c - P_t) - (\pi_c - \pi_t) \right] \tag{6-2}$$

in which A is the surface area of the capillary through which filtration may occur, and L_p is the filtration coefficient of the capillary lining, which has the dimensions (volume) (unit area of filtering surface)$^{-1}$ (unit of pressure)$^{-1}$ (time)$^{-1}$. The direction of net fluid movement J_v, as stated, reverses from the arteriolar to the venous end of the capillary.

It had long been accepted that the Starling forces were such that normally an interstitial pressure existed that was slightly positive to atmospheric pressure, and which contributed to the return of fluid from interstitium back to the vascular compartment. In a series of ex-periments involving the subcutaneous implantation of perforated cap-sules in various sites in the dog and subsequently measuring the pressures of the fluid within the capsules, however, Guyton (8) has demonstrated that interstitial hydrostatic pressure is invariably slightly negative to atmospheric pressure in nonedematous animals. By inserting a needle through the skin and then through a perforation of the capsule into its cavity, he consistently obtained negative values in normal tissues, which averaged −6.4 mm Hg. In edematous states, by contrast, the interstitial fluid pressures were always positive. Presumably the same situation exists in man. Our tissues thus normally remain "dry" as a result of a mean intravascular oncotic pressure that exceeds the mean hydrostatic pressure within the capillary bed. Such a situation, of course, is not incompatible with the large volume of ultrafiltration at the arterial end and reabsorption of interstitial fluid at the venous side of the capillary bed, since these movements depend only upon local imbalances of the Starling forces (equation 6-1), which can still apply despite a mean negative value of the hydrostatic pressure of interstitial fluid.

A number of factors can alter this delicate balance to produce an excess of interstitial fluid: (1) vasodilatation of the arteriole increases the hydrostatic filtering pressure in the capillary bed and may increase the area for filtration per capillary or actually open up previously unperfused capillary beds; (2) a decrease in concentration of plasma proteins or an increase in the concentration of proteins in interstitial fluid reduces the net osmotic force favoring reabsorption of fluid from interstitium to capillary; (3) an increase in venous pressure reduces the return of fluid to the capillary at its venous side; and (4) a decrease in interstitial fluid hydrostatic pressure which plays more of a role, however, in determining sites of edema and less of a role in producing edema. Under many circumstances, one or more of these factors can act to increase interstitial fluid volume, as indicated in Table 6-1.

Most of the entries in Table 6-1 are self-explanatory. There has, however, been no earlier comment on the protein content of the interstitial fluid. Capillaries are not totally impermeable to plasma proteins, and some protein leaks continuously into the interstitium. This usually amounts to about 1.0 gm/dl of interstitial fluid, as compared with a circulating protein concentration of 7.0 gm/dl of plasma. The effective osmotic pressure of the plasma proteins is thus diminished by the opposing oncotic pressure of soluble proteins in the interstitial fluid; it is the $\Delta \pi = \pi_c - \pi_t$ that is important.

Yet another factor, however, must be considered, namely, the per-

TABLE 6-1   *Factors Contributing to Edema Formation*

I.   ARTERIOLAR DILATATION
   A. Inflammation
   B. Heat
   C. Toxins
   D. Neurohumoral Excess or Deficit

II. REDUCED EFFECTIVE OSMOTIC PRESSURE
   A. Hypoproteinemia
      1. Malnutrition
      2. Cirrhosis
      3. Nephrotic syndrome
      4. Protein-losing gastroenteropathy

   B. "Leaky" Capillary Endothelium
      1. Inflammation
      2. Burns
      3. Trauma
      4. Allergic or immunologic reaction

   C. Lymphatic Obstruction

III. INCREASED VENOUS PRESSURE
   A. Congestive Heart Failure
   B. Thrombophlebitis
   C. Cirrhosis of Liver

IV. SODIUM RETENTION
   A. Excessive Salt Intake
   B. Increased Tubular Reabsorption of Sodium
      1. Reduced renal perfusion
      2. Increased renin–angiotensin–aldosterone secretion

---

meability of the capillary membrane to the plasma proteins. A membrane that is totally impermeable to a given solute is said to have a reflection coefficient, σ, equal to 1.0 for that solute. A solute that passes through a membrane so freely that its concentration in the filtrate is the same as in the perfusing fluid has a σ equal to 0 for that membrane. The effective osmotic pressure $\Delta\pi$, which controls reabsorption of interstitial fluids back into capillaries, is thus determined not only by the absolute difference in concentration of each protein in capillary lumen and interstitium but also by the concentration difference, which must be multiplied by the appropriate reflection coefficient for that protein in that part of the capillary bed. Thus $\Delta\pi_{\text{actual}} = \sigma\Delta\pi_{\text{theoretical}}$ for each protein involved.

The normal, small leakage of plasma proteins into the interstitial fluids is compensated by their return to the vascular compartment via the lymphatics. This keeps the protein concentration in interstitial fluids low and preserves a net oncotic pressure force, which favors return of interstitial fluid to the capillaries. When capillary permeability to plasma proteins increases excessively, as it may with injury from burns, toxins, allergies, inflammation, and so on, then the $\Delta\pi$ may decrease as the reflection coefficient of capillary membranes falls toward zero, with an increase in concentration of plasma proteins in the interstitial fluids. Lymphatic obstruction similarly diminishes $\Delta\pi$, and the edema of elephantiasis following chronic infection with *Filaria bancrofti* is due to such a local lymphatic blockage.

GENERALIZED EDEMA OR ANASARCA

Thus far the discussion has dealt only with factors that may produce edema in circumscribed portions of the body, for example, at the site of a bee sting, hives, a burn, localized cellulitis, or a region with blocked lymphatic or venous drainage. In all instances, the local accumulation of interstitial fluid, recognized as edema, has occurred at the expense of a transiently reduced intravascular volume. The effective intravascular volume is speedily reconstituted to normal by a compensatory renal retention of salt and water, and no fluid accumulation occurs beyond the local edema.

Quite a different picture emerges when fluid loss into the interstitial spaces is large, chronic, and generalized, as in the nephrotic syndrome, hepatic cirrhosis, and congestive heart failure. In these conditions it is not local tissue changes, which only produce a circumscribed, limited zone of edema. Rather it is an inadequacy of the circulation itself which is primarily at fault.

Edema of the nephrotic syndrome

The purest example of such generalized edema is perhaps the nephrotic syndrome. In this condition, the damaged glomerular capillaries leak protein into the urine with resultant hypoproteinemia. When the serum albumin concentration falls to 2.5 gm/dl of plasma or less, edema generally appears. The fall in serum proteins, of which albumin, being the smallest molecule, contributes most to the oncotic pressure, has two major and related effects.

1. Reduction of the intravascular volume. As noted in Chapter 3, the volume of each body fluid space is determined by the quantity of a specific solute, distribution of which is limited largely to that space. In the case of the intravascular volume, the unique solute is the serum albumin. Albumin comprises 4 to 5 gm of the total 7 gm of proteins/dl of plasma. Furthermore, since it is a smaller molecule than most of the circulating globulins, albumin normally contributes more than 80% of the protein oncotic pressure of the plasma. When serum proteins are lost through the kidneys, the plasma volume is reduced. In response to this reduction in intravascular volume, and to a decrease in renal perfusion, a sequence of intrarenal adjustments occurs, such that the renin–angiotensin mechanism is activated, aldosterone biosynthesis and secretion are stimulated, as is antidiuretic hormone secretion, and the kidneys retain sodium and water.

2. Increase of interstitial fluid volume. Associated with the drop in serum protein concentrations, there is a reduction in the net oncotic pressure that tends to draw fluid from interstitial spaces back into the vascular compartment, and edema fluid accumulates. This fluid must come initially from the intravascular plasma, which further compromises the circulation and increases the stimulus for renal retention of sodium and water. The retained sodium and water cannot, however, correct the inadequacy of the circulating intravascular volume. The retained salt and water simply leak into the interstitial spaces and increase the edema; the primary defect, too little serum protein, persists; more sodium and water are retained; and more and more edema fluid accumulates. Finally, the gradual rise in interstitial hydrostatic pressure limits further edema.

Though the increase in interstitial fluid is general, edema tends to appear first where tissue turgor is normally lowest. Periorbital edema, facial puffiness, and swelling of the fingers in the morning may be the earliest signs of edema. After arising and being upright most of the day, the patient may note that his periorbital and facial edema has disappeared toward evening, while his feet and ankles have become puffy, often making it difficult to put on his shoes. Gravity has redistributed the excess interstitial fluid.

Because the pulmonary vasculature is perfused at low pressures (about 5 mm Hg) the oncotic pressure of the plasma proteins suffices to keep the lungs free of edema, even when serum protein concentrations are markedly reduced. Patients with the nephrotic syndrome may, however, become dyspneic, as a result of pleural effusion. The parietal pleural surface, perfused at systemic vascular pressures, not the visceral pleura, is the source of the effusion. If left ventricular failure supervenes, from hypertension or some other cause in the presence of hypoproteinemia, pulmonary interstitial or alveolar edema may be aggravated by the reduction in plasma oncotic pressure.

Edema of cirrhosis
The edema of cirrhosis of the liver involves at least two etiologic factors, and these may be combined in varying degrees. First, the cirrhotic liver has generally lost much of its hepatocellular functions, including the ability to synthesize serum albumin. Thus, as in the nephrotic syndrome, the plasma oncotic pressure is too low, and the plasma volume is reduced. This produces renal retention of sodium and water with edema, but without correcting the plasma volume deficit. Second, the cirrhotic process obstructs the intrahepatic portion of the portal venous system. The resulting increased hydrostatic pressure of the portal vein not only causes esophageal varices, but also reduces the amount of interstitial fluid returned to the portal venous system. There is an accumulation of interstitial fluid within the tissues drained by the portal system, which include, of course, the viscera. The ascites seen in cirrhotic patients is the clinical manifestation of this sequestration of interstitial fluid in the abdominal cavity. The portal capillary bed is often more permeable to serum albumin in portal hypertension; thus albumin, given intravenously, will enter the ascitic fluid rapidly to further enlarge the swollen belly.

Cardiac edema
The cause of edema in congestive heart failure has been the topic of many studies, and yet all aspects of this condition are not fully understood. There is clearly no reduction in intravascular volume; the dilated veins attest to a full venous system, and the elevated venous pressure reduces the return of interstitial fluid to the vascular compartment. The reduced cardiac output is, however, sensed on the arterial side through baroreceptors and by the renal juxtaglomerular

apparatus as a reduced perfusion pressure. This again sets off at least the renin–angiotensin–aldosterone-antidiuretic hormone axis to effect sodium and water retention. The high systemic and often pulmonary, venous pressure sequesters the retained fluid in the interstitial spaces without improving cardiac function, and so the stimulus for more fluid retention continues and the amount of edema increases. Only by increasing cardiac output can the vicious cycle be broken and the edema decrease spontaneously.

Less well understood are the congestive states associated with high cardiac output, as with anemia or cor pulmonale. So-called high out-put cardiac failure, however, like low output failure, is associated with a decreased blood flow to the kidneys, and this may be the com-mon denominator in sodium-retaining states associated with heart failure. A reduced perfusion of the kidneys, that is, even a small re-duction in filtration per nephron, promotes reabsorption of an in-creased percentage of filtered sodium and hence increases sodium retention, at least temporarily. This purely renal mechanism may also operate in cirrhosis and the nephrotic syndrome; in both conditions plasma volume is contracted and renal perfusion is thereby com-promised.

The conditions associated with generalized edema thus seem to rep-resent persistent overactivity of a normal regulatory mechanism that had great survival value to our forebears. Acute blood loss and diar-rheal or sweat losses reduce intravascular volume and perfusion pres-sure. This triggers the renin–angiotensin system as indicated in Figure 3-5. The angiotensin, through its direct vasoconstrictor effect on vas-cular smooth muscle, sustains blood pressure and simultaneously in-duces biosynthesis of aldosterone, which in turn signals the kidneys to retain sodium and water and thus replenish the dangerously reduced vascular volume. With hypoproteinemia or cardiac failure the same deficit is sensed, and salt and water retention results. But instead of correcting the circulatory deficit the retained fluid accumulates in the interstitial spaces. Edema occurs, but the stimulus for salt and water retention persists.

References

1. Starling, E. H. Physiological factors involved in the causation of dropsy. Lancet, May, 1896.

2. Starling, E. H. The fluids of the body. University of Chicago Press, Chicago, 1909, pp. 67–68.

3. Krogh, A., Landis, E. M., and Turner, A. H. The movement of fluid through the human capillary wall in relation to venous pressure and to the colloid osmotic pressure of the blood. J. Clin. Invest. 11:63–95, 1932.

4. Landis, E. M. Capillary pressure and capillary permeability. Physiol. Rev. 14: 404–481, 1934.

5. Pappenheimer, J. R. Passage of molecules through capillary walls. Physiol. Rev. 33:387–423, 1953.

6. Landis, E. M. and Pappenheimer, J. R. Exchange of substances through the capillary walls. *In:* Handbook of physiology. Circulation, Washington, D.C., Am. Physiol. Soc., Sect. 2, Vol. 2, 1963, pp. 961–1034.

7. Gauer, O. H., Henry, J. P., and Behn, C. The regulation of extracellular fluid volume. Ann. Rev. Physiol. 32:547–595, 1970.

8. Guyton, A. C., Granger, H. J., and Taylor, A. E. Interstitial fluid pressure. Physiol. Rev. 51:527–563, 1971.

7
Diuretics

INTRODUCTION

Diuresis is an increase in urine flow. Any agent that promotes an increased flow of urine is a diuretic. Water is thus the most common diuretic. Clinically, diuretics are used in most instances to reduce the extracellular fluid volume. The clinical effectiveness of a diuretic lies in its ability to enhance urinary excretion of sodium. This relieves edematous states caused by nephrotic syndrome, cirrhosis or heart failure. Today, however, the commonest use of diuretics is in the treatment of hypertension.

Many agents can increase the excretion of sodium but only a few are used in practice. With the large volume of glomerular filtrate in the normal adult, some 25,000 mEq of sodium are filtered daily, of which less than 1% is excreted. Agents that increase the glomerular filtration rate by affecting the renal vasculature or by increasing the perfusion pressure—increasing cardiac output or systemic blood pressure—generally increase sodium excretion. Only those substances with a direct action on the kidney are regarded as diuretics. Xanthine diuretics increase cardiac output, renal blood flow, and glomerular filtration rate, as do the adrenal corticosteroids, but neither are effective diuretics. Certain prostaglandins that increase renal blood flow may markedly enhance sodium excretion (1). If analogs can be made that are not destroyed as rapidly as the natural hormones and that are effective orally, then a new class of diuretics may become available.

The clinical stalwarts today, however, are all agents that in one way or another, inhibit the reabsorption of sodium in the nephron. They may be classified according to the site of their major action along the nephron. To the extent that their mode of action is known, they may also be classified as (1) osmotic diuretics, (2) inhibitors of urinary acidification, (3) inhibitors of sodium and/or chloride transport, and (4) aldosterone antagonists. Studies of the action of the various diuretics have contributed substantially to our understanding of renal physiology, which in turn has led to tailor-made diuretics with carbonic anhydrase inhibitory activity or aldosterone antagonism, to cite two examples.

OSMOTIC DIURESIS

Osmotic diuretics are of more heuristic than practical value. Recently they have been reintroduced for the treatment. of cerebral edema and acute renal failure. Any solute of relatively low molecular weight that is freely filtered at the glomerulus, but poorly reabsorbed through the tubular epithelium may serve as an osmotic diuretic. Glucose, urea, and mannitol are the most common agents. When present in sufficient amounts in the tubular fluid, they interfere with the reabsorption of water and, hence, of sodium chloride in the proximal tubule and in the loop of Henle.

The proximal tubule is highly permeable to water. As solutes, chiefly sodium and chloride, are reabsorbed in this segment of the nephron, water follows rapidly, so that about 70% of the glomerular filtrate is normally reabsorbed isotonically in the proximal tubule. A high permeability of the cells lining the proximal tubule to water and to solutes is necessary to accomplish this large, rapid reabsorption. Such high permeability, however, prevents the establishment of osmotic gradients or large specific solute gradients between the luminal and peritubular fluids. When large amounts of a poorly reabsorbable solute are present in the glomerular filtrate, they osmotically oppose the reabsorption of water in the proximal tubule. The high water and salt permeability of the epithelium precludes a drop in luminal sodium concentration below some 100 mEq/liter of tubular fluid. At this concentration no net reabsorption of sodium occurs, since its outward transport of sodium from luminal fluid is just balanced by passive leakage of sodium from peritubular fluid to lumen. In the absence of net solute reabsorption water reabsorption also stops. Sodium chloride-containing fluid is presented to the loop of Henle in an increased volume directly proportional to the quantity of poorly reabsorbable, osmotically active solute filtered through the glomeruli.

Normally about 10% of filtered water and 15% of filtered sodium chloride are reabsorbed in the loop of Henle. The water leaves the descending limb of the loop as it passes down into the hypertonic medullary interstitium. Sodium chloride is reabsorbed passively, it is thought, in the thin ascending limb of Henle's loop, and actively in the thick ascending segment of the loop.

During osmotic diuresis both water and salt reabsorption are hindered. Experimental studies have demonstrated a marked reduction in medullary hypertonicity during osmotic diuresis. In hydropenic rats the tonicity may drop from more than 2000 to about 400 mOsm/kg of water during an osmotic diuresis induced by mannitol (2). This loss of hypertonicity in the medullary interstitium reduces the osmotic force drawing water from the descending limb of Henle's loop, and less water is reabsorbed.

Conditions are unfavorable for sodium reabsorption as well. In the descending limb of the loop, the solute concentration of the luminal fluid increases as water is drawn out until the osmolality of the luminal fluid matches that of the medullary interstitium. Thus, deep within the medulla, the osmolalities of luminal fluid and peritubular fluid are usually very high and are thought to be equal. But within the tubule sodium chloride contributes nearly all the osmolality, whereas in the interstitium, urea and sodium chloride contribute about equally to the high osmolality. This affords a gradient for outward passive diffusion of sodium chloride from the thin ascending limb of the loop, which appears to possess the requisite high permeability to sodium (3). With the reduction in hypertonicity of the medullary interstitium associated with osmotic diuresis, this gradient-favoring reabsorption of sodium is diminished; less sodium leaves the tubule.

The lower hypertonicity of the medullary interstitium during osmotic diuresis diminishes reabsorption of both water and sodium chloride. The increased medullary blood flow during osmotic diuresis is the major factor dissipating the hypertonicity of the medullary interstitium—a "washout" effect. Infusion of hypertonic mannitol solutions directly into a renal artery reduces the vascular resistance in the kidney (4) by means that are not entirely clear. This reduced vascular resistance is thought to increase blood flow in the vasa recta and thus "wash out" the hypertonicity of the medullary interstitium during osmotic diuresis.

Increased absolute amounts of sodium chloride and of water are delivered to the thick ascending limb of the loop of Henle as a result of their impaired reabsorption in the proximal tubule and in the thin segments of Henle's loop. Active chloride reabsorption in the thick ascending segment is not impaired, and sodium chloride reabsorption, without an accompanying reabsorption of water, proceeds as usual, so the fluid delivered to the distal convoluted tubule is increased in volume, but may have its sodium concentration reduced to usual levels of some 50 to 70 mEq/liter. Whether these levels constitute a gradient limitation for sodium chloride reabsorption is not at present known, but during modest osmotic diuresis the usual sodium concentrations may be achieved. Since the total volume of salt and water reaching the thick ascending limb is increased during osmotic diuresis, the absolute amount delivered to the distal convoluted tubule and collecting ducts is also increased, as is urine flow and sodium excretion. With a large osmotic load the concentration of sodium in the fluid emerging from the thick ascending limb rises to 70 to 90 mEq/liter or higher, despite the fact that more sodium and chloride are reabsorbed in this segment; the active reabsorptive process is simply overwhelmed by the quantities of sodium chloride reaching this segment.

The reabsorptive capacities of the distal convoluted tubule and of the collecting ducts are also swamped by the flow of fluid, and little further modification of urine composition is achieved during the rapid transit of the urine through these segments. The result is that, during either hydropenia with maximal activity of antidiuretic hormone or water diuresis in the absence of antidiuretic hormone, the urine concentration in brisk osmotic diuresis approaches that of the plasma, about 300 mOsm/kg of water (Fig. 7-1), and the urine sodium concentration is generally about 70 to 90 mEq/liter of urine.

The magnitude of diuresis achieved with an osmotic diuretic may be considerable: 100 gm of mannitol injected intravenously into a normal hydropenic subject increases urine flow within minutes, and volumes of 8 to 10 ml/minute are attained within an hour. With

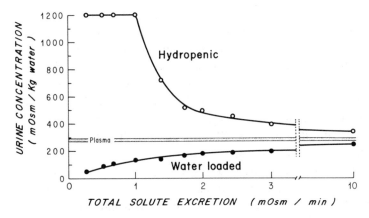

Fig. 7-1 Effect of osmotic diuresis on urine concentration in the hydropenic subject (upper) and water-loaded subject (lower). (Represented from data kindly made available by J. D. Crawford.)

larger amounts of mannitol, 20–30% of filtered water and 15% of filtered sodium are excreted during the height of the diuresis. Even larger excretion rates can be attained. In the dog, for example, as much as 65% of filtered water and 30% of filtered sodium can be delivered into the urine acutely if large concentrations of mannitol are infused rapidly. The inhibition of water and sodium reabsorption in the proximal convoluted tubule and in the loop of Henle contribute about equally in producing such massive diuresis (5).

Glucose and urea are the most common solutes associated clinically with osmotic diuresis, the former in uncontrolled diabetes mellitus, when high blood sugar leads to quantities of glucose in proximal tubular fluid that exceed the reabsorptive capacity of the epithelium, and the latter, when the blood urea is elevated as a result of very high rates of protein catabolism or fewer filtering glomeruli. Foreign solutes such as mannitol and glycerol have been used to produce an osmotic diuresis. The essentially nonreabsorbed hexose mannitol is highly effective, as noted, but its inability to penetrate cell membranes prevents its absorption from the intestines, and it must, therefore, be administered intravenously. Even the administration of sodium salts in large amounts can produce an osmostic diuresis, but clearly this would not decrease the content of sodium in the body—the goal in the use of diuretics.

Because of their slow passage across the blood-brain barrier, mannitol, urea, and glycerol are used to reduce cerebral edema. To be effective they must be administered in large amounts. While in the body they may cause considerable expansion of extracellular fluid volume at the expense of the volume of intracellular fluid. The acute effects of this increase in extracellular fluid volume and, with it, of intravascular volume must be carefully considered if such agents are to be used in patients with marginal cardiac compensation.

When urine flow is brisk after an osmotic diuretic has been administered, the sodium concentration in the urine is generally fixed in the range of 70 to 90 mEq/liter. Thus, the ratio of water to sodium (plus potassium, strictly speaking) in the urine is greater than in the extracellular fluids, and the tendency is for the concentration of sodium in the serum to rise. This tendency is counteracted by at least two factors: (1) transfer of intracellular water to the extracellular fluid in response to high concentrations of the osmotically active agent in the latter and (2) thirst from the increased serum osmolality, leading to water intake. The serum sodium may thus be low, high, or normal during osmotic diuresis, depending on the balance, on the one hand, of water intake and water transfer from intracellular to extracellular fluids—both tending to lower serum sodium concentration—and, on the other hand, of the tendency of the high water-to-sodium ratio in the urine to elevate the concentration of sodium in serum.

INHIBITION OF URINARY ACIDIFICATION

Urinary acidification is accomplished by the secretion of hydrogen ions in exchange for sodium ions reabsorbed from the tubular fluid. The secreted hydrogen ion is generated within the tubular epithelial cells from the ionization of water, leaving a hydroxyl ion behind. In the presence of CO_2 and the enzyme carbonic anhydrase, this hydroxyl ion is rapidly converted to bicarbonate. It is this bicarbonate that accompanies the reabsorbed sodium ion back into the body fluids (see Chapter 4). Inhibition of carbonic anhydrase reduces hydrogen ion secretion and sodium bicarbonate reabsorption.

Following early reports that sulfanilamide could produce a metabolic acidosis associated with an alkaline urine and an increased excretion of bicarbonate, it was found that N-unsubstituted sulfonamides were able to inhibit carbonic anhydrase, an enzyme present in large concentrations in the kidney. This knowledge led to the synthesis of a series of heterocyclic sulfonamide inhibitors of this enzyme, of which the most useful has been acetazolamide—see review by Maren (6).

Because acetazolamide is quantitatively absorbed from the intestines, it is effective by oral administration. Its renal clearance in dogs is approximately equal to its glomerular filtration rate, but its clearance is decreased by probenecid, an agent that inhibits secretion of organic acids in the proximal tubule, which suggests some secretion of acetazolamide at this site.

Within minutes after the acute administration of acetazolamide the urine pH rises, as does excretion of bicarbonate, sodium, and potassium. The fractional excretion of filtered bicarbonate may rise from its usual level of less than 1% to levels as high as 30%. With this, some 2–5% of filtered sodium and an even larger proportion of filtered potassium may be excreted. But a concomitant moderate reduction in the glomerular filtration rate of about 20% does occur. The main site of action of acetazolamide is in the proximal tubule, where most hydrogen ion secretion occurs. Hydrogen ion secretion in the distal tubule and collecting duct is also inhibited. The increased potassium excretion is a consequence of the delivery of the large amount of unreabsorbed sodium and bicarbonate from the proximal tubule into the distal nephron. The bicarbonate ion in this segment acts as a poorly reabsorbable anion that, together with the large amount of sodium in the tubular fluid, enhances the electrical negativity of luminal fluid and thus draws potassium into the urine.

Acetazolamide is only a weak diuretic clinically. Continued administration of the drug produces a self-limiting response. The initial loss of bicarbonate in an alkaline urine results in a hyperchloremic acidosis with reduced plasma bicarbonate concentration. When the serum bicarbonate concentration has fallen, so that the small quantities of filtered bicarbonate can be largely reabsorbed utilizing what minimal, noninhibited carbonic anhydrase activity persists, the effects of acetazolamide wane. Thus, despite continuous administration of the drug, the reaction of the urine reverts to acidic, and urinary sodium, potassium, and ammonium return to control values (Fig. 7-2).

Whereas the diuretic effect of acetazolamide on renal excretion of bicarbonate is self-limited, its inhibitory effect on the secretion of aqueous humor is more persistent, and the agent has been used to treat chronic glaucoma. Since, however, it tends to increase urinary alkalinity and at the same time inhibits citrate excretion, there is

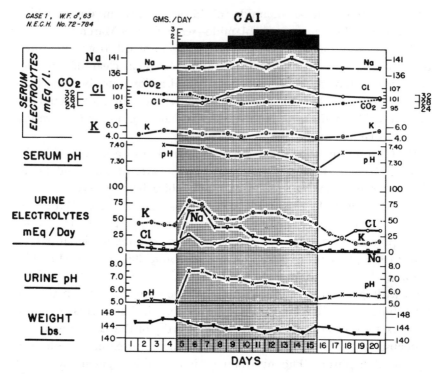

Fig. 7-2 Effect of Diamox on serum electrolyte concentrations, urinary electrolyte excretion, body weight, and urine and serum pH. Note that sodium and potassium excretion increased, without a change in urine chloride, as hyperchloremic acidosis developed in the serum. Reprinted, by permission from the *New England Journal of Medicine* (18).

some risk of intrarenal calcification from its chronic use. The hyperchloremic acidosis mobilizes skeletal calcium, which is excreted into an alkaline urine in the absence of the solubilizing effect of urinary citrate on calcium. This combination of factors slightly increases the risk of deposition of calcium as calculi or nephrocalcinosis.

INHIBITION OF SODIUM AND CHLORIDE REABSORPTION
The major modern diuretics fall into this category. Organic mercurials were the sole members of this group until chlorothiazide was synthesized in an attempt to produce a more potent inhibitor of carbonic anhydrase. The result, in the mid-1950's, was the beginning of the de-

velopment of several potent agents in this category. Although all these diuretics inhibit sodium and chloride reabsorption, they are chemically a diverse group of compounds. This is evident from the chemical formulae shown in Figure 7-3.

Mercurial diuretics were the first of the potent diuretics, but now they are largely of historical interest. Their renal action was discovered soon after the introduction of organic mercurials in the treatment of syphilis, and for years they were the mainstay of diuretic programs. The toxic mercuric ion in these compounds was combined with an organic compound, usually theophylline. Because of poor intestinal absorption and intestinal irritation they were generally injected intramuscularly, but when a rapid diuretic effect was desired, they

Fig. 7-3 Structural formulas of commonly used diuretics.

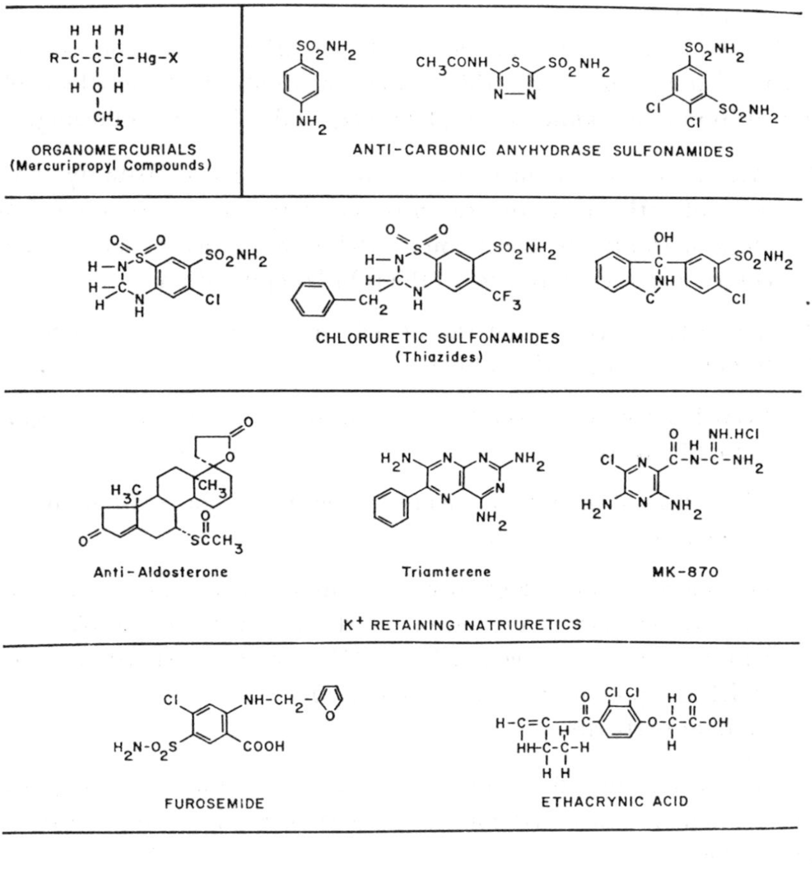

were often administered intravenously despite the very small risk of an acute sensitivity reaction with vascular collapse. Even with intravenous administration, onset of diuresis was delayed some 30 to 40 minutes, peak effects were not seen for 2 to 4 hours, and the effects persisted over several hours. Organic mercurials increase the excretion of sodium, chloride, and usually potassium and ammonium. The urine during diuresis generally becomes acid, and a systemic, hypokalemic alkalosis results. Because systemic alkalosis itself inhibits the diuretic effect of mercurials, their action is self-limited.

There has been much interest in the mechanism of action of mercurial diuretics. Not all organic mercurials are diuretics. Parachloromercuribenzoate (PCMB), a potent sulfhydryl inhibitor, is not a diuretic. In fact, PCMB promptly reverses the diuretic action of other organic mercurials. It had been thought that small amounts of free mercuric ions liberated from organic mercurials in an acid urine might account for their diuretic effect (7).

Burg's studies (8, 9) of the action of mercurial diuretics on isolated, perfused fragments of the thick ascending limb of Henle's loop obtained from rabbit kidneys have, however, established the following:

1. Merslyl, an organic mercurial diuretic, inhibits reversibility about 50% of active chloride reabsorption in the thick ascending limb without significant effects on electrical resistance or sodium and chloride conductivities across the tubular epithelium.

2. This effect occurs when the mercurial diuretic is exposed to the luminal surface of the tubule.

3. PCMB promptly reverses the inhibition of chloride transport caused by mersalyl.

4. The action of mersalyl is unaffected by the pH of perfusate over a range of 6.0 to 7.4.

5. Free mercuric ions ($HgCl_2$) in the luminal perfusate, unlike mersalyl, cause marked depression of the transtubular electrical potential that is not reversed by PCMB, whereas mercuric cysteine, which is a potent diuretic *in vivo,* has no effect when added to the luminal perfusate.

From these findings, Burg concluded that the organic mercurial itself, rather than free mercuric ion, is responsible for its characteristic diuretic effect.

Although the organic mercurials' major site of action is the luminal surface of the thick ascending limb of the loop of Henle, they gain access to the tubular urine largely by secretion in the proximal tubule. By inhibiting sodium chloride reabsorption in the thick ascending limb, mercurial diuretics interfere with both the concentrating and diluting capacities of the kidney. See review by Cafruny (10).

The *benzathiadiazine diuretics,* of which chlorothiazide was the first effective example, were synthesized in a conscious effort to produce a stronger carbonic anhydrase inhibitor. Although still possessing some carbonic anhydrase inhibitory activity, these compounds produce a large chloruresis that indicates another major mechanism of action. In fact, they are also secreted in the proximal tubule, where they partially inhibit carbonic anhydrase, but their major site of action is more distal. Curiously, they inhibit maximal dilution of the urine without interfering with concentrating ability. This suggests a major site of action just distal to the thick ascending limb, perhaps in the first portion of the distal convoluted tubules.

The benzathiadiazine diuretics were the first potent orally effective diuretics. Chlorothiazide, administered in large amounts intravenously, causes a marked increase in the urinary excretion of sodium, chloride, potassium, and bicarbonate acutely. Excretion of sodium, chloride, and bicarbonate after intravenous administration may rise to as much as 10% of the filtered load, and potassium excretion may increase to a level exceeding the quantity filtered. With the usual diuretic doses, excretion of sodium, chloride, and potassium increases, but the effects on bicarbonate excretion are inconstant. Despite the demonstrable inhibitory effect of these compounds on carbonic anhydrase activity, the most common disturbance in the body fluid composition associated with their chronic oral administration is a hypokalemic, metabolic alkalosis. Unlike mercurial diuretics, the action of the benzathiadiazine diuretics is not affected by the acid–base status of urine or body fluids, and severe hypokalemia can result that is particularly dangerous to a patient who is also receiving digitalis. The duration of action is some 6 to 48 hours. See review by Beyer (11).

The commonest use of the benzathiadiazine diuretics today is not in the treatment of edema, but as an adjunct in the management of arterial hypertension. This effect again depends largely on producing a modest sodium depletion in the nonedematous hypertensive patient. Such reduction in extracellular fluid volume tends to reduce blood pressure and renders the hypertension more responsive to reduction by other antihypertensive agents. Since diazoxide, a benzathiadiazine derivative, has a prompt and potent antihypertensive effect when administered intravenously, but is nondiuretic, it is postulated that the other compounds of this class may also have some direct relaxing effect on vascular smooth muscle, which contributes to their antihypertensive action.

Seemingly paradoxically, thiazide diuretics have been used successfully to diminish the severity of polyuria and, hence, also of polydipsia in diabetes insipidus. The sustained mild reduction in extracellular fluid volume created by the initial negative sodium balance interferes with maximal urine dilution and may reduce urine volumes by 30–40%. In diabetes insipidus such a reduction in daily urine volume may be sufficient to relieve the annoying polyuria (12).

The most potent of the oral diuretics are *furosemide* and *ethacrynic acid,* which were introduced almost simultaneously in the mid-1960's. The two compounds are chemically unrelated; ethacrynic acid is a derivative of phenoxyacetic acid, and furosemide is a sulfamylbenzene derivative of anthranilic acid (see Fig. 7-3). Both drugs are rapidly absorbed when given orally; their diuretic effect is apparent in minutes and persists for 1 to 3 hours. Each is secreted by the proximal tubule, but only about one-third of the drug is excreted in the urine, the remainder being excreted in the gut, probably via the bile. At peak effect, 20 to 30% of filtered sodium and chloride may be excreted. In usual diuretic doses there is no constant effect on bicarbonate excretion. See review by Goldberg (13).

It is clear that the major site of action of both compounds is in the thick ascending limb of Henle's loop, where they strongly inhibit active chloride reabsorption (14, 15). Ethacrynic acid administered to dogs is excreted in a chemically modified form in the urine; one major excretion product is ethacrynic-cysteine. When this combination was perfused through isolated rabbit tubules, it was more than 100 times as potent an inhibitor of chloride transport as ethacrynic acid itself. Complexed with cysteine ethacrynic acid is generally less reactive chemically and less toxic than in its uncombined form. Thus, ethacrynic acid–cysteine, or perhaps other such complexes, would seem to be effective, acting from the luminal side of the thick ascending limb, to block active chloride reabsorption. Furosemide acts in the uncombined form. Neither diuretic exhibited an effect from the peritubular side of the isolated tubule segments (14, 15). Since the capacity for sodium chloride reabsorption in the thick ascending limb of the loop is considerable, amounting to as much as 20–40% of filtered sodium chloride, inhibition of reabsorption at this site can produce a very large diuresis. There are slight differences in the action of these two agents in different species, but in man they are the most powerful diuretic agents available. The inhibitory action of both agents on the thick ascending limb of the loop inhibits both the concentrating and diluting ability of the kidneys. They are thought to have minor inhibitory effects in the proximal tubule as well. In usual diuretic dosages neither seems to have an effect on the renal vasculature or intrarenal distribution of blood flow, as once claimed; direct inhibitory effects on membrane transport have been documented. The molecular mechanism of their action remains unknown. Both agents may produce profound potassium depletion if used chronically without adequate potassium supplementation.

ALDOSTERONE ANTAGONISTS

Three agents are generally included in this class of diuretics: spironolactone, amiloride, and triametrene. Only the spirolactones are true aldosterone antagonists; spironolactone is the compound of this group of true antagonists in general use. The spirolactones were developed as a result of the observation that progesterone is a naturally occurring aldosterone antagonist, which suggested that other, structurally similar, nonhormonal compounds might also compete with aldosterone.

Aldosterone is the potent steroidal hormone from the adrenal cortex that stimulates reabsorption of sodium in the distal convoluted tubule and collecting duct. It is responsible for the reabsorption of the last bit of sodium from the urine in sodium-retaining states, lowering urinary sodium losses often to 1 or 2 mEq/day. Spirolactones are steroidal analogs that compete with aldosterone for its physiologic binding sites in the cytosol and nuclei of responsive cells. By preventing the initial hormonal binding, they block the sequence of reactions in which the hormonal effect depends (16). The affinity of spironolactone for the aldosterone-binding sites is, however, only about one-thousandth that of the hormone itself. Thus, spironolactone is a relatively weak antagonist of aldosterone. It must be administered in large amounts orally, since it is poorly absorbed from the intestines. Since its action is simply to counteract the effects of aldosterone, it has no diuretic effect on adrenalectomized animals or subjects with Addison's disease. Furthermore, the portion of filtered sodium reabsorption modulated by aldosterone is normally small, and in edematous states associated with reduced renal perfusion and glomerular filtration, even a larger fraction of filtered sodium is reabsorbed at sites proximal to that affected by aldosterone. Thus, inhibition of aldosterone activity in such circumstances is not likely to produce a significant diuresis, and it does not.

The major use of spironolactone is in conjunction with other diuretics that are more potent and act at a more proximal site. Inhibition of the effect of aldosterone then prevents reabsorption of the sodium in the distal tubules and collecting ducts that had not been reabsorbed proximally. More important often than the modest effect spironolactone has on the excretion of sodium is the inhibitory effect it has on potassium and hydrogen ion secretion. The increased aldosterone secretion in the sodium-retaining edematous states primes the sodium-reabsorptive capacity of the distal tubule and collecting ducts. When potent diuretics deliver more sodium to these distal sites, sodium reabsorption does increase, and with it there is an increased electrical negativity of the luminal fluid that draws potassium into the urine and may account for the very large potassium losses and severe potassium depletion that results from the use of such potent diuretics. Blocking the action of aldosterone on the renal tubule cells with spironolactones prevents such large losses of potassium. In fact, renal ability to excrete potassium may be so compromised by spironolactones that, if potassium supplements are continued with the aldosterone blockers, serious hyperkalemia with potassium intoxication can ensue. Acid excretion (titratable acid and ammonium) is also inhibited by spironolactone.

Amiloride and *triamterene* are largely antikaliuretic agents, though they produce a modest natriuresis as well. Thus, they are similar to spironolactone in the effect they produce and in their distal site of action. Unlike the spirolactones, however, their effects occur irrespective of the presence or absence of aldosterone or other adrenal corticosteroids. Both agents are effective when administered orally.

Amiloride is a pyrazinoyl compound, and triamterene is a pteridine derivative, related chemically to folic acid, but without antifolate activity; known antifolates do not possess diuretic activity either. The two compounds thus are not chemically related, nor do their modes of action seem to be similar, although the end results of their actions on the distal nephrons are.

In the toad bladder, which reabsorbs sodium actively, amiloride at low concentrations (10^{-6}–10^{-5} M) applied to the urinary surface inhibits sodium transport almost instantaneously but reversibly (17). The inhibitory action of amiloride is reversed by simply rinsing the urinary surface with Ringer's solution. From the opposite, serosal side the amiloride has no effect on sodium transport. Similar results have been obtained in the isolated rabbit cortical collecting tubule (9). Amiloride (10^{-5}M), applied to the fluid perfusing the lumen, inhibited sodium reabsorption and potassium secretion and reversed the transtubular epithelial potential from -35V with the lumen negative to a small positive potential of $+5$mV. The latter potential was assumed to result from some persistent hydrogen ion secretion as it decreased toward zero when acetazolamide was added to the bath or CO_2 was eliminated from the bathing solution. By contrast, amiloride had no effect on the active reabsorption of chloride in the thick ascending limb of the loop of Henle.

Triamterene also inhibits sodium transport by the isolated toad bladder, but only when it is added to the serosal side; the action is slow and does not seem to be completely reversible. See review by Goldberg (13).

XANTHINE DIURETICS

Largely for the sake of completeness this class of mildly diuretic agents deserves mention. Included in the group are caffeine, theobromine, and theophylline and the related aminouracils amisometradine and chlorazanil. The most common representative clinically is aminophylline, the salt of theophylline-ethylene diamine. These drugs are used as adjunctive agents in the treatment of edema resistant to other diuretic regimes. Aminophylline administered intravenously shortly after a mercurial diuretic would often result in diuresis when each agent separately had failed. Though they have been employed for many years, little is known about the mechanism of action of these compounds. They possess several extrarenal effects—increasing cardiac output, stimulating the central nervous system, and dilating the bronchi. The increased cardiac output with enhanced renal blood flow and increased glomerular filtration rate may account for the modest increase in excretion of sodium, chloride, and water that intravenous aminophylline induces. Some studies suggest, however, that the diuretic effect persists after the blood flow and filtration rate have returned to control levels, which would indicate a direct tubular action. Since the

TABLE 7-1   *Sites of Action of Diuretics in the Nephron*[a]

DIURETIC	PROXIMAL TUBULE	LOOP OF HENLE; THICK ASCENDING LIMB MEDULLARY	CORTICAL	NEPHRON DISTAL
Acetazolamide	+			±
Amiloride				+
Aminophylline	+			
Chlorothiazide	±		+	
Ethacrynic acid	±	+	±	
Furosemide	±	+	±	
Mercurials		+	±	
Spironolactone				+
Triamterene				+

[a] A + indicates major site of action; a ± indicates site of minor action or of weak evidence for site of action.

xanthines can inhibit phosphodiesterase, the enzyme responsible for the inactivation of cyclic adenosine 3′,5′-monophosphate, there is a suspicion that somehow this action of the xanthines may account for their diuretic effect; the suspicion remains, however, unconfirmed.

Table 7-1 summarizes the major sites of action of the diuretics just discussed, and Table 7-2 indicates their effects on the excretion of sodium, potassium, chloride, and bicarbonate.

TABLE 7-2   *Effects of Diuretics on Electrolyte Excretion*[a]

DIURETIC	Na	Cl	K	HCO_3	MAXIMAL FILTERED Na EXCRETED %
Acetazolamide	↑	—	↑	↑	5
Amiloride	↑	—	↓	↑	3
Aminophylline	↑	↑	↑	↑	2
Chlorothiazide	↑	↑	↑	↓	10
Ethacrynic acid	↑	↑	↑	↓	25
Furosemide	↑	↑	↑	—	25
Mercurials	↑	↑	↑	↓	20
Spironolactone	↑	—	↓	↑	2
Triamterene	↑	—	↓	↑	2

[a] The ↑ and ↓ indicate increased or decreased excretion, respectively; the — indicates no or an inconstant effect.

References

1. Lee, J. B., McGiff, J. C., Kannegiesser, H., Aykent, Y. Y., Mudd, J. G., and Frawley, T. F. Prostaglandin A_1: antihypertensive and renal effects. Ann. Int. Med. 74:703–710, 1971.
2. Gottschalk, C. W. Micropuncture studies of tubular function in the mammalian kidney. The Physiologist 4:35–55, 1961.
3. Imai, M. and Kokko, J. P. Sodium chloride, urea, and water transport in the thin ascending limb of Henle. J. Clin. Invest. 53:393–402, 1974.
4. Goldberg, A. H. and Lilienfield, L. S. Effects of hypertonic mannitol on renal vascular resistance. Proc. Soc. Exper. Biol. Med. 119:635–642, 1965.
5. Gennari, F. J. and Kassirer, J. P. Osmotic diuresis. New Eng. J. Med. 291:714–720, 1974.
6. Maren, T. H. Carbonic anhydrase: chemistry, physiology, and inhibition. Physiol. Rev. 47:595–781 1967.
7. Levy, R. I., Weiner, I. M., and Mudge, G. H. The effect of acid-base balance on the diuresis produced by organic and inorganic mercurials. J. Clin. Invest. 30:1089–1104, 1951.
8. Burg, M. B. and Green, N. Effect of mersalyl on the thick ascending limb of Henle's loop. Kidney Int. 4:245–251, 1973.
9. Burg, M. B. The mechanism of action of diuretics in renal tubules. *In* Recent advances in renal physiology and pharmacology, L. G. Wesson and G. M. Fanelli, Jr., eds. University Park Press, Baltimore, pp. 99–109, 1974.
10. Cafruny, E. J. The site and mechanism of action of mercurial diuretics. Pharm. Rev. 20:89–111, 1968.
11. Beyer, K. H. The mechanism of action of chlorothiazide. Ann. N.Y. Acad. Sci. 71:363–379, 1958.
12. Earley, L. E. and Orloff, J. The mechanism of antidiuresis associated with the administration of hydrochlorothiazide to patients with vasopressin-resistant diabetes insipidus. J. Clin. Invest. 41:1988–1997, 1962.
13. Goldberg, M. The renal physiology of diuretics. Handbook of physiology—renal physiology, Berliner, R. W. and Orloff, J., eds. Am. Physiol. Society, Washington, D.C. pp. 1003–1031, 1973.
14. Burg, M. and Green, M. Effect of ethacrynic acid on the thick ascending limb of Henle's loop. Kidney Internat. 4:301–308, 1973.
15. Burg, M., Stoner, L., Cardinal, J., and Green, N. Furosemide effect on isolated perfused tubules. Am. J. Physiol. 225:119–124, 1973.
16. Fanestil, D. D. Mode of spirolactone action: competitive inhibition of aldosterone binding to kidney mineralocorticoid receptors. Biochem. Pharmacol. 17:2240–2242, 1968.
17. Bentley, P. J. Amiloride: A potent inhibitor of sodium transport across the toad bladder. J. Physiol., London. 195:317–331, 1969.
18. Leaf, A., Schwartz, W. B., and Relman, A. S. Oral administration of a potent carbonic anhydrase inhibitor (Diamox®): I. Changes in electrolyte and acid-base balance. N. Eng. J. Med. 250:759–764, 1954.

8

Acute Renal Failure

The term *acute renal failure* refers to a diverse group of clinical states associated with acute suppression of renal function. Acute renal failure is often, but not always associated with oliguria—24-hour urine volumes of 400 ml or less—and, rarely, with anuria—total cessation of urine output. Azotemia is a regular feature of acute renal failure.

Conditions associated with acute renal failure are generally subclassified as prerenal, renal, and postrenal. This classification helps practitioners think about the problem in an orderly way, which is important, since many of the conditions causing suppression of renal function are reversible if recognized and treated specifically. This is particularly true with respect to postrenal factors.

POSTRENAL ACUTE RENAL FAILURE

Obstruction of the urinary collecting system anywhere from the calyces to the urethral meatus can cause postrenal acute renal failure. Obstruction above the bladder must, however, occur bilaterally unless there is only one functioning kidney. Renal reserve is so large that a single normally functioning kidney is compatible with a lifetime of optimal health. Kidney stones—calcium, urate, or cystine—are major causes of obstruction of the upper urinary tract, though they rarely cause simultaneous bilateral obstruction. This occurs more commonly when one kidney has lost its function gradually from disease and the ureter of the opposite kidney is then obstructed by a stone. In addition to stones, blood clots and sloughed papillae from papillary necrosis may obstruct the ureters. Retroperitoneal fibrosis may surround and compress the ureters. Diffuse, retroperitoneal malignancies may cause such fibrosis, but the fibrosis is more often benign and may result from the long-term use of methysergide maleate (Sansert) for the treatment of migraine.

Urethral strictures in the male resulting from the use of silver nitrate instillations and instrumentation in the treatment of gonorrhea were common causes of urinary obstruction in the past. Prostatic hypertrophy is the major cause of urinary obstruction in the elderly male. The increased hydrostatic pressure within the collecting system may suppress renal function, even though urine volume may not be reduced. Catheterization of the bladder following attempted normal voiding reveals a considerable residual urine volume in the bladder. Relief of the obstruction by indwelling catheter or prostatectomy may yield a dramatic improvement as illustrated by the two cases summarized in Table 8-1. It is advisable to decompress an overexpanded bladder slowly; too rapid emptying may cause a diffuse and alarming bleeding from the surface of the bladder. Some patients who suffer sufficient tubular damage from the long period of partial obstruction have renal sodium wasting to such a degree that loss of extracellular fluid volume and vascular collapse may occur upon relief of obstruction unless supplementary sodium intake is provided.

Neurogenic bladder, with loss of afferent sensory sensation as in tabes dorsalis or diabetic pseudotabes, may result in chronic overdistention of the bladder and obstructive uropathy. Other types of neurologic deficits may have similar results.

It is essential in all unexplained cases of acute renal failure to rule out obstruction. This can usually be done by appropriate radiologic procedures. Radiopaque stones, calcium or cystine can be visualized without contrast media, but this is not the case with radiolucent uric acid stones or blood clots. If, on catheterization of the bladder, no urine is obtained, then the obstruction may be higher up. It may then be necessary to cystoscope and insert catheters up the ureters. Gen-

TABLE 8-1   *Two Cases of Prostatic Obstruction*

A. J. M., age 70, M. G. H. #1020751

Uremia. $K = 6.6$, $CO_2 = 17$ mM, BUN $= 60$ mg/dl, hemoglobin $= 9.3$ gm/dl. Blood pressure 200/80. Edema, cardiac enlargement, pulmonary congestion.

Catheterized: diuresis 15 liters in 24 hours

DATE	BUN
7/12	60
Catheterized	
7/13	27
7/14	12 lungs clear, edema-free
	blood pressure 150/70

B. I. G., age 65, M. G. H. #236

Seizures, uremia, Hb $= 7.3$ gm/dl, BUN $= 175$ mg/dl, $CO_2 = 16$ mM Heart greatly enlarged, pulmonary vessels engorged.

Catheterized: diuresis 30 liters in 5 days

		CREATININE	
DATE	BUN	SERUM	CLEARANCE
	----- mg/dl -----		liters/24 hr
6/24	175	16	
Catheterized			
6/28	46	7.4	17
8/4	35	3.3	27
10/15	37	4.0	25
Prostatectomy			
10/24	24	2.3	43
11/13	14		

on 7/16 lungs clear, heart normal size and shape

---

erally, only one ureter need be probed, since the finding of one patent ureter in the presence of two kidneys excludes obstruction as the cause of renal failure. Furthermore, bullous edema of the ureteral mucosa may follow instrumentation and itself produce temporary ureteral obstruction. Ultrasound to detect a dilated collecting system above a point of obstruction is proving to be a useful noninvasive diagnostic procedure.

In the presence of obstructive uropathy, examination of the urine is not diagnostic. A small amount of protein may be present, but with compression of the ureters from without, the urine may be unremarkable. Red blood cells and crystals may accompany obstruction with stones or tumor, and often the presence of infection makes itself evident with bacteria and white cells in the fresh urine. Red cell casts are not present; their occurrence is indicative of intrarenal pathology.

PRERENAL ACUTE RENAL FAILURE

Prerenal acute renal failure results from diminished perfusion of the kidneys. This may be the consequence of heart failure with reduced cardiac output. Alternatively, if extracellular, or vascular volume is insufficient, as a result of sodium depletion or blood loss, then even with a normal heart, perfusion of the kidneys may be inadequate to sustain normal kidney function. The kidneys, with a combined weight in the adult of about 300 gm, receive an abundant blood supply of about 1200 ml/minute, or 20–25% of the cardiac output. With loss of vascular volume or with cardiac failure, the large blood flow to the kidneys may be sharply reduced. Interestingly, even in so-called high-output heart failure, as with anemia or cor pulmonale, the circulation to the kidney is decreased.

If the pressure in the afferent glomerular artery falls below 60–70 mm Hg, then glomerular filtration ceases and no urine is formed. Short of total cessation of glomerular filtration, varying degrees of decrease in glomerular filtration rate occur. Dilation of the afferent glomerular arteriole and constriction of the efferent arteriole tend to sustain glomerular filtration in the presence of decreased renal blood flow, but there is a limit to the compensatory adjustment, and the absolute level of filtration falls. Prerenal failure ensues with a disproportionate elevation of the blood urea nitrogen (BUN) compared with the level of serum creatinine. Normally, the BUN is about 10 to 15 mg and creatinine 1.0 mg/dl serum. As the reduced renal perfusion diminishes the volume of filtrate per glomerulus, less urea and creatinine are filtered. But the slower trickle of filtrate allows more time for smaller molecules, such as urea, to diffuse back into the blood. Creatinine, being a larger, less diffusible molecule, mostly remains in the luminal fluid and is excreted. The increased back-reabsorption of urea causes its concentration in the blood to increase disproportionately to that of creatinine. BUN/creatinine ratios of 20 to 1 or greater are the expectation in prerenal acute renal failure. It must always be remembered, however, that, though the rate of creatinine production is quite constant, the rate of urea production depends on the rate of protein catabolism. With acute illness, often in association with fever, increased tissue destruction, and a catabolic state, the production of urea may increase markedly and contribute significantly to a disproportionate increase in the blood level of urea. A common clinical condition associated with both prerenal acute renal failure and increased protein catabolism is bleeding into the upper gastrointestinal tract, as may occur from peptic ulcers or esophageal varices.

In addition to the absolute reduction of blood flow to the kidneys in prerenal azotemia, there may be a redistribution of the blood flow in the kidneys. From the "washout" of the inert gas krypton-85, Barger and associates (1) have concluded that, with reduced perfusion of the kidneys, there is a redistribution of the blood flow away from the outer cortical nephrons and toward the nephrons in the inner cortex and juxtamedullary regions. Similar results come from the injection into the renal arteries of a pulse of radioactive microspheres of a size that will lodge in the glomerular capillaries (2). Not all investigators concur in this evidence, however, for other techniques indicate a uniform, albeit decreased, perfusion of all parts of the kidney (3, 4).

There is one very characteristic finding in the scanty urine found in prerenal azotemia. Although routine examination is unremarkable (though there may be slight proteinuria), chemical analysis reveals a very low sodium content and concentration, frequently less than 5 mEq/liter. Generally, 20 mEq of sodium/liter of urine is taken as the upper limit in this condition.

By definition, prerenal acute renal failure must be promptly reversible upon reestablishing normal intravascular volume, blood pressure, and cardiac output. If the hypoperfusion of the kidneys is too severe or prolonged, however, then correction of the circulatory state may not be associated with a return of normal kidney function. An ischemic injury to the kidney has supervened, and we are dealing with the major cause of intrarenal acute renal failure.

INTRARENAL ACUTE RENAL FAILURE

Intrarenal causes of acute renal failure are manifold. Acute glomerulonephritis and vasculitis may present with acute suppression of renal function. The cause of renal failure is generally attributed to the inflammatory or immunologic process affecting the glomeruli diffusely, interfering with their normal function. Red blood cells are likely to be abundant in the urine, and careful examination of the urine sediment often reveals red blood cell casts. In severe terminal hepatic disease, usually with cirrhosis, an acute renal failure may occur, the so-called hepatorenal syndrome. Distinctive features of this syndrome are: virtual absence of sodium from the urine, as in prerenal renal failure, and absence of renal pathology. This last point has been dramatically demonstrated by transplanting the kidneys of patients dying with uremia from hepatorenal syndrome into appropriate recipients and observing prompt function of the donor kidney in its new environment. This suggests that the renal failure is the result of a functional disorder, most likely a redistribution of a reduced renal blood flow away from cortical nephrons, which thereby impedes glomerular filtration. Bilateral renal artery occlusion from blood clots or from atheromatous plaques freed into the bloodstream during aortic catheterization can also acutely suppress kidney function.

Ischemic and toxic injuries

After considering these causes of intrarenal acute renal failure, one is left with a large category of patients who develop acute renal failure from acute tubular necrosis, which is thought to result from two major causes: injury to the kidneys from ischemia or from nephrotoxic substances.

Ischemic acute renal failure, often called "acute tubular necrosis," is an all too common occurrence in our hospitalized, very sick patients. It is generally accepted that the blood supply to normal kidneys can be blocked for up to about 30 minutes without sustained damage to the kidneys. Often, in the course of surgery, acute hemorrhage, heart failure, shock, trauma, dehydration, or sepsis, a period of hypotension of sufficient severity and duration to produce ischemic renal failure occurs. This hypotensive period is often noted, but surprisingly commonly, the acute renal failure is discovered only when marked oliguria or an unexplained rise in concentrations of BUN and serum creatinine occurs. As mentioned, a prerenal deficit in renal perfusion may progress to acute tubular necrosis if the ischemia becomes too marked or prolonged. When such organic damage is inflicted on the kidney, correction of blood volume, blood pressure, and cardiac output no longer promptly reestablishes renal function. Dysfunction of the damaged kidneys persists. Red cells, tubular cells, casts, and cellular debris appear in the scanty urine, and the concentration of sodium, which had been very low, generally rises to levels of 40 to 70 mEq/liter or higher, indicating tubular damage and inability to conserve sodium.

Normal kidneys can tolerate considerable intravascular hemolysis or rhabdomyolysis and excrete the hemoglobin or myoglobin with only transient reductions in glomerular filtration rate. In conjunction with extracellular volume depletion and hypoperfusion of the kidneys, however, the same degree of free hemoglobin or myoglobin in the serum will result in typical acute renal failure. In addition to the other features mentioned, free hemoglobin or myoglobin should be detectable in the scanty urine during the early phase of acute renal failure in such cases. Mismatched blood transfusions, disseminated intravascular coagulopathies, massive malarial infestation (black water fever), and a variety of hemolysins may be responsible for intravascular hemolysis. Rhabdomyolysis is most commonly due to trauma, but an increasing number of nontraumatic causes of rhabdomyolysis are being reported; these include extreme exertion, hyperthermia, sepsis, prolonged seizures, potassium depletion, phosphate depletion, alcoholism, and drug abuse. Muscle swelling and tenderness, high levels of muscle creatine phosphokinase in the serum, and myoglobinuria are special features of these causes of acute renal failure.

A host of diverse chemicals have been implicated as nephrotoxins. A partial list is given in Table 8-2. Many other substances may cause idiosyncratic reactions in the sensitized individual. Furthermore, many chemicals that have accepted medical uses are, unfortunately, potentially nephrotoxic, for example, several antibiotics, analgesics, vascular and renal contrast media, and antiseptics. Almost every medicament is a potential toxin, and a surprising number wreak their havoc on the kidneys. When administered under conditions of dehydration and reduced renal perfusion, their nephrotoxic effects may be accentuated.

Pathology

The pathology of acute tubular necrosis has been a source of considerable uncertainty among morphologists. Following the discovery of acute renal failure associated with crush injuries incurred during the bombing of London in the Second World War, Lucké (5) summarized the pathologic features of the oliguric renal disorder—which we would refer to today as acute ischemic tubular necrosis—as destructive

TABLE 8-2 *A Partial List of Nephrotoxins*

A.	**METALS AND IONS**	**C.**	**ORGANIC COMPOUNDS**
	mercuric chloride		carbon tetrachloride
	uranium		chloroform
	lead		methyl alcohol
	gold		phenol
	chromium		toluene
	cadmium		ethylene glycol
	bismuth		oxalic acid
	arsenic		
	phosphorus	**D.**	**MEDICATIONS**
	chlorate		mephenesin
			phenacemide
			quinine
B.	**ANTIBIOTICS**		versene
	methicillin		methoxyflourine
	colistimethate		
	neomycin	**E.**	**MISCELLANEOUS**
	polymyxin		pesticides
	gentamicin		poisonous mushrooms
	sulfonamides		cantharides
	cephaloridine		contrast media

changes affecting the tubular epithelium of the distal nephron. He coined the term *lower nephron nephrosis* for this entity. Often, however, pathologists were unable to find any pathologic changes in kidneys of patients dying in uremia with acute renal failure, or perhaps they found only a few mitotic figures in the tubular epithelial cells indicative of a regenerative process in progress at the time of death.

The pathology of acute tubular necrosis was clarified by the studies of Jean Oliver and associates, who used acid maceration and a careful microdissection technique to separate individual nephrons from kidneys of patients dying of acute renal failure (6). They found the characteristic pathology to consist of patchy regions of necrosis of the renal tubular epithelium, which seemed to occur randomly throughout the length of the nephron. There was no preference for the distal nephron, and the term *lower nephron nephrosis* quietly slipped into disuse.

Oliver and his associates, furthermore, distinguished between the renal lessons produced by chemical injury and by ischemia. Nephrotoxins produce patchy tubular necrosis, but the basement membrane of the renal tubules is spared. Ischemic damage to the kidneys also results in patchy necrosis of renal tubular epithelium, but rupture through the tubular basement membrane also occurs, often with communication between the peritubular capillaries and the lumen of the nephron. Oliver gave this lesion the name *tubulorrhexis* and attributed to it the hematuria and occasional red blood cell cast seen with ischemic renal damage. He further indicated that patients whose primary renal insult was from a nephrotoxic agent often might show tubulorrhexis on postmortem examination, the systemic effects of the nephrotoxin having produced vomiting and diarrhea with dehydration or vascular collapse, hypotension, and shock. Thus, the depressed individual who ingests mercuric chloride (sublimate of mercury) in a suicide attempt develops bloody diarrhea, vomiting and shock. His kidneys at postmortem will likely show the ischemic changes of tubulorrhexis as well as necrosis of tubular epithelial cells.

Pathophysiology

Although there is now agreement regarding the pathology of the kidney damaged by acute tubular necrosis, as seen at postmortem or on biopsy, controversy still rages over the pathogenesis of the suppression of kidney function, and the usual accompanying oliguria. Possible primary causative factors are limited in general to glomerular or tubular disorders. Glomerular filtration may be impaired because of inadequate blood flow or because of either insufficient filtration pressure or impermeability of the filtering membranes of the glomeruli, despite adequate blood flow. The tubules may contribute to the suppression of renal function by increased reabsorption of luminal fluid through damaged tubular epithelium or by obstruction by casts, cellular debris, or cell swelling. All these possibilities have been entertained and, in fact, demonstrated in a variety of experimental models of acute renal failure in animals. Nephrotoxic acute renal failure produced in animals by injections of mercuric chloride, uranyl nitrate, or chromate, on the one hand, or ischemic insults on the other, produced by clamping a renal artery, infusing norepinephrine into the renal arteries, inducing hemorrhagic shock, or injecting glycerol intramuscularly, have provided many models for study. It is likely that each of the possible etiologic factors may be present or absent, and each differs in its degree of contribution to pathogenesis in the different models cited. In each model several factors undoubtedly contribute to the renal failure. These will be briefly considered, in the hope, not of adding further confusion, but at least of providing the interested reader with references to pursue.

During the first epoch of micropuncture studies, A. N. Richards (7) noted, by direct microscopic examination of a frog kidney poisoned with mercuric chloride, that filtration through the glomeruli persisted, as evidenced by passage of a dye into the proximal tubule, but neither dye nor urine emerged from the ureter. Richards concluded that in this circumstance the glomerular filtrate was all reabsorbed through the damaged tubular epithelium. Such total reabsorption of glomerular filtrate as a factor in acute renal failure has been both denied and demonstrated. After injection of ^{14}C-inulin directly into a tubular lumen via micropuncture in one kidney damaged by ischemia or uranyl nitrate, significant excretion of the radioactive inulin has been observed in the urine from the contralateral normal kidney, establishing increased permeability of the renal tubular epithelium in the experimental kidney (8, 9, 10).

Casts and cellular debris are invariably present in all forms of experimental acute renal failure, but whether they obstruct the tubules sufficiently to account for the suppression of renal function has been argued. In acute renal failure in rats following mercuric chloride poisoning, Oken and associates (11, 12) carefully measured the intratubular fluid pressure within the proximal tubules of surface nephrons. They reasoned that, if renal failure were caused by tubular obstruction, the pressure of fluid within the tubule proximal to the site of obstruction should be elevated. In fact, they found pressures to be low, which excluded tubular obstruction, they thought. Subsequently, Arendhorst, Finn, and Gottschalk (13) demonstrated that ureteral obstruction, or obstruction of individual tubules, causes a fall in intraluminal fluid pressure proximal to the obstruction within 24 hours after its onset. The fall in pressure was thought to result from constriction of the afferent glomerular arteriole, which would reduce glomerular filtration. This intrarenal response to obstruction occurs on an individual nephron basis via an unknown feedback loop, perhaps involving the juxtaglomerular apparatus of individual nephrons.

The importance of tubular obstruction in acute renal failure may have been underestimated because of the infrequency with which obstruction is observed by conventional histologic examination of kidney sections from patients or experimental animals with acute renal failure. The nephron is long and tortuous, but it need be occluded at only one point to stop functioning. This point of obstruction may be out of the field of section so that the observer sees only the patent lumens. Following temporary ischemia a wide range of hydrostatic pressures has been measured in proximal tubules, with many values considerably higher than those observed in normal kidneys (8), a finding compatible with tubular obstruction. After uranyl nitrate damage such a dispersal of pressures was not observed (10), which is consistent with other evidence that tubular obstruction is not important in this model of acute renal failure.

Much more attention has been given to the possibility that impaired glomerular filtration is the primary disorder in this group of conditions. This is so in spite of the fact that, except in the very early stages of experimental renal injury (14), the glomeruli have been regarded as normal even when renal function is severely depressed. Therefore, failure of filtration has been postulated to be a disorder of function rather than of structure.

Recently, however, Cox and associates (15) demonstrated that, in the failure of renal function following prolonged infusion of high levels of norepinephrine into one renal artery of the dog, there occurs a striking alteration in the appearance of the visceral surface of the glomerular tuft, as seen by scanning electron microscopy. The normal finely fenestrated branching and interdigitation of the projections from the epithelial cells that make up the "foot processes" were lost, and the epithelial cells seemed to be fused together with loss of the normal filtration slits. By infusing very large volumes of saline into their experimental animals, these investigators were able to increase the blood flow to the experimental kidney well above normal, and yet the kidney produced no urine. They suggested that the morphologic changes observed in the glomeruli might account for the failure of filtration. Such changes in the fine structure of the glomeruli are not generally present in other models of acute renal failure.

Some investigators have found diminished renal blood flow, but others have observed little if any reduction in total renal blood flow in their experimental models of acute renal failure. Conventional means of measuring renal blood flow, such as the clearance of para-aminohippurate (PAH), are of no value in the damaged kidney, since a fall in clearance could be the result of impaired extraction of PAH by injured renal tubules. By combining the Fick principle with measurements of arterial–venous differences, Cournand and associates (16, 17) and Phillips and associates (18) found renal blood flow in dogs to be reduced following a period of renal ischemia. Sheehan and Davis (19) noted a similar reduction in renal blood flow persisting after cor-

rection of the systemic circulation and referred to this as renal ischemia with failed reflow.

For some time it was assumed that reduced renal blood flow was the
factor responsible for suppressed renal function following an ischemic
or a toxic insult. Catecholamines were suggested as a possible cause
for the persistent renal ischemia, but acute renal failure may persist
for 2 or 3 weeks after correction of the circulatory failure that initiated the renal failure, and there should be no stimulus for such a
protracted elevation of catecholamine levels in the blood. The renin–
angiotensin system has also been considered a cause of persistent renal
hypoperfusion in acute renal failure. Levels of renin in peripheral
blood do not, however, correlate with the presence of acute renal failure in man (20, 21); immunization of rats against hog renin failed to
protect them from mercuric chloride- or glycerol-induced acute renal
failure (22); and injection of renin antibodies into experimental animals failed to protect them against acute renal failure (23).

These studies do not exclude an intrarenal action of the renin–
angiotensin system during acute renal failure. When the renin–
angiotensin system was suppressed (as demonstrated by a reduction
in renal renin concentration in rats) by maintaining rats on a high potassium intake for several weeks, the animals were partially protected
from the acute nephrotoxic effects of mercuric chloride injections
(24). Renal renin has also been depleted in rats by long-term salt loading, after which the rats were almost completely protected from acute
renal failure when challenged with glycerol-induced myoglobinuria
(25), mercury poisoning (26), or dichromate poisoning (27). Infusion
of a synthetic competitive inhibitor of angiotensin (1-sarcosine, 8-
alanine angiotensin II) protects rat kidneys from the effects of hemorrhagic hypotension (Frega, personal communication). Such experiments
suggest, but do not establish, an intrarenal role for the renin–
angiotensin system in the genesis of acute renal failure.

Recently, a number of studies using newer methods of measuring
renal blood flow have yielded disparate values in experimental models
of acute renal failure. Direct measurements of blood flow through the
renal arteries with magnetic flow meters indicate that total renal
blood flow may not be as markedly reduced during acute renal failure
as other, less direct methods had led investigators to believe. Levels of
60–100% of the control rate of renal blood flow may be present, although the kidneys are not functioning (15, 28).

Early on, Trueta and colleagues (29) suggested that total renal blood flow might have little meaning in view of the arteriovenous shunts that Trueta postulated to be present in the juxtamedullary glomeruli. The existence of such shunts, however, was challenged by Homer Smith (30), and today it is generally accepted that no arteriovenous shunts occur in normal or acutely damaged kidneys. Although no shunts of the conventional kind occur in the kidneys, it has been claimed that intrarenal redistribution of blood flow does take place. The "washout" of the inert gases krypton-85 and xenon-133, injected directly into a renal artery, has been used to assess the total and regional blood flow within the kidney. This method was applied in acute renal failure by Hollenberg and associates (31, 32), who interpreted the loss of the rapid component to indicate decreased cortical perfusion with no alteration or with an absolute increase in deeper cortical and outer medullary blood flow. Though the method has provided much useful information regarding the distribution of blood flow in the normal kidney, its application to the diseased kidney is open to serious criticism.

It has been a puzzling feature of experimental acute renal failure that, in some models at least, renal blood flow may be essentially normal or only slightly reduced, but glomerular filtration, as measured by conventional whole kidney clearance techniques, is essentially suppressed. It has been postulated that a slight increase in vascular resistance in the afferent glomerular arteries might be just offset by a corresponding dilatation of efferent glomerular arterioles such that total renal vascular resistance and, hence, blood flow were unaffected, but hydrostatic pressure within the glomerular capillaries was so reduced that filtration could no longer be sustained. No available evidence favors such an explanation. Many micropuncture studies have reported discrepancies between single-nephron glomerular filtration rates of superficial cortical nephrons and whole kidney glomerular filtration rates. The former may be normal or only slightly reduced in the presence of marked suppression of the latter (8–10, 33–36). Such results may be due to unrepresentative sampling of the nephron population, tubular obstruction, or back-diffusion of the filtered inulin. When afferent and efferent glomerular arteriolar hydrostatic pressures have been directly measured, the hydrostatic pressure gradient across the glomerular capillary was not changed, but total glomerular permeability was reduced from control levels (10, 37).

As mentioned above, there are experimental animal models to support every proposed scheme for the pathogenesis of acute renal failure. Obstruction of tubules and reabsorption of tubular urine through damaged tubular epithelia seem to be the causes of experimental post-ischemic acute renal failure (44). What the actual situation is in human acute renal failure due to ischemic or nephrotoxic injury remains to be determined.

MANAGEMENT

The principle of management of acute renal failure is to sustain the life of the patient while the self-limited pathologic process heals itself. It is not the role of this text to describe therapy, but practice here is based entirely on physiologic principles and therefore merits consideration in a discussion of pathophysiology. In general, procedures aimed at promoting survival during the period of renal shutdown include

1. Immediate care
   A. Correct blood and fluid deficits
   B. Correct electrolyte disturbances
   C. Treat sepsis

2. Maintenance
   A. Maintain normal hydration
   B. Minimize azotemia
   C. Prevent hyperkalemia
   D. Avoid overmedication

In the absence of renal function, the problem of how much fluid the patient should receive requires informed consideration. Once fluid deficits, if any, are corrected, then a state of fluid balance should be maintained. Overhydration overloads the cardiovascular system, with the danger of acute pulmonary edema. Underhydration may delay the return of kidney function. Fluid balance requires replacement of fluid losses. In addition to the small urinary losses in the oliguric patient, there is a continuous "insensible loss" of fluid via skin, lungs, and stool, to which must be added any abnormal drainages or extrarenal losses. Table 8-3 presents pertinent data and the calculations of the fluid requirements of an anuric patient with acute renal failure.

TABLE 8-3   *Calculation of Water Requirements in Patient with Acute Renal Failure*

PATIENT PPW   MALE   AGE 43   MGH   83 44 51

A. Interval of anuria	13 days
B. Initial weight	86 kg
C. Weight on 13th day	79 kg
D. Loss of weight	7 kg
E. Total body water, initial, 60% body weight	51 liter
F. Initial BUN	15 mg/dl
G. BUN on 13th day	215 mg/dl
H. BUN	2 gm/liter
I. Total increase in urea nitrogen	102 gm
J. Protein catabolism (6.25 × urea nitrogen)	638 gm
K. Lean tissue loss (4.55 × protein)	2.9 kg
L. Weight loss—lean tissue loss	4.1 kg
M. Fat equivalent (lean tissue loss × 0.9)	3.7 kg
N. Average daily protein catabolism	49 gm
O. Calories derived from protein (gm × 4)	196 cal
P. Average daily fat catabolism	284 gm
Q. Calories derived from fat (gm × 9)	2565 cal
R. Water from fat oxidized (gm × 1.07 + gm × 10%)	4329 ml
S. Water from protein oxidized (gm × 0.41 + gm × 3)	2175 ml
T. Total water of catabolism	6504 ml
U. Average daily water catabolism	500 ml
V. Water from 100 gm of I.V. glucose daily	100 ml
W. Daily water of metabolism	600 ml
X. Estimated daily insensible fluid loss	1000 ml
Y. Total daily exogenous water requirement	400 ml

It can be seen that in this patient a daily fluid intake of only 400 ml was required to meet his insensible loss of water of 1000 ml/day. The balance of his water needs was met by the catabolism of body tissues, protein, and fat, plus the 100 gm of glucose he received each day. This individual lost a half kilogram per day, this being expected in an adult whose state of hydration is kept normal during an oliguric period. If this water of oxidation had been ignored and 1.0 liter of water given daily, he would have been overhydrated by some 5.72 liters, sufficient to dilute his serum sodium from its normal value of 140 mEq/liter to 125 mEq/liter [140 × (47.40/53.12)]. If he had been hydrated to maintain a constant body weight of 86 kg throughout the anuric period, 7 liters of excess water would have been formed, diluting his serum sodium even further and possibly threatening his cardiac competence.

To reduce the severity of the azotemia, it is important to reduce the rate of protein catabolism while kidney function is suppressed. Catabolism of tissue proteins liberates not only urea as an end product, but sulfuric acid, phosphate, uric acid, organic acids, phenols, guanidine, potassium, and so on, at least some of which contribute to the uremic syndrome. Survival studies of normal subjects on a life raft by J. L. Gamble (38) indicated that glucose has a marked sparing effect on protein catabolism in the fasting individual. To produce a further significant protein-sparing effect, total nonprotein calories must be increased to nearly 2000/day. Since such caloric intake is generally not tolerated by uremic patients, physicians until recently had to be content to administer only 100 gm (400 calories) of glucose daily.

Recent studies have shown that man is able to recycle and reutilize amino nitrogen in the endogenous production of amino acids (39). This has led to the use of very low protein diets of some 8 to 12 gm of high-quality protein to reduce the azotemia in chronic renal failure (40, 41). The counterpart in acute renal failure has been the introduction of renal failure fluids (42) in which a mixture of essential amino acids with 30% glucose is given slowly intravenously over each 24-hour period. This treatment not only diminishes the rate of rise of the BUN, but apparently also even hastens the healing of the acute renal damage. It would seem that when the ketoacids of the eight amino acids essential for man become commercially available, it will be possible to provide a totally nitrogen-free nourishment that should be optimal for the anephric state.

With tissue damage, infection, and catabolism of body protein, intracellular potassium is liberated into the extracellular fluids. With suppression of renal function this potassium cannot be excreted, and hyperkalemia occurs, with all of its attendant hazards to the neuromuscular conducting systems, especially those of the heart. The rate at which hyperkalemia develops depends on the extent of tissue injury and the rate of protein catabolism. With crush injuries and burns, potassium concentrations may rise rapidly to dangerous levels, producing cardiac arrhythmias and finally arrest. The electrocardiogram is a rapid and useful method of monitoring the adverse effects of hyperkalemia on the heart. Elevation and peaking of the T-wave is the earliest electrocardiographic evidence of cardiac embarrassment from the elevated serum potassium concentration.

Hyperkalemia may pose an immediate threat to life and constitute a true medical emergency. Treatment is based on driving extracellular potassium back into cells and subsequently removing the excess of potassium from the body. To shift potassium from extracellular to intracellular fluids, two maneuvers are effective:

1. Glucose together with insulin administered intravenously deposits glucose as glycogen within the liver, and this obligates an accompanying intracellular movement of potassium. Each gram of glycogen in the liver obligates 3 ml of intracellular fluid with its usual high concentration of potassium, ~160 mEq/liter.

2. Alkalinization of the extracellular fluids shifts potassium into cells, and acidosis has the opposite effect. Sodium bicarbonate is infused intravenously in amounts sufficient to raise the pH of extracellular fluids, which generally has fallen, due to metabolic acidosis associated with failure of kidney function.

Both these procedures provide only temporary benefit, since the intracellular potassium again leaks into the extracellular fluids when the glycogen is metabolized or as metabolic acidosis again supervenes. Steps must, therefore, be taken to remove potassium from the body. Sodium-substituted cation exchange resins such as sodium polystyrene sulfonate may be administered orally or by enema. In the bowel, sodium is exchanged for potassium, which is then removed with passage of the resin. In practice, 1 gm of resin may be expected to remove 1.0 mEq of potassium. This is not much, but the quantity of potassium that must be removed from the extracellular fluid to protect the heart is not large. When ion exchange resins are not effective in controlling hyperkalemia, dialysis, either peritoneal or hemodialysis, may be required. Dialysis by either route against a potassium-free fluid should control hyperkalemia if the procedure is not delayed too long.

The intravenous injection of calcium provides a pharmacologic means of promptly reversing the toxic cardiac effects of hyperkalemia. As noted previously, hypercalcemia counteracts the effects of hyperkalemia on the neuromuscular conducting systems.

In the past—and still all too frequently—patients with acute renal failure have developed toxicity from overmedication with drugs that depend on renal excretion for their removal from the body. The fate of most drugs is either to be metabolized to an inactive form in the liver and the metabolites excreted or to be excreted unchanged by the kidneys; a few compounds are removed via lungs or bowel. When the kidneys fail, removal of many drugs is impaired. This simple and obvious fact is still too often overlooked, and usual daily doses continue to be administered, with potentially or actually disastrous consequences.

COURSE OF ACUTE RENAL FAILURE
Acute renal failure due to ischemic or nephrotoxic injury is a self-limiting condition. If the patient survives, a gradual healing of the renal injury occurs as the injured nephrons reepithelialize their tubular epithelium. Characteristically, patients are oliguric (< 400 ml urine/day) for a variable period lasting on the average about 10 days. Very rarely, complete anuria occurs, but this is more characteristic of blockage of the excretory passageways. In a minority, perhaps 10–20% of recognized cases, a nonoliguric acute failure develops (43). But since the condition must represent a continuum of increasing renal injury, it is likely that more nonoliguric cases occur, but simply pass unnoticed. The elevations of BUN and of serum creatinine indicate that the effective glomerular filtration rate is profoundly depressed in all recognized instances. When normal 24-hour urine volumes persist, the urine is coming from a very limited filtration surface and passing through damaged tubules that possess decreased reabsorptive or secretory activity. This accounts for the levels of sodium in the urine of usually some 40 to 80 mEq/liter irrespective of the state of hydration and of the extracellular fluid volume.

When urine flow resumes in the oliguric patient and reaches levels of more than 1000 ml daily, the BUN and serum creatinine may continue to rise for several more days. This occurs because glomerular filtration is returning to tubules that have not regained their full functional integrity and are serving chiefly as simple conduits for the filtered volume. Alternatively, recovery of tubule cells may have reached a state in which back-reabsorption of filtrate is decreasing and some of the filtrate reaches the renal pelvis and is excreted. Only when the urine formed comes from a usual large volume of filtrate and abnormal back-reabsorption no longer occurs do the kidneys effectively clear urea and creatinine, bringing their concentrations in the serum down to normal levels.

As urine flow returns to normal and the glomerular filtration rate increases, a few patients develop a true renal sodium-wasting syndrome with loss of extracellular fluid volume of threatening magnitude until sodium reabsorptive capacity is regained by the new renal tubule cells. During this interval sodium replacement must be diligently managed.

In patients with extensive rhabdomyolysis there is often a rapid decline of serum calcium concentration to values as low as 5 to 6 mg/dl of serum within a few days of onset of acute renal failure. This is due to calcium deposition in the damaged muscle (45). During recovery of the kidneys this calcium is mobilized, and some 20 to 25% of patients will have hypercalcemia, though several months may pass before the calcium deposits are completely cleared from the muscles.

With simple nephrotoxic injury, regeneration of tubular epithelial cells takes place over the intact basement membrane, and normal renal function should be restored. With disruption of the basement membrane in ischemic injury, some fibrosis and distortion of the renal tubule may occur during recovery, resulting in a permanent reduction in renal function. Most patients who survive acute renal failure of either ischemic or nephrotoxic origin recover all or most of their renal function. Failure to completely recover is often attributable to intercurrent urinary tract infection. Maximal recovery may take as long as a year; urinary concentrating ability is the function slowest to return.

The mortality from acute renal failure remains unfortunately high, at about 60%, despite many important improvements in management. This is because sicker and older patients are kept alive by respirators, heart pacers, and all the modern technology of medicine, and in these patients, acute renal failure often supervenes. The persistent high mortality reflects the severity of the underlying disease responsible for the acute renal failure.

References

1. Barger, A. C. and Herd, J. A. The renal circulation. New Eng. J. Med. 284: 482–490, 1971.
2. Logan, A., Jose, P., and Eisner, G. Intracortical distribution of renal blood flow in hemorrhagic shock in dogs. Circ. Res. 29:257–266, 1971.

3. Wallin, J. D., Rector, F. C., and Seldin, D. W. Measurement of intrarenal plasma flow with antiglomerular basement membrane antibody. Am. J. Physiol. 221:1621–1628, 1971.

4. Rouffignac, C. de. Do similar factors control the glomerular filtration rate of superficial and juxtamedullary nephrons? Proc. VIth Int. Cong. Nephrol., Abs. of Symposia, pp. 47–48, 1975.

5. Lucké, B. Lower nephron nephrosis. The renal lesions of the crush syndrome, of burns, transfusion and other conditions affecting the lower segments of the nephrons. Military Surgeon 99:371–396, 1946.

6. Oliver, J., MacDowell, M., and Tracy, A. The pathogenesis of acute renal failure associated with traumatic and toxic injury: Renal ischemia, nephrotoxic damage and the ischemic episode. J. Clin. Invest. 30:1397–1440, 1951.

7. Richards, A. N. Direct observations of change in function of the renal tubule caused by certain poisons. Trans. Assoc. Amer. Physicians 44:64–67, 1929.

8. Eisenbach, G. M. and Steinhausen, M. Micropuncture studies after temporary ischemia of rat kidneys. Pflügers Arch. 343:11–25, 1973.

9. Tanner, G. A., Sloan, K. L., and Sophasan, S. Effects of renal artery occlusion on kidney function in the rat. Kidney Int. 4:377–389, 1973.

10. Blantz, R. C. The mechanism of acute renal failure after uranyl nitrate. J. Clin. Invest. 55:621–635, 1975.

11. Flanagan, W. J. and Oken, D. E. Renal micropuncture study of the development of anuria in the rat, with mercury-induced renal failure. J. Clin. Invest. 44:449–457, 1965.

12. Flamenbaum, W., McDonald, F. D., DiBona, G. F., and Oken, D. E. Micropuncture study of renal tubular factors in low dose mercury poisoning. Nephron 8:221–234, 1971.

13. Arendhorst, W. J., Finn, W. F., and Gottschalk, C. Nephron stop-flow pressure response to obstruction for 24 hours in the rat kidney. J. Clin. Invest. 53:1497–1500, 1974.

14. Suzuki, T. and Mostofi, F. K. Electron microscopic studies of acute tubular necrosis. Early changes in the glomeruli of rat kidney after subcutaneous injection of glycerin. Lab. Invest. 23:8–14, 1970.

15. Cox, J. W., Baehler, R. W., Sharma, H., O'Dorisio, T., Osgood, R. W., Stein, J. H., and Ferris, T. F. Studies on the mechanism of oliguria in a model of unilateral acute renal failure. J. Clin. Invest. 53:1546–1558, 1974.

16. Cournand, A., Riley, R. L., Bradley, S. E., Breed, E. S., Noble, R. P., Lauson, H. D., Gregerson, M. F., and Richards, D. W. Studies of the circulation in clinical shock. Surgery 13:964–995, 1943.

17. Lauson, H. D., Bradley, S. E., and Cournand, A. The renal circulation in shock. J. Clin. Invest. 23:381–402, 1944.

18. Phillips, R. A., Dole, V. P., Hamilton, P. B., Emerson, K., Jr., Archibald, R. M., and Van Slyke, D. D. Effects of acute hemorrhagic and traumatic shock on renal function of dogs. Am. J. Physiol. 145:314–336, 1946.

19. Sheehan, H. L. and Davis, J. C. Renal ischemia with failed reflow. J. Path. Bact. 78:105–120, 1959.

20. Del Greco, F., and Krumlovsky, F. Renin activity in acute renal failure. Brit. Med. J. 4:304, 1970.

21. Ochoa, E. Finkielman, S., and Agrest, A. Angiotension blood levels during the evolution of acute renal failure. Clin. Sci. 38:225–231, 1970.

22. Flamenbaum, W., Kotchen, T. A., and Oken, D. E. Effect of renin immuniza-

tion on mercuric chloride and glycerol-induced renal failure. Kidney Internat. 1:406–412, 1972.

23. Oken, D. E., Cotes, S. C., Flamenbaum, W., Powell-Jackson, J. D., and Lever, A. F. Active and passive immunization to angiotensin in experimental acute renal failure. Kidney Int. 7:12–18, 1975.

24. Flamenbaum, W., Kotchen, T. A., Nagle, R., and McNeil, J. S. Effect of potassium on the renin–angiotensin system and mercuric chloride-induced acute renal failure. Am. J. Physiol. 224:305–311, 1973.

25. Thiel, G., McDonald, F. D., and Oken, D. E. Micropuncture studies of the basis for protection of renin-depleted rats from glycerol-induced acute renal failure. Nephron 7:67–79, 1970.

26. Flamenbaum, W., McDonald, F. D., DiBona, G. F., and Oken, D. E. Micropuncture study of renal tubular factors in low dose mercury poisoning. Nephron 8:221–234, 1971.

27. Henry, L. N., Lane, C. E., and Kashgarian, M. Micropuncture studies of the pathophysiology of acute renal failure in the rat. Lab. Invest. 19:309–314, 1968.

28. Riley, A. L., Alexander, E. A., Midgal, S., and Levinsky, N. G. The effect of ischemia on renal blood flow in the dog. Kidney Int. 7:27–34, 1975.

29. Trueta, J., Barclay, A. E., Daniel, P. M., Franklin, K. J., and Prichard, M. M. L. Studies on the renal circulation. Blackwell, Oxford, 1947.

30. Smith, H. The kidney. Oxford University Press, 1951, pp. 15 and 816.

31. Hollenberg, N. K., Epstein, M., Rosen, S. M., Basch, R. I., Oken, D. E. and Merrill, J. P. Acute oliguric renal failure in man: evidence for preferential renal cortical ischemia. Medicine 47:455–475, 1968.

32. Hollenberg, N. K., Adams, D. F., Oken, D. E., Abrams, H. L., and Merrill, J. P. Acute renal failure due to nephrotoxins: renal hemodynamics and angiographic studies. N. Eng. J. Med. 282:1329–1334, 1970.

33. Bank, N., Mutz, B. F., and Aynedjian, H. S. The role of "leakage" of tubular fluid in anuria due to mercury poisoning. J. Clin. Invest. 46:695–704, 1967.

34. Biber, T. U. L., Mylle, M. B., Gottschalk, C. W., Oliver, J. R., and MacDowell, M. C. A study by micropuncture and microdissection of acute renal damage in rats. Am. J. Med. 44:664–705, 1968.

35. Henry, L. N., Lane, C. E., and Kashgarian, M. Micropuncture studies of the pathophysiology of acute renal failure in the rat. Lab. Invest. 19:309–314, 1968.

36. Flamenbaum, W., MacDonald, F. D., DiBona, G. F., and Oken, D. E. Micropuncture study of renal tubular factors in low dose mercury poisoning. Nephron 8:221–234, 1971.

37. Daugharty, T. M., Ucki, I. F., Mercer, P. F., and Brenner, B. M. Dynamics of glomerular filtration in the rat. V. Response to ischemic injury. J. Clin. Invest. 53:105–116, 1974.

38. Gamble, J. L. Physiological information from studies on the life raft ration. The Harvey Lecture Series 42:247–273, 1946–1947.

39. Walser, M., Coulter, A. W., Dighe, S., and Crantz, F. R. The effect of ketoanalogues of essential amino acids in severe chronic uremia. J. Clin. Invest. 52:678–690, 1973.

40. Giordano, C. Use of exogenous and endogenous urea for protein synthesis in normal and uremic subjects. J. Lab. Clin. Med. 62:231–246. 1963.

41. Giovannetti, S. and Maggiore, Q. A low-nitrogen diet with proteins of high biological value for severe chronic uremia. Lancet 1:1000–1003, 1964.

42. Abel, R. M., Beck, C. H., Jr., Abbott, W. M., Ryan, J. A., Jr., Barnett, G. O.,

and Fischer, J. E. Improved survival from acute renal failure after treatment with intravenous essential L-amino acids and glucose. N. Eng. J. Med. 288:695–699, 1973.

43. Vertel, R. M. and Knochel, J. P. Nonliguric acute renal failure. JAMA 200: 598–602, 1967.

44. Finn, W. F., Arendhorst, W. J., and Gottschalk, C. W. Pathogenesis of oliguria in acute renal failure. Circulation Research 36:675–681, 1975.

45. Akmal, M., Goldstein, D. A., Telfer, N., Wilkinson, E., and Massry, S. G. Resolution of muscle calcification in rhabdomyolysis and acute renal failure. Ann. Internat. Med. 89:928–930, 1978.

9

Chronic Renal Failure

INTRODUCTION

We have seen that the kidney has several important functions. It regulates the volume and concentration of the body fluids. It maintains acid–base balance, excreting excesses of acid or alkali after their initial effects have been countered by the action of buffers and the lungs. It preserves the concentration in the body fluids of critical solutes such as potassium, phosphate, and magnesium within narrow limits. It excretes the waste products of metabolism and many other noxious substances that may have been purposefully or inadvertently ingested. It is the major source of erythropoietin. It regulates blood pressure by elaborating renin, which in turn produces angiotensin, the most potent known vasomotor agent and an initiator of adrenal cortical synthesis of aldosterone.

All these vital functions are liable to suffer when the kidneys are progressively destroyed by disease processes. The chronic renal failure we discuss here is largely independent of the kind of disease process that has damaged the kidneys. It does not matter whether the initial disease was glomerulonephritis, polycystic kidney disease, pyelonephritis, hereditary nephritis, nephrosclerosis, amyloidosis, or some other condition, chronic renal failure is the same functional end state. It is true that some stigmata of the primary disease process may persist, but often when the patient is first seen with far-advanced renal failure it is difficult or impossible to identify the disease process responsible for the damage even by tissue examination.

AZOTEMIA

Azotemia, the accumulation of nitrogenous waste products, chiefly urea, in the blood is the hallmark of renal failure. Examination of the process whereby azotemia develops as the kidneys fail is informative. Figure 9-1 shows the relationship between glomerular filtration rate (GFR) measured as the clearance of inulin and the blood urea nitrogen concentration (BUN) in a group of patients with chronic renal

Fig. 9-1 The relationship of blood urea nitrogen (BUN) to glomerular filtration rate (inulin clearance). Although this figure includes some observations obtained from patients with acute glomerulonephritis, the general relationship, x • y = k, as discussed here in relation to chronic renal failure, is still clearly valid. The average value for BUN × GFR = 1098 is indicated by the curve (1).

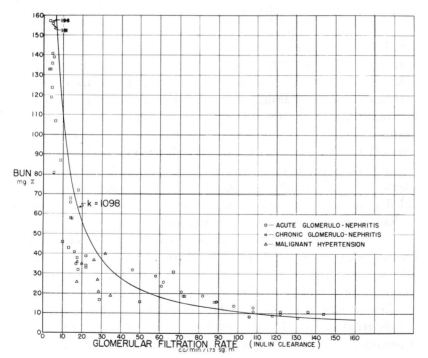

failure. The dotted line is a rectangular hyperbola, $x \cdot y = k$, calculated from the mean product of BUN $\times$ GFR. It is clear from these data that the BUN is determined chiefly by the glomerular filtration rate. This is not surprising when one considers the physiologic meaning of $x \cdot y = k$. Since x equals glomerular filtration rate and y, BUN concentration, their product, our constant k, is the quantity of urea nitrogen filtered through the glomeruli per unit of time. If we ignore for the moment the relatively fixed fraction of the filtered urea that diffuses back into the body during the subsequent passage of the filtered fluid down the renal tubules, then $x \cdot y$ represents the rate at which urea is excreted from the body. In the steady state the quantity excreted equals the quantity formed. It is just the seemingly inefficient operation of the kidney with its high filtrate and reabsorbate volumes that allows urea, and other substances that depend largely on filtration for their excretion, to be carried normally at low concentrations in the body fluids. Thus, an individual with early, minimal renal disease may have an inulin clearance of 100 ml/minute and sustain a BUN concentration of 10 mg/dl. Reexamination of the same individual years later may show that the relentless progression of the disease has reduced his glomerular filtration rate to only 10 ml/minute. He still maintains the rate of urea excretion equal to its rate of production, but now at the expense of a BUN concentration of 100 mg/dl. Thus, though we generally regard elevated blood urea nitrogen as an unfavorable condition, as indeed it is, it affords, nevertheless, an automatic means of maintaining a rate of urea excretion equal to its rate of production. So the term *urea retention* applied to chronic renal failure is in a sense a misnomer; only that urea is retained that is necessary to raise its concentration enough to make x times y equal a constant. Over the months or years that renal function is gradually deteriorating, the daily increment of "retained urea" is very small, and the patient remains essentially in a steady state so far as the formation and excretion of urea are concerned.

Figure 9-1 tells us further that azotemia in chronic renal failure does not arise as a result of an increased back-diffusion of urea through leaky tubules. If this were the case, points representing elevated BUN concentrations would appear on the right side of the figure. Glomerular filtration rate, not tubular reabsorption, accounts for the uremia of chronic renal failure. The normal individual reabsorbs some 50–60% of the filtered urea. With forced water diuresis the back-reabsorption

of urea may fall to about 30% of that filtered. As renal failure supervenes and the urine volume becomes an increasing fraction of the glomerular filtrate, however, the back-reabsorption of urea diminishes.
Thus, in far-advanced renal failure, the high levels of BUN exist despite the fact that the urea clearance approaches the inulin clearance,
so that no detectable back-reabsorption of urea is occurring. This is
discussed further below.

Up to this point we have been talking as if the rate of urea formation were constant in any individual and equal from one person to
the next. This is not, of course, the case. Except in periods of rapid
tissue growth or destruction the rate of urea formation is determined
by the level of dietary protein. Within given socioeconomic groups
the average amount of protein in the diet may stay fairly constant, but
there are marked individual variations. Hence, instead of one average
rectangular hyperbola representing the data, there should be an entire
family of them, each representing a given rate of urea formation or of
protein catabolism. This is shown schematically in Figure 9-2, in
which rectangular hyperbolae with higher values of k indicate diets
of higher protein content.

This brings us to a consideration of the value of the BUN as an index of kidney function. The nature of the rectangular hyperbola is
such that the rise in BUN with early decreases in the glomerular filtration rate is at first so gradual as to be an insensitive index of renal
function. Further, we rarely know the precise amount of dietary protein an individual patient is ingesting or his metabolic status. Thus,
a given BUN value may be associated with a fairly good glomerular
filtration rate in a patient with a high protein diet, or it may represent a severely compromised filtration rate in a patient whose diet is
low in protein.

For these reasons we need an indicator that more faithfully represents glomerular filtration rate. The serum creatinine concentration is
such an indicator. It is at least independent of protein intake and, unless the patient is eating a lot of meat broth, it is largely unaffected
by exogenous sources. Inescapably, however, it shows the same insen-
sitivity to early decreases in glomerular filtration rate as the BUN.
Clinically we must, therefore, measure the rate of creatinine excretion
in the urine as well as the plasma level. From the resulting calculated
value of the creatinine clearance we can quite accurately estimate how
much a patient's renal function has been damaged from the ravages of

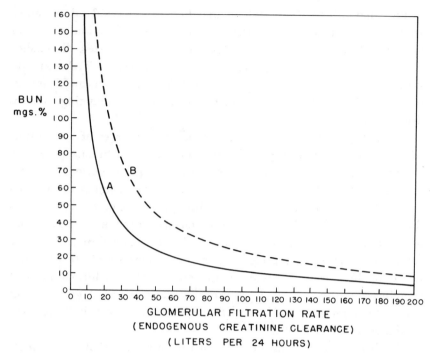

Fig. 9-2 The relationship of blood urea nitrogen (BUN) to glomerular filtration rate (creatinine clearance) as a function of protein catabolism. Curve B represents a higher rate of catabolism than curve A. For each level of GFR a higher level of BUN exists for a higher rate of protein catabolism. (1).

his illness. Urinary creatinine originates from the spontaneous breakdown of muscle phosphocreatine. It is, therefore, an index of lean body mass that normally remains quite constant from day to day in the same person. With advancing renal failure, loss of appetite and cachexia with wasting of muscle mass result in a gradual decrease in the rate of creatinine excretion. This tends to keep the serum creatinine level from rising with progression of renal failure as rapidly as it would otherwise. By combining serum with urine creatinine determinations and calculating the creatinine clearance, however, one can assess the status of renal function with sufficient accuracy for all clinical purposes.

The creatinine clearance in chronic renal failure is one of the functional measurements that correlates well with the structural changes that are occurring, that is, fibrosis, distortion of the normal renal architecture, and a reduction in the number of functioning nephrons. In a sense the creatinine clearance indicates the proportion of nephrons still functioning. By x-ray one sees the gross counterpart of these changes in the small, contracted kidneys with loss of cortical substance.

There have been many attempts to identify the toxic compound in uremia. In the past, small organic molecules and ions, which may accumulate in the body fluids when the excretory function of the kidneys declines, were blamed for the loss of appetite, nausea, vomiting, lassitude, weight loss, anemia, itching, twitching, bleeding tendency, and so forth, that characterize the uremic syndrome. Impetus to this search has come from the appreciation that dialysis, which removes some molecules from the body fluids, will prevent signs and symptoms of uremia and allow indefinite prolongation of life. Recently, more refined analytical methods have made possible the pursuit of this chimera among small polypeptides. A considerable number of compounds potentially implicated in the toxicity of uremia can be listed (Table 9-1). As yet, however, no single compound has been found that, on administration, reproduces the clinical picture of uremia. It is more likely that this symptom complex can be attributed to a multitude of disturbances resulting from renal failure rather than to a single re-

TABLE 9-1 *Some Organic Compounds that Accumulate during Uremia*

Acetoin	Methylguanidine
Aliphatic amines	B_2-Microglobulin
Amino acids	"Middle molecues"
Aromatic amines	Myoinositol
2,3-Butylene glycol	Natriuretic hormone (?)
Creatinine	Other guanidines
Cyclic AMP	Oxalic acid
Diamine oxidase	Parathyroid hormone
Gastrin	(and fragments?)
Glucagon	Phenols
B_2-Glucoprotein	Polyamines
Glucuronic acid	Pyridine derivatives
Growth hormone	Renin
Guanidinosuccinic acid	Retinol-binding protein
Indoles	Ribonuclease
Lipochromes	Urea
Mannitol	Uric acid

tained compound. Nevertheless, the level of urea in the body is used as a yardstick for the retention of compounds that may contribute to the toxicity of this state. All substances that, like urea, are normally present in the body fluids at low concentrations and are excreted in the urine at high concentrations tend to accumulate as renal function fails. Thus creatinine, phosphate, potassium, organic acids, guanidine, phenols, and others, all increase in concentration in the blood, and the rise in BUN serves as a rough guide to the severity of the uremic state and as an objective measure of the patient's response to therapy.

Whether the accumulation of urea itself contributes to the disturbances is still a matter of conflicting reports. To assess this factor, patients with renal failure have been dialyzed against solutions with and without urea. The indications are that urea does contribute to the disturbances of the uremic state. When added to the dialyzate, urea causes headache, fatigue, nausea, vomiting, glucose intolerance, and bleeding tendency, but not all the features of the uremic syndrome.

ACIDOSIS

In view of the key role the kidneys play in preserving acid–base balance in the body, it is not surprising that, with failure of their function, disturbances in this realm arise. Because the average diet yields an acid residue of some 50–100 mEq/day, renal failure is almost invariably associated with acidosis. All three of the kidney's mechanisms for excreting acid and preserving bicarbonate are impaired, but often to varying degrees (2, 3).

With early renal failure no disturbance of acid–base regulation may be apparent, but with glomerular filtration reduced to one-third or less of normal, some acidosis is often present. This may be a hyperchloremic acidosis due to failure of ammonia production, bicarbonate reabsorption, or both. In the former case the urinary pH may indicate nearly maximal acidity ($\sim$4.7), whereas in the latter a relatively alkaline urine (pH > 6.0) is found despite systemic acidosis. It may be useful to trace the sequence of events leading to hyperchloremic acidosis in each instance.

With failure of complete reabsorption of bicarbonate, sodium bicarbonate is lost in the urine. This reduces the concentration of bicarbonate in the renal reabsorbate and in the body fluids. The loss of sodium leads to some contraction of extracellular fluid volume with an increase in serum chloride concentration. Since sodium and chloride exist in nearly equivalent amounts in most natural foods, the loss of some sodium with bicarbonate leads to hyperchloremia; ingestion of sodium chloride and excretion of sodium bicarbonate must result in an increase in the concentration of chloride in the extracellular fluids equivalent to the fall in bicarbonate. Since the urine is relatively alkaline, little sodium can be conserved by renal production of ammonium.

When ammonia-producing activity is the earlier casualty of renal disease, hyperchloremia may again characterize the resulting acidosis, but a urine of maximal acidity may be formed. In such cases acids formed during metabolism, largely sulfuric acid but also organic acids, react, with plasma bicarbonate to depress it. Since glomerular filtration is not yet too severely reduced, the anions of these "undetermined acids" are largely excreted. Like sulfate, they are generally poorly reabsorbable once filtered. Because of the inadequate ammonia production, they cannot be excreted as their ammonium salts but instead obligate excretion of fixed cation, largely sodium. Thus, H_2SO_4 is formed in the body from the oxidation of sulfur-containing amino acids, but Na_2SO_4 is excreted. The retained hydrogen ions cause acidosis. Since chloride is more readily reabsorbed than sulfate, it is not lost in proportion to sodium. Again the nearly equivalent amounts of sodium and chloride in most foods, together with the obligatory loss of sodium with other anions in the urine in this condition, result in hyperchloremia. The requirement to preserve extracellular fluid volume prevents correction of the hyperchloremia by excretion of neutral sodium chloride in the urine. With advancing renal disease and declining glomerular filtration rates, hyperchloremia recedes as other anions are retained.

With more advanced renal failure about one-half of patients are unable to reabsorb all the filtered bicarbonate at normal plasma concentrations of this anion (see Figure 9-3) (2). Wastage of bicarbonate in an alkaline urine results in a fall in the serum bicarbonate, and a metabolic acidosis ensues. These patients exhibit the renal disorder of proximal renal tubular acidosis. In this condition bicarbonate reabsorption in the proximal tubule is depressed, and the presence of this anion defeats the action of hydrogen ion secretion in the distal nephron to acidify the urine, resulting in urinary loss of bicarbonate. Once concentrations of bicarbonate in the glomerular filtrate are sufficiently reduced, however, essentially all of this anion can be reabsorbed and the urine can be acidified.

The other half of patients with chronic renal failure who are not

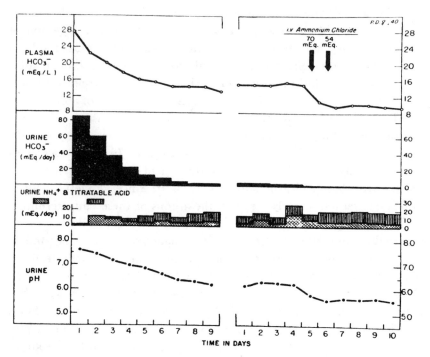

Fig. 9-3 Plasma bicarbonate concentration, urine pH, and daily excretion of bicarbonate, ammonium, and titratable acid in patient P. D. Observations began the day after acidosis had been corrected and treatment with alkali had been stopped. The break in the middle of the observations indicates an interruption of 7 days. See text for details. Reprinted from (2) with permission of the *Journal of Clinical Investigation.*

bicarbonate wasters (see Figure 9-4) still characteristically become acidotic because ammonia production is not augmented sufficiently to meet the need for hydrogen ion excretion, even when urine acidification is maximal.

Years ago Henderson and Palmer (4) found that patients with terminal renal failure and acidosis excreted as acid a urine as did those with normal kidneys in adjacent beds on the wards of the Massachusetts General Hospital. When they measured the titratable acid and ammonium content of the patients with renal failure, however, they found these to be severely deficient for the acidotic state of the patients. The acid urine formed was the result of the small quantity of buffer that the urine contained. This allowed even the small quantity of hydrogen ion that was secreted to convert the small amount of buffer to its acid form and thus depress urinary pH.

Generally, the acidotic patient with chronic renal failure also has a depression of serum chloride concentration. Because of the reduced glomerular filtration rate in this condition sulfate, phosphate, and other anions are retained in the body fluids, as is urea. These anions gradually displace chloride, causing its low concentrations in the serum. It should be clear that it is the failure to excrete the hydrogen ion of sulfuric and phosphoric acids, not the retention of their anions, that causes the acidosis of renal failure.

It is thought that the hydrogen ion has a direct depressing effect on neuromuscular irritability. Patients with chronic renal failure may have very low serum calcium concentrations without manifesting overt

Fig. 9-4 Plasma bicarbonate concentration, urine pH, and daily excretion of bicarbonate, ammonium, and titratable acid in patient R. M. Observations began the day after acidosis had been corrected and treatment with alkali had been stopped. Reprinted from (2) with permission of the *Journal of Clinical Investigation*.

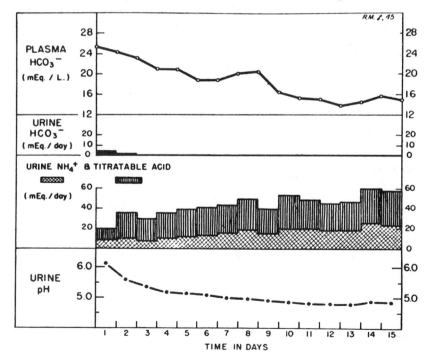

tetany. The drop in serum pH is insufficient to produce a significant increase in the ionization of calcium in the serum. The increased hydrogen ion concentration protects against the effects of the low serum calcium. Thus, care must be taken to avoid correcting the acidosis too rapidly, or what was manifest only as muscular twitches and occasional muscle cramps in such a patient may be converted into overt seizures.

Patients with chronic renal failure often seem to stabilize their acidotic state for long periods of time, though measurements of their hydrogen ion "balance" indicate that they should be continuously accumulating hydrogen ion (5). The same phenomenon has been demonstrated in normal subjects rendered acidotic by administration of ammonium chloride (6). It is thought that the skeleton serves as a major store of buffer under such circumstances and that a gradual loss of its mineral stores accompanies such buffering (7). Almost every patient with chronic renal failure of months' to years' duration shows some demineralization of his skeleton by x-ray examination, and such patients have been shown to be in a negative calcium balance that can be rectified by correcting the acidosis (7).

It is likely that another factor also contributes to the seemingly fixed low concentrations of bicarbonate in the serum in chronic renal failure. The low serum calcium concentrations commonly associated with this condition (see below) induce a secondary hyperparathyroidism. But parathyroid hormone inhibits proximal reabsorption of bicarbonate in the kidney, leading to reduced serum bicarbonate concentrations (8, 9). To the extent that proximal tubular functions are not already impaired by the disease process affecting the kidneys, and the proximal tubule is, therefore, still able to respond to its normal hormonal regulators, the secondary hyperparathyroidism of chronic renal failure contributes to the associated acidosis.

SODIUM WASTING

The kidney in chronic renal failure is a "salt-losing kidney." It may be necessary to stress the kidney's sodium-conserving ability by placing the patient on a low sodium diet to bring out this functional defect; Figure 9-5 compares the response of a normal subject to that of a patient with chronic glomerulonephritis. Both individuals were placed on a 200-mg sodium diet. The change in weight, the daily urine vol-

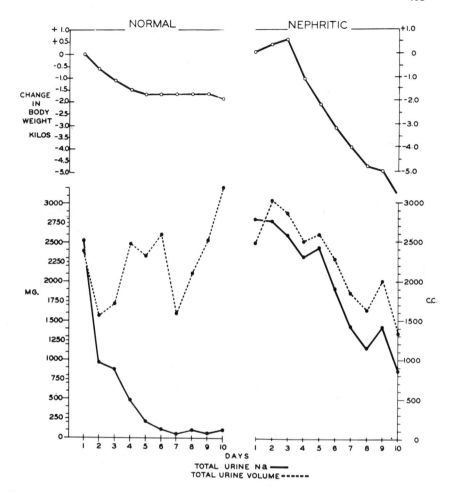

Fig. 9-5 A comparison of the response of a normal subject and a patient with chronic renal failure to a 200-mg sodium diet. Urinary volume, urinary sodium excretion, and changes in body weight are shown (1).

ume, and sodium excretion are shown. The normal subject was in negative sodium balance for the first four days, losing approximately 5 gm of sodium in his urine during this period. This is the amount of sodium in some 1.5 liters of extracellular fluid and corresponds well to the loss in body weight. After this initial period the urinary sodium losses became vanishingly small and the body weight of this normal subject stabilized.

By contrast the nephritic patient was unable to conserve body sodium under similar circumstances. Even on the 10th and last day of the study, his urine contained considerable sodium. Note that, in contrast to the normal subject, in whom renal sodium excretion was totally independent of urine volume, in the nephritic patient the decrease in sodium excretion that occurred was accomplished at the expense of a drop in urine volume. As a consequence of renal salt wasting, extracellular fluid volume was reduced by about 6 liters, as indicated by the loss of body weight. The study was of necessity terminated and saline infused intravenously to prevent impending vascular collapse.

To varying degrees all patients with chronic renal failure waste sodium, as did the patient whose response is depicted in Figure 9-5. The sodium wasting may disappear abruptly when such a patient suffers a bout of acute congestive heart failure. The sudden reduction in cardiac output presumably causes a further sharp reduction in glomerular filtration rate, and with this, sodium reabsorption becomes more nearly complete.

Sodium wasting in chronic renal failure may result in a vicious cycle that can be life threatening. Loss of sodium with attending reduction in extracellular fluid volume and intravascular volume, further reduces the glomerular filtration rate. This aggravates the uremia. The patient becomes sicker with anorexia, nausea, and perhaps vomiting, which prevents sodium intake while renal salt wasting persists. Often replacement of sodium may be a life-saving measure in breaking such a cycle of events. In fact, it is generally true that increasing the sodium intake of any patient with chronic renal failure improves whatever function remains, provided his cardiovascular system can tolerate the added extracellular fluid volume. In the many patients who have associated hypertension, the possibility of aggravating the hypertension or producing congestive heart failure rules out supplementary salt intake.

There has been much discussion of the cause of sodium wasting in chronic renal failure. The argument generally centers around the question of whether the intrinsic reabsorptive ability of the renal tubule is impaired or whether the conditions under which the kidneys operate are such as to preclude normal sodium reabsorption even by normal renal tubules. These are questions to which a definite answer is difficult to achieve experimentally. Although there may be some loss of intrinsic renal sodium reabsorptive ability in chronic renal failure, the important role of osmotic diuresis in causing sodium wasting is generally acknowledged. Platt (10) pointed out that the high blood urea levels result in a marked increase in the amount of this solute filtered per nephron. Furthermore, the well-known hypertrophy of the few remaining glomeruli and nephrons in the kidneys of these patients may further aggravate the situation. The large amount of solute filtered per glomerulus may interfere with water reabsorption in the proximal tubule and thus obligate large amounts of sodium to remain in the urine.

Another aspect of this same problem can be sensed by considering urine volumes in chronic renal failure. Up to virtually terminal stages, patients with chronic renal failure maintain urine volumes in the normal range of 1 to 2 liters/day. Often they have mild polyuria with urine volumes of 3 liters or more. This urine output arises from a volume of glomerular filtrate that may be one-tenth or less that of the normal kidney. If one considers the microscopic picture of the diseased kidney with most glomeruli fibrosed, and recalls that the low glomerular filtration rate reflects a proportionate decrease in the number of functioning nephrons, then one must conclude that, at least in the terminal portions of the nephron, the flow of urine is at least 10 times more rapid than in the normal kidney. The fact that the few remaining nephrons often show considerable hypertrophy only increases this flow. It is not surprising that such high rates of flow might interfere with tubular reabsorptive processes. (Conversely, one could argue that impaired tubular reabsorptive capacity left solute in the luminal fluid, obligating water also to remain and thus producing the high rates of urine flow and the normal urine volumes.)

Another view is that the ability of the surviving nephrons to excrete increasing amounts of sodium as the glomerular filtration rate falls represents a homeostatic function mediated by a natriuretic factor. The sodium in the diet must be excreted regardless of how many functioning nephrons remain. A normal adult with glomerular filtration rate of 120 ml $(min)^{-1}$ who ingests 10 gm of salt daily can sustain sodium balance by excreting 0.7% of the filtered sodium. With the glomerular filtration rate reduced to 10 ml $(min)^{-1}$, 8% of the filtered sodium must be excreted to sustain sodium balance, since there are no significant extrarenal means of removing sodium in the absence of diarrhea or sweating. Natriuretic activity has been reported in the urine of uremic patients with high fractional excretions of filtered sodium (31). This view does not explain the continued loss of sodium manifest by many nephritic patients on low sodium intakes, such as that shown in Fig. 9-5, unless a chronically elevated natriuretic factor in a uremic patient requires many days to shut off. Recently evidence has been presented (36) that strongly supports this possibility. By a very gradual reduction in sodium intake patients with chronic renal failure and markedly reduced glomerular filtration rates were able to adapt to very low sodium intakes. They achieved sodium balance while ingesting a mean of only 5.0 ± 2.9 (S.D.) mEq of sodium daily—a very low sodium intake—without other change in renal function. Thus, it seems that the sodium-wasting tendency of chronic renal failure may result from several influences which effect a high fractional sodium excretion, including osmotic factors, tubules damaged by disease and natriuretic factors.

Whatever its cause, this situation gives rise to another constant feature of chronic renal failure, the presence of isosthenuria. This is the fixation of urine concentration in a range approaching that of serum. Expressed in terms of the common determination of specific gravity, this range is 1.008 to 1.012. In terms of the more valid freezing point determination, values of 250–400 mOsm/liter are obtained. In response to a period of water deprivation, on the one hand, or of forced water intake, on the other, both the concentrating and diluting ability are seriously curtailed in the chronically diseased kidney. Concentrating ability is usually lost earlier or at least is more easily recognized. Generally, concentrating ability is severely limited by the time the BUN rises above 50 mg/dl in chronic renal failure.

The specific gravity of the urine can be a useful index of its concentration, provided the limitations of this method are understood. This measurement reflects the weight of solute in a given volume of urine and can vary greatly for the same molar concentrations of different solutes (see Fig. 9-6) (11). In concentrating the urine it is the osmotic activity of the solute (measured conveniently by the freezing point depression method), not its weight, that is physiologically important. So it is not surprising that there is only a rough correlation between the measurements of specific gravity and of osmolarity, as shown in Figure 9-7. The osmolarity is the only true indicator of the reabsorptive activity of the renal tubules.

One may ask whether other important solutes of the body are lost

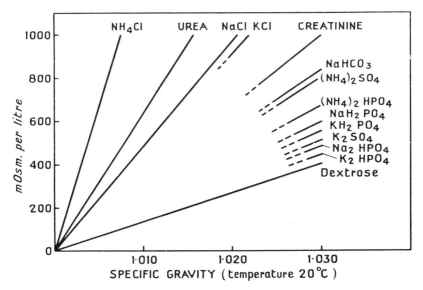

Fig. 9-6 The relationship of the concentration of various solutes (mOsm/liter) in aqueous solution to the specific gravity of the resultant solution. Reprinted from (11) with permission of *The Lancet*.

excessively in the relative diuresis of chronic renal failure. The expectation might be that all solutes normally present at high concentrations in the plasma and at low concentrations in the urine would be "wasted." Actually, sodium and chloride are the only ones whose loss causes a significant disturbance. It is probably true that many kidneys waste glucose in chronic renal failure, but the quantities are minuscule (12) and would usually go undetected in regular clinical tests.

CALCIUM AND PHOSPHORUS METABOLISM

The calcium and phosphate levels in the serum (normal values for calcium are 8 to 10.5 and for phosphorus 3 to 5 mg/dl or 2.0 to 2.5 and 1.0 to 1.7 millimolar, respectively) depend on a delicate balance between absorption of these ions from the gut, their deposition in or resorption from bone, and their excretion via the kidney. These processes are regulated by several hormones and vitamin D and are affected by the acid–base status as well. It is not surprising that with renal failure complex disorders in calcium and phosphorus metabolism may occur.

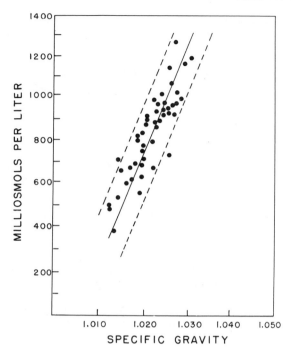

Fig. 9-7 The relationship of the total osmotic activity (mOsm/liter, measured by freezing point depression) and the specific gravity of urine. Reprinted from (30) with permission of W. B. Saunders Company.

As the glomerular filtration rate falls the serum phosphorus rises, for the same reasons that the concentration of urea in the blood increases. Unlike urea, however, tubular reabsorption of phosphate is controlled by parathyroid hormone, which acts predominantly in the proximal tubule to reduce the amount of filtered phosphate which is reabsorbed. This action of parathyroid hormone decreases the rate of rise of serum phosphorus as glomerular filtration rate declines. A normal adult with a glomerular filtration rate of 150 liters/24 hours and a serum phosphorus of 4 mg/dl can excrete 1000 mg of phosphorus with 80% of filtered phosphate reabsorbed. If the glomerular filtration rate falls to 25 liters/day the same amount of phosphates can be excreted by the diseased kidneys at the same serum concentration only if the tubular reabsorption of filtered phosphate is reduced to zero by the action of parathyroid hormone. Further reduction in glomerular filtration rate will allow the same rate of phosphate excretion only at the expense of an increase in concentration of serum phosphorus. But the latter will decrease serum ionized calcium and elevate further the levels of parathyroid hormone (32). Only by reducing the phosphate intake can a rising level of serum phosphate and its sequelae, be avoided as glomerular filtration rate fails (33). The parathyroid hormone acts directly on bone to cause resorption of calcium and phosphate. Since the phosphate added from this source to the extracellular fluids cannot be disposed of through the usual renal route without further elevating serum phosphorus, the serum ionized calcium concentration cannot increase and continues to stimulate parathyroid activity. This secondary hyperparathyroidism is one of the factors leading to dissolution of the skeletal system, predominantly of the long bones or peripheral skeleton as compared with the axial skeleton, which may even show areas of osteosclerosis.

Another physiologic disturbance that may affect calcium and phosphorus balance is chronic acidosis. As discussed, acidosis also results in a dissolution of bone, perhaps with buffering of hydrogen ions in the skeleton. The negative calcium balance associated with chronic acidosis in renal failure has been demonstrated (7).

The demineralization of the skeleton in chronic renal failure is apparently aggravated by a diminished absorption of calcium from the gut. When the renal route for excretion of phosphate is blocked by the reduced glomerular filtration rate, more phosphate is excreted into the gastrointestinal tract. This increased intestinal phosphate was thought to bind dietary calcium in relatively insoluble calcium phosphate salts that prevented absorption of ingested calcium (13). It has subsequently been shown in studies of calcium absorption by isolated intestinal segments that the rates of calcium transport are nearly independent of the concentration of phosphate within the luminal fluid, over a considerable range (14). Thus, to explain the diminished intestinal absorption of calcium on the basis of increased phosphate in the intestinal contents is probably an oversimplification.

It has long been known that the hypocalcemia and the decreased absorption of calcium from the intestines are resistant to usual amounts of vitamin D, but can often be improved with very large doses of this vitamin. DeLuca and associates (15) and Kodicek and associates (16) have found that the active form of vitamin D is not calciferol (vitamin D_3), as had been assumed, but more polar metabolites of calciferol. Thus, they have found that 25-hydroxycholecalciferol, which is formed from calciferol in the liver, undergoes further hydroxylation to 1,25-dihydroxycholecalciferol in the kidney, becoming the active form of vitamin D. Presumably, the loss of the renal step in the metabolism of vitamin D in chronic renal failure is the important element in the vitamin D resistance associated with this condition. In fact, daily treatment of uremic patients for 6–10 days with small doses of 1,25-dihydroxycholecalciferol is reported to increase serum calcium and phosphorus with an increased intestinal absorption of calcium (17).

In a series of elegant studies Wasserman (18) has demonstrated that vitamin D affects intestinal absorption of calcium by inducing synthesis of a calcium-binding protein in the intestinal mucosa. In the uremic experimental animal it has now been demonstrated that synthesis of this binding protein is impaired in response to calciferol (19). But the role of this protein in calcium absorption remains unclear. Further studies in progress should complete this exciting story and, it is hoped, provide effective therapy to bypass the disturbance in the metabolism of vitamin D in chronic renal failure.

The sum of these effects is to cause demineralization of the skeleton. Some degree of demineralization accompanies chronic renal failure in virtually all instances. Radiologic evidence of this can usually be seen most readily in the hands, where there is general loss of density and coarsening of trabeculae of bone. Here also the subperiostal reabsorption of cortical bone that is characteristic of hyperparathyroidism, whether primary or secondary, can be seen in the metacarpal and phalangeal bones. The axial skeleton may be spared these changes and in some cases even show increased radiologic density, as mentioned. The reason for such regional differences in skeletal calcification is not understood, and there remain many unresolved controversies and unsettled facts in this problem. Although some disturbance of calcium metabolism nearly always exists in patients with chronic renal failure, the skeletal manifestations are usually not clinically symptomatic. A rare patient may, however, develop florid skeletal disturbances that dominate the clinical picture of his renal failure (20).

Evidence is accumulating that a high level of parathyroid hormone in the body fluids may contribute to the uremic syndrome in addition to its well-recognized role in the renal osteodystrophy. Massry and associates (34) have indicated that the high concentrations of parathyroid hormone may play a role in the central nervous system derangements, the peripheral neuropathy, the increased arterial, corneal, skin, joint, and other soft tissue calcification, impotency, and probably other adverse effects of uremia.

There is also tantalizing evidence from animal experiments that limiting phosphate intake can even prevent progression of renal disease. Rats with subtotal nephrectomies fed a diet sufficiently restricted in phosphate to prevent accumulation of this ion, suffered no progressive deterioration of renal function, whereas animals allowed ad lib phosphate intake had progressive loss of renal function associated with extensive soft tissue calcification, which included the kidneys (35). This suggests that sufficient curtailment of dietary phosphate with judicious use of the active form of vitamin D may not only reduce the skeletal manifestations of uremia, but actually delay progression of renal failure. Much further study will be required to ascertain the relevance of such findings to renal disease in man.

ANEMIA

Another regular accompaniment of chronic renal failure is anemia. The hematocrit is often between 20 and 35%. A roughly inverse correlation has been found between the blood urea concentration and the hemoglobin level. Sometimes anemia may be the first indication that severe renal failure has occurred.

Bleeding tendencies manifested by spontaneous nose bleeds, menorrhagia, and sometimes gastrointestinal bleeding may contribute to the anemia. Classically, however, the anemia is normochromic and normocytic. The number of circulating reticulocytes in the peripheral blood is low or normal and the bone marrow is hypoplastic, showing general depression of the red cell series. The cause of bone marrow suppression in uremia is not known. It is possible that a deficiency of erythropoietin, a peptide hormone, produced chiefly in the kidney, that stimulates production of red blood cells (21), may accompany the destruction of renal parenchyma in chronic renal failure. Deficiency of this hormone probably makes an important contribution to the anemia of renal failure (22).

In addition to suppression of marrow activity, there is an increased rate of destruction of red blood cells in the peripheral blood (23). The half-life of red cells in uremic patients is shortened, and red cells from a normal donor infused into a uremic recipient also have a considerable shortening of their half-life. Thus, the red cell of the uremic patient is abnormal, and the abnormality can be conferred upon normal cells, presumably by some factor(s) in the uremic patient.

OTHER DISTURBANCES

Bleeding tendency

It is estimated that 17–20% of patients with chronic renal failure have some problem with bleeding during their illness. Bruising, as well as external blood loss, occurs. Nose bleeds and gastrointestinal bleeding are the most common manifestations of the abnormal bleeding tendency, which undoubtedly results from a number of factors. Thrombocytopenia (a platelet count of less than 30,000/cu mm, as opposed to normal values of 200,000) may be a cause of bleeding in chronic renal failure, but it occurs only in about 5% of patients with abnormal bleeding. Since the platelets have normal survival time, depression of their production in the marrow seems likely. With dialysis or recovery from renal failure the platelet deficiency corrects itself.

Most investigators agree that a qualitative rather than quantitative disturbance of platelets leads to bleeding. A defect in platelet adhesiveness in azotemic renal failure occurs that is related to the serum creatinine level. In one series, all patients manifesting bleeding had serum creatinine levels greater than 5 mg/100 cc. Although all who were bleeding had markedly reduced platelet adhesiveness, not every patient with such impaired platelet adhesiveness was bleeding. Normally, adenosine diphosphate (ADP) releases platelet factor 3, which in turn activates the clotting sequence. The release of factor 3 is inhibited by uremic plasma, and this seems to be the major cause of the bleeding tendency in chronic renal failure. There is evidence suggesting that guanidinosuccinic acid, which increases many fold in the plasma of uremic patients, may be the dialyzable factor that inhibits normal release of platelet factor 3 (24).

Hypertension

Hypertension also characterizes most cases of chronic renal failure, although some patients, that is, most with amyloidosis, are never found to be hypertensive during their disease. Relative renal ischemia with activation of the renal–angiotensin system contributes to the development of hypertension in some patients. The kidneys normally elaborate antihypertensive substances, such as the prostaglandins (25), and loss of these substances may also contribute to the hypertension. The inability to adjust sodium content of the body fluids may lead to over-expansion of the extracellular fluid volume and thus increase blood pressure. This may occur with a high salt intake, although the failing kidney, as mentioned above, is generally a salt "waster," so that patients who at an earlier stage of their renal disease may have manifested the nephrotic syndrome with massive edema generally enter a "dry stage" as the kidneys fail and chronic renal failure develops. There are exceptions to this rule, and cases of amyloidosis and diabetic glomerulosclerosis may show all the features of the nephrotic syndrome through the terminal stage of uremia. The prolonged hypertension often takes its toll on cardiac function, and left-sided congestive heart failure with pulmonary congestion is a common feature of terminal chronic renal failure.

Patients with renal function so reduced as to require dialysis to preserve life almost all develop hypertension. In about three-fourths of these patients, reduction of salt intake or removal of extracellular fluid by dialysis controls the hypertension (26). Hypertension in this group is thus the consequence of overloading the extracellular fluid volume by overexpanding the vascular volume. The remaining patients continue to have hypertension even after any excess of sodium has been removed by dialysis. In this group, nephrectomy corrects the hypertension. The removal of the source of excessive renin–angiotensin activity is necessary for control of hypertension in these patients.

Ionic disturbances

Disturbances in the concentration and content of several ions in the body fluids may be responsible for important features of chronic renal failure. Retention of magnesium and high concentrations in the serum may contribute to the drowsiness and depressed sensorium of some patients and even to the terminal coma. Elevated levels of serum magnesium (> 2.5 mEq/liter) are, however, inconstant findings, and low levels (< 1.5 mEq/liter) may also be encountered. The low levels may contribute to the increased neuromuscular irritability so common in these patients. They are probably found most often in patients who, because of anorexia, have a poor food intake and, because of diarrhea, may become depleted of magnesium.

The concentration of potassium in patients with chronic renal failure may likewise be abnormally high (> 5.5 mEq/liter) or low (< 3.5 mEq/liter). This again depends on the factors that determine the balance between intake and output of this ion. The urinary excretion of potassium in chronic renal failure tends to be fixed and independent of the intake (27). Secretion of potassium into the bowel also contributes to removal of potassium from the body in renal failure. Thus, a patient whose intake exceeds this rate of excretion may quickly become dangerously hyperkalemic, whereas a patient who is eating poorly and perhaps in addition having diarrhea may become severely hypokalemic. Severe acidosis, acute infection with a catabolic response, excessive potassium intake prescribed by a physician, or an acute complication causing oliguria can all result in rapid development of life-threatening hyperkalemia in these patients. About half the patients with chronic renal failure sustain normal levels of serum potassium until terminal oliguric stages.

Both hyperkalemia and hypokalemia interfere with normal neuromuscular conduction, and both cause fatal cardiac arrhythmias if sufficiently severe.

Neurologic dysfunction

Disorders of neuromuscular function are manifold in chronic renal failure. Almost all patients show some increased neuromuscular irritability manifested by coarse tremors, involuntary jerking of extremities, and small-muscle twitchings. Rarely, large-muscle cramps or frank tetany with a positive Chvostek's sign are found in association with hypocalcemia and can be corrected specifically by the administration of calcium. Usually the disturbances cannot be directly traced to an imbalance of any single body constituent. In fact, there may be very low levels of ionized calcium in the serum without overt tetany, presumably because of the concomitant depression of the nervous system by the increased concentration of hydrogen ions, and other associated derangements.

With poor kidney function, drugs that depend on renal excretion for their removal from the body may accumulate in the body fluids and exert toxic effects, often on the nervous system. With the increased consumption of medicines by the public this can be no small factor in uremic disturbances. Even penicillin, when used in the high dosages recommended in certain therapeutic regimens, may produce seizures, and patients with chronic renal failure are prone to intoxication at much lower doses than normal individuals (28). The same applies to many commonly used medicines, for example, digitalis, salicylates, and long-acting barbiturates.

In patients with far-advanced renal failure we are coming increasingly to recognize a peripheral neuropathy. This is a mixed motor and sensory neuritis (29). Its early manifestation, a prolonged conduction time in peripheral nerves, is not uncommon. Its florid form, with severe localized muscle weakness (usually in the extremities), sensory disturbances, and often considerable pain, occurs less frequently. However, with prolongation of the lives of patients suffering chronic renal failure, the incidence of this overt disturbance seems to be on the increase. No specific factor has been implicated as the cause of this uncommon but troublesome disturbance.

Many other derangements associated with chronic renal failure could be mentioned, but the major features of this syndrome have been considered. What has been said, it is hoped, will help readers recognize the patient with chronic renal failure from the disturbances he manifests. He is likely to appear chronically ill and thin with muscle wasting because of the anorexia, nausea, and vomiting that interfere with his state of nutrition. He is pale from anemia and may have a sallow, yellowish-brown hue. This discoloration was once attributed to retention of urochromes, but light adsorption spectroscopy of the skin indicates the pigmentation to be largely melanin. He may show subcutaneous ecchymoses over exposed parts of the body, reflecting his increased susceptibility to bruising. His skin and mucous membranes are likely to be dry and his subcutaneous tissue turgor poor as a result of sodium wasting. In addition to its dryness, his skin may be excoriated, and he may scratch himself frequently. Secondary hyperparathyroidism seems related to the itching, since parathyroidectomy may promptly relieve this distressing symptom. A closer look at his skin may reveal tiny whitish crystals plugging the sweat glands, the so-called urea frost that results from high concentrations of urea in body fluids. This close approach is likely to make one aware of the uremic or uriniferous odor of the patient's breath; bacterial splitting of salivary urea contributes to its ammoniacal character. He has slow, deep respirations, the characteristic Kussmaul breathing of acidosis. Coarse twitches of his extremities may be seen and, rarely, frank tetany or seizures from the deranged ionic composition of extracellular fluids. His sensorium may be depressed, and he is often apathetic, but when aroused, is rational and well oriented. These are some of the features that together indicate that a patient's underlying problem is chronic renal failure, whatever the original disease process may have been that progressively destroyed his kidneys.

References

1. Leaf, A. and Newburg, L. H. Significance of the body fluids in clinical medicine. Charles C Thomas, Springfield, Ill., 1955, p. 72.
2. Schwartz, W. B., Hall, P. W., Hays, R. M., and Relman, A. S. On the mechanism of acidosis in chronic renal failure. J. Clin. Invest. 38:39–52, 1959.
3. Seldin, D. W. and Wilson, J. D. Renal tubular acidosis. In J. B. Stanbury, J. B. Wyngaarden, and D. S. Fredrickson, eds. Metabolic basis of inherited disease. 2nd ed. McGraw-Hill, New York, 1966, pp. 1230–1246.
4. Palmer, W. W. and Henderson, L. J. A study of the several factors of acid excretion in nephritis. Arch. Intern. Med. 16:109–131, 1915.
5. Goodman, A. D., Lemann, J., Lennon, E. J., and Relman, A. S. Production, excretion and net balance of fixed acid in patients with renal acidosis. J. Clin. Invest. 44:495–506, 1965.
6. Lemann, J., Jr., Lennon, E. J., Goodman, A. D., Litzow, F. R., and Relman, A. S. The net balance of acid in subjects given large loads of acid or alkali. J. Clin. Invest. 44:507–517, 1965.
7. Litzow, J. R., Lemann, J., Jr., and Lennon, E. J. The effect of treatment of acidosis on calcium balance in patients with chronic azotemic renal disease. J. Clin. Invest. 46:280–286, 1967.
8. Hellman, D. E., Au, W. Y. W., and Bartter, F. C. Evidence for a direct effect of parathyroid hormone on urinary acidification. Am. J. Physiol. 209:643–650, 1965.
9. Muldowney, E. P., Donohue, J. F., Carrol, D. V., Powell, D., and Freaney, P. Parathyroid acidosis in uremia. Quart. J. Med. 61:321–342, 1972.
10. Platt, R. Structural and functional adaptation in renal failure. Brit. Med. J. 1:1313 and 1372, 1952.
11. Isaacson, L. C. Urinary osmolality and specific gravity. Lancet 1:72–73, 1959.
12. Hawkins, J. A., MacKay, E. M., and Van Slyke, D. D. Glucose excretion in Bright's disease. J. Clin. Invest. 8:107–121, 1930.
13. Liu, S. H. and Chu, H. I. Studies of calcium and phosphorus metabolism with special reference to pathogenesis and effects of dihydrotachysterol (A. T. 10) and iron. Medicine 22:103–161, 1943.
14. Stanbury, S. W. and Lumb, G. A. Metabolic studies of renal osteodystrophy. Medicine 41:1–31, 1962.
15. DeLuca, H. F. Vitamin D—1973. Am. J. Med. 52:1–12, 1974.
16. Kodicek, E. The story of vitamin D from vitamin to hormone. Lancet 1:325–329, 1974.
17. Brickman, A. S., Coburn, J. W., and Norman, A. W. Action of 1,25 dihydroxycholecalciferol, a potent, kidney-produced metabolite of vitamin D, in uremic man. New Eng. J. Med. 287:891–895, 1972.

18. Wasserman, R. H., Corradino, R. A., and Taylor, A. N. Vitamin D-dependent calcium-binding protein. J. Biol. Chem. 243:3978–3986, and 3987–3993, 1968.

19. Avioli, L. V., Lee, S. W., Birge, J., Slatopolsky, E., and DeLuca, H. F. The nature of the defect in intestinal calcium absorption in chronic renal disease. J. Clin. Invest. 48:4a, 1969.

20. Stanbury, S. W., Lumb, G. A., Nicholson, W. F. Elective subtotal parathyroidectomy for renal hyperparathyroidism. Lancet 1:793–799, 1960.

21. Jacobson, L. O., Goldwasser, E., Fried, W., and Plzak, L. Role of the kidney in erythropoiesis. Nature 179:633–634, 1957.

22. Fried, W. Erythropoietin. Arch. Int. Med. 131:929–938, 1973.

23. Loge, J. P., Lange, R. D., and Moore, C. V. Characterization of anemia associated with chronic renal insufficiency. Am. J. Med. 24:4–18, 1958.

24. Stein, I. M., Cohen, B. D., and Kornhauser, R. S. Guanidinosuccinic acid in renal failure and experimental azotemia. New Eng. J. Med. 280:926–930, 1969.

25. Hickler, R. B., Birbari, A. E., Qureshi, E. U., and Karnovsky, M. L. Purification and characterization of vasodilator and antihypertensive lipid of rabbit renal medulla. Trans. Assoc. Am. Phys. 79:278–283, 1966.

26. Vretes, V., Cangiano, J. L., Berman, L. B., and Gould, A. Hypertension in end-stage renal disease. New Eng. J. Med. 280:978–981, 1969.

27. Leaf, A. and Camara, A. A. Renal tubular secretion of potassium in man. J. Clin. Invest. 28:1526–1533, 1949.

28. Bennett, W. M., Singer, I., and Coggins, C. H. A guide to drug therapy in renal failure. JAMA 230:1544–1553, 1974.

29. Asbury, A. K. Uremic polyneuropathy. Arch. Neurol. 8:413–428, 1963.

30. Dunstan, H. P. and Corcoran, A. C. Functional interpretation of renal tests. Med. Clin. N. Am. 39:947–956, 1955.

31. Bourgoignie, J. J., Hwang, K. H., Ipakachi, E., and Bricker, N. S. The presence of a natriuretic factor in urine of patients with chronic uremia. J. Clin. Invest. 53:1559–1567, 1974.

32. Bricker, N. S. and Fine, L. G. The trade-off hypothesis: current status. Kidney Internat. 13 (Suppl. 8):55–58, 1978.

33. Slatopolsky, E., Caglar, S., Gradowska, L., Canterbury, J. M., Reiss, E., and Bricker, N. S. On the prevention of secondary hyperparathyroidism in chronic experimental renal insufficiency in the dog. J. Clin. Invest. 50:492–500, 1971.

34. Massry, S. G. Is parathyroid hormone a uremic toxin? (editorial) Nephron 19 (3):125–130, 1977.

35. Ibels, L. S., Alfrey, A. C., Haut, L., and Huffer, W. E. Preservation of function in experimental renal disease by dietary restriction of phosphate. N. Eng. J. Med. 298:122–126, 1978.

36. Danovitch, G. M., Bourgoignie, J., and Bricker, N. S. Reversibility of the "salt-losing" tendency of chronic renal failure. N. Eng. J. Med. 296:14–19, 1977.

10

The Clinical and Physiological Significance of the Serum Sodium Concentration

Flame photometry has made the serum sodium concentration one of the simplest, most readily available, and most frequently measured constituents of the body fluids. Interpretation of this measurement is often, however, confused. It is not always appreciated that a given concentration of the serum sodium may be consistent with several different functional states. Only when this measurement is combined with other clinical information about the patient is its full significance obtained. The purpose of this chapter is to explore the physiologic states associated with alteration of the serum sodium concentration so that the most information may be extracted from this determination. The chapter is intended to review, emphasize, and extend aspects of the regulation of the volume and concentration of the body fluids presented in Chapter 3.

THE NORMAL SERUM SODIUM CONCENTRATION

In health the serum sodium concentration is kept within narrow limits, usually 136–143 mEq/liter, despite large individual variations in intake of salt and water. Since serum normally has a water content of

93%, the sodium concentration expressed more rigorously per liter or kilogram of serum water is about 7% higher than those values. The constancy of the serum sodium concentration is a consequence of two facts: the salts of sodium comprise the major osmotically active solutes in the serum, and the body zealously preserves the total solute concentration of the serum, in health, within narrow limits of about 275–290 mOsm/kg of water. In fact, there is reason to believe that the slight variation in serum sodium concentration found in the same individual when measured on successive mornings in the fasting state largely represents variation in the measurement rather than in the individual—so precisely is this concentration maintained.

Chapter 3 described how the constancy of serum osmolality is preserved through the thirst–neurohypophyseal–renal axis. A rise in serum osmolality of only 1–2% is sufficient to release antidiuretic hormone from the neurohypophysis with resultant concentration of the urine and conservation of body water. Furthermore, this same stimulus affecting an adjacent area of the hypothalamus leads to thirst that motivates drinking. The combination of increased water intake and renal conservation of water reduces the osmolality of body fluids. But dilution of body fluids inhibits release of antidiuretic hormone (ADH) with resultant excretion of a dilute urine hypotonic to the serum. Such water diuresis normally rids the body promptly of an excess water, the serum sodium and solute concentrations increase, ADH is again released, and the urine volume diminishes as the urinary solute concentration rises. The constant vigilance of this double negative feedback loop (Fig. 3-9) keeps the total solute concentration, and thus sodium concentration, within the narrow normal limits despite large daily fluctuations in ingestion of water and salt.

Since all cells of the body are highly permeable to water, this mechanism that regulates the tonicity of the extracellular fluids likewise sets the tonicity of the intracellular fluids. Although the solutes that contribute to intracellular osmolality are different, or are at different individual concentrations inside and outside of cells, their sum must add up to the same total solute concentration. Stated more rigorously, there is a single prevailing chemical potential of water throughout the intracellular and extracellular fluids; the only exceptions are in organs, like the kidney, that produce anisosmolar secretions.

It is generally agreed that no osmotic gradients can exist between cells and the extracellular fluids bathing them, with the exceptions mentioned—the energy costs in pumping water out of leaky cells would be prohibitive. Net movement of water across cell membranes occurs only secondary to transport of solutes and in response to the osmotic gradients established by such solute transport, that is, the absorption of water from the gut or the reabsorption of glomerular filtrate from the lumen of the nephron. Nevertheless, there has been much discussion in the literature about the possible intracellular binding of water or of the major solutes sodium and potassium. Such binding would affect activity and osmotic coefficients of intracellular solute and water. With so many macromolecules, and membrane surfaces, charged and uncharged, in cells, there must be some constraints on the freedom of motion of water molecules and solutes. Molecules of DNA can, for example, limit the freedom of water molecules to move in response to their thermal energy. The degree to which intracellular water takes on an "ice-like configuration" and thus has a decreased osmotic coefficient (i.e., lower vapor pressure) is still under investigation. Methods of obtaining such information about the state of intracellular water and solutes are still imperfect. Classic methods have involved measurements of the swelling or shrinking of tissues placed in solutions of different osmolality and comparisons of the behavior with that expected for a perfect osmometer. Except perhaps in the case of red cells, the corrections necessary for the extracellular fluid content of the tissue and for the reflection coefficients of the solutes used in the bathing medium have made this a very indirect and cumbersome approach. More recently, nuclear magnetic resonance techniques that can focus on the freedom of mobility of water molecules or on sodium or potassium ions have been applied to this problem, but the results are as yet controversial. Attempts to measure the activity of intracellular ions directly with special electrodes reversible to sodium or potassium ions have been reported. The technical problems associated with the small dimensions of such electrode surfaces, junction potentials, polarization of surfaces by intracellular proteins, interference by other intracellular ions, compartmentation, and heterogeneity of the intracellular compartments have made such measurements very difficult. Nevertheless, preliminary, though often conflicting, results have been obtained (see Appendix).

For the present discussion, the actual activity and osmotic coefficients for intracellular solutes and water, respectively, are not as important as the question of whether in health or disease changes might occur that would either release significant amounts of "bound" water or remove "free" water. For example, it has often been suggested that in a variety of morbid states extracellular sodium might disappear into cells, where it would become osmotically inactive and thus free water to dilute the body fluids. It has been postulated also that solvent water might diminish or increase as a result of changes in the binding of water by macromolecules within cells. Such shifts probably do not occur to a significant degree during life. Though sodium may accumulate in cells under certain circumstances, it obligates nearly as much water when intracellular as when occupying its more usual extracellular site. Only at the surface of bone, when sodium ions are incorporated into the crystalline matrix, does such a major change of activity coefficient occur, but sodium salts sequestered in bone are not released in response to the osmolality of the body fluids. Figure 10-1 shows plasma osmolality plotted against the sum of exchangeable sodium and potassium divided by total body water, measured by isotope dilution techniques in patients with very large differences in serum sodium and osmolality (1). The linearity of these relations suggest that in this diverse group of patients significant variations in activity coefficients or osmotic coefficients were not occurring. More data on this very important, but technically difficult problem are needed.

In summary, the important fact is that osmotic equality exists between extracellular and intracellular fluids—a single chemical potential for water prevails throughout the body fluids (except in kidneys and sweat glands). The solutes contributing to this uniform osmolality differ in extracellular and intracellular fluids. It is unlikely that during life acute changes can occur in the activity coefficients of the salts of the major ions (sodium and potassium) or in the solvent properties of water sufficient to change the serum sodium concentration appreciably.

HYPERNATREMIA

An elevation of the serum sodium concentration above 145 mEq/liter, hypernatremia, always indicates too little water for the quantity of solute in the body. The important clinical distinction is whether this relative water deficit has arisen despite normal renal conservation of water or as a consequence of failure of such conservation. Small volumes of maximally concentrated urine indicate the former, whereas a copious, dilute urine establishes the latter.

The finding of dilute urine in the presence of hypernatremia

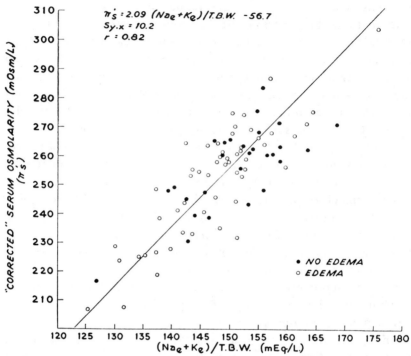

Fig. 10-1 The relation between the "corrected" serum osmolarity and the ratio of (Na_e + K_e)/ total body water. Reprinted from (1) with permission of the *Journal of Clinical Investigation.*

means either neurohypophyseal insufficiency with lack of antidiuretic hormone or a disorder of the renal tubules that prevents them from responding normally to the hormone. Potassium depletion (2), hypercalcemia (3, 4), certain drugs (e.g., lithium (5), and demethylchlortetracycline (6), or intrinsic renal disease may interfere with normal renal concentrating ability and usually are readily recognized, if kept in mind. Under these conditions, administration of vasopressin results in little, if any, further increase in urinary concentration. On the other hand, a urine hypotonic to the serum in the presence of hypernatremia and a response to exogenous antidiuretic hormone are the *sine qua non* for the diagnosis of diabetes insipidus resulting from neurohypophyseal insufficiency.

Usually the patient with diabetes insipidus, or one of the other conditions mentioned above, has a serum sodium concentration within normal limits. As long as the thirst mechanism remains intact, the tonicity of the body fluids is protected, but at the expense of a marked polydipsia and polyuria. Hypernatremia should not, therefore, be expected in uncontrolled diabetes insipidus, although it may be present in slight degree. Usually, only under the stress of enforced restriction of fluid intake does the defect in renal concentrating ability manifest itself as hypernatremia. Such fluid restriction may be deliberately induced under observation for diagnostic purposes, but it may occur involuntarily after surgery or trauma to the head when the state of consciousness prevents the normal response to thirst. Serious dehydration may then develop rapidly unless adequate measures are taken to replace the water losses.

When large amounts of poorly reabsorbable solutes are filtered into the renal tubules, they obligate the excretion of large amounts of water and ions. Considerable quantities of sodium may be lost in the urine during such an osmotic diuresis. Since the sodium concentration of the urine during an osmotic diuresis is less than its concentration in the extracellular fluids, the loss of water is relatively greater than that of sodium, and hypernatremia results if water intake is restricted. Hypernatremia has been reported in uncontrolled diabetes mellitus in which an osmotic diuresis resulted from heavy glycosuria (7). Hyponatremia may also, however, be found in uncontrolled diabetes mellitus if the fluid intake is maintained and the large sodium and water losses are replaced only by water.

The hypernatremia seen in comatose patients maintained on a high intake of protein and salt by gastric tube is a variant of this situation. The resulting large load of urea and salt to be excreted may increase the obligatory renal losses of water sufficiently to produce negative water balance and hypernatremia. The hypernatremia may be associated with either considerable or only minor reductions of extracellular fluid volume, depending on how much salt is replaced in the tube feedings. Since fairly normal urine volumes are elaborated under such circumstances, the volume of liquids administered daily may seem sufficient to meet usual fluid requirements; hypernatremia in these circumstances may be severe before it is recognized. Special attention should, therefore, be given to the water requirements of the comatose patient who cannot respond to the sensation of thirst. Although a considerable literature exists regarding a causal association between cerebral disturbances and hypernatremia, in my experience all such cases have resolved themselves into those with neurohypophyseal damage, and consequent inability to conserve water, or those simply due to underestimation by physicians of the fluid requirements of the confused or unresponsive patients.

Rarely, one encounters a patient who has lost both thirst and neurohypophyseal function. Although conscious, he may suffer a profound hypernatremia without thirst and without clinical evidence of depletion of body fluid volume. One such patient suffered bouts of mental confusion and hyperpyrexia with a serum sodium concentration of 170–180 mEq/liter that responded to the administration of water. Only with a carefully followed schedule of fluid intake and judicious use of vasopressin can the extremes of hypernatremia or hyponatremia be avoided in such a patient. Responsibility for the management of such a case gives one a profound respect for the normal mechanisms that continuously and unobtrusively preserve the serum sodium concentration within its normal narrow limits.

The rare case of nephrogenic diabetes insipidus should also be mentioned as a cause of hypernatremia. Failure of the renal tubule to respond to antidiuretic hormone, rather than lack of hormone, is the defect here, but without other evidence of renal dysfunction (8). In infancy this condition may give rise to the clinical picture of the so-called water baby. Persistent dehydration with hypernatremia results in irritability, low-grade fever, retarded growth, and permanent damage to the brain if the condition remains unrecognized and untreated with provision of adequate water.

Slight hypernatremia has been described in association with primary excess of sodium-retaining hormones, as in Cushing's syndrome (9) or hyperaldosteronism (10). More commonly, serum sodium concentration in these conditions is at the upper limit of normal, and a hypokalemic alkalosis coexists. There is no entirely satisfactory explanation at present of how an excess of adrenocortical hormones causes such resetting of the "osmostat" at higher concentrations of solute in the body fluids. An action of corticosteroids to depress the sensitivity of the osmoreceptors or to inhibit release of antidiuretic hormone from the hypothalamus has been suggested. Moreover, an effect of corticosteroids to decrease distal tubular reabsorption of solute-free water (11) would increase the tendency to hypernatremia.

A high intake of sodium does not normally produce hypernatremia. It does create a state of expanded extracellular fluid volume, which increases glomerular filtration rate, reduces sodium reabsorption in the proximal tubule, and inhibits secretion of aldosterone—conditions highly favorable for excretion of the excess salt load. In fact, hypernatremia is frequently associated with renal conservation of sodium, a situation termed by Peters (12) the "dehydration reaction." This occurs when reduction of extracellular fluid volume attends the water deficit, causing the hypernatremia, and results in some decrease in glomerular filtration rate and stimulation of aldosterone output (13).

The treatment of all the disorders associated with hypernatremia involves the administration of sufficient water to dilute body solutes down to normal concentrations. Reduction of salt and solute intake may be helpful in reducing obligatory water losses. When neurohypophyseal insufficiency is a factor in the water deficit, administration of antidiuretic hormone may be very useful, as reviewed elsewhere (14), or in some cases thiazide diuretics (15) or chlorpropamide (16) may help to reduce the urinary water losses.

It is important to be aware of the magnitude of the water deficit that a given elevation of serum sodium concentration signifies. In an 80-kg male with a serum sodium of 170 mEq/liter who had received only isotonic, saline-containing solutions during a stormy postoperative period, the quantity of water required to lower his serum sodium concentration to 140 mEq/liter is some 10 liters. This assumes that a normal total body water content, ~60% of body weight was present. Thus

$$48\,\frac{170}{140} - 48 = 58.3 - 48$$
$$= 10.3 \text{ liters of water needed}$$

It is evident that simply adding another liter or two of salt-free dextrose solutions to the fluids administered daily falls far short of correcting the hypernatremia, especially if the patient is febrile and incurring considerable "insensible water losses." One might plan to replace half the calculated water deficit the first day and on subsequent days gradually replace the balance of the deficit.

HYPONATREMIA

Reduction of the serum sodium concentration below 130 mEq/liter, hyponatremia, is frequently encountered in clinical medicine. Although very low concentrations usually bear serious prognostic import, concentrations of less than 100 mEq/liter are compatible with life and even with recovery. The prognosis is usually that of the underlying disease, of which hyponatremia may be just one manifestation. Clinically, the symptoms resulting from the low sodium concentration per se are often difficult to unravel from those of the primary illness, which may be quite serious. When a "pure" dilutional hyponatremia was induced in normal subjects by excessive water administration, as discussed below (17), symptoms, attributable to dysfunction in the central nervous system, were not severe or characteristic, even with serum sodium concentrations as low as 117 mEq/liter. Difficulty concentrating, anorexia, headache, apathy, nausea, and vomiting were the only symptoms manifested. From clinical observations one is justified in anticipating that coma and perhaps generalized convulsions would result from more profound dilution than that induced experimentally in these subjects.

Severity of symptoms depends, not only on the degree of hyponatremia, but also on the rapidity of its development. The lowest serum sodium I have encountered was in a patient whom my House Staff informed me had a serum sodium concentration of 88 mEq/liter! Expecting to see a comatose patient, I was supported in my disbelief of the reported serum sodium when I was introduced to a woman sitting comfortably beside her bed. A blood specimen I drew and analyzed myself, however, had a serum sodium concentration of only 92 mEq/liter. Severe hyponatremia had developed so gradually in this woman as to leave her virtually symptom-free. It is perhaps the transient disequilibrium between intracellular and extracellular tonicity, particularly with reference to the central nervous system, that accounts for the symptoms of hyponatremia. A corollary of this is that correction of hyponatremia should be accomplished at a pace that does not create disequilibrium in the opposite direction from too rapid an increase in tonicity of the extracellular fluids.

Since cell membranes afford no absolute barrier to penetration by water, the low serum sodium concentration, with its associated reduction in the total solute concentration of the serum, must be reflected in an equal hypotonicity of intracellular fluids. Such an adjustment of intracellular fluids could be accomplished by either of two means: loss or osmotic inactivation of intracellular solute, which reduces intracellular tonicity without affecting cell volume; or net gain of cellular water, which dilutes intracellular solute and increases cell volume. Experimentally, hyponatremia of short duration has not been associated with negative balances of potassium (17), and it is unlikely that any intracellular solutes other than the salts of potassium could be lost from cells in quantities sufficient to avoid dilution and cell swelling. Furthermore, studies of the volume of distribution *in vivo* of a large water load indicate equal distribution over the total body water and thus establish a net gain of intracellular water and exclude significant osmotic inactivation of intracellular solute in response to the dilution of the extracellular fluids (18). Many *in vitro* studies have demonstrated that, at least acutely, cells behave as osmometers, taking up water and swelling in response to dilution of their bathing medium.

Since the symptoms of hyponatremia suggest interference largely with function of the central nervous system, it is noteworthy that Yannet (19) reported some years ago that the brain's response to dilution of the extracellular fluids is an exception to the general statement that cells imbibe water and swell. From direct tissue analyses in experimentally induced hyponatremia he found that brain tissue did in fact lose potassium and that brain cells may, therefore, respond to dilution of extracellular fluids with a small gain of intracellular water and little swelling. Although the amounts of potassium lost from this tissue were apparently too small to affect external balances, or were taken up by other tissues, this response by the brain may have special significance. Enclosed as it is within its nonexpansible bony confines, a response by the brain similar to that of other tissues might result in a serious increase of intracranial pressure after every large ingestion of fluid!

Although hyponatremia always indicates a relative excess of water over solute in the body, it occurs clinically under three entirely different circumstances. These will be discussed separately.

Hyponatremia without circulatory insufficiency

The prototype of this clinical situation was initially recognized in experiments on human beings (17). A long-acting preparation of vasopressin was administered so as to maintain continuous antidiuresis in normal subjects after a control period of constant water and salt intake, as shown in Figure 10-2. The antidiuretic effect of the hormone is indicated by the abrupt rise in urinary concentration and fall in urine volume. As expected, the retained water produced a gain in

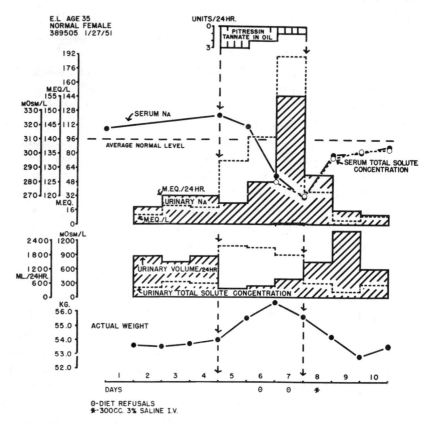

Fig. 10-2 The effect of a long-acting preparation of antidiuretic hormone on water and sodium excretion in a normal subject. Reproduced from (17) with permission of the *Journal of Clinical Investigation.*

body weight and a dilution of serum sodium and of total solute concentration. Unexpected, however, was the intense diuresis of sodium and chloride that regularly occurred about the third day of vasopressin administration in these studies. A rise in glomerular filtration rate and suppression of aldosterone output (20) have been found at the time of the saline diuresis. In addition, reabsorption of sodium chloride and water in the proximal tubule is reduced because of dilution of serum proteins in the peritubular capillaries, as discussed on page 29, Chapter 2. The mechanism of the increased sodium excretion is summarized in Figure 10-3. It appears that the body was making its normal response to overexpansion of the effective extracellular fluid volume by excreting sodium, but that the exogenous vasopressin was preventing the concomitant normal water diuresis. This interpretation is supported by the prevention, at least temporarily, of the sodium diuresis by administration of sodium-retaining hormones (17), which establishes that the sodium loss is not the consequence of interference with renal tubular function by the hypotonicity of body fluids.

Subsequent and more protracted studies in animals demonstrated that, with continued administration of vasopressin, a steady state develops in which water and sodium balances are reestablished, but hyponatremia persists (21). The urinary concentration falls, despite continued administration of vasopressin, for hypotonicity appears to interfere directly with the antidiuretic action of this hormone (22). The increased renal and medullary blood flow associated with the expansion of body fluids results in a "washout" of the hypertonic medullary interstitium, also diminishing the effect of the hormone. Furthermore, the hyponatremia directly stimulates aldosterone secretion, preventing further renal sodium wasting (61). An essentially normovolemic state exists; urine volume and sodium excretion reflect the intake of water and sodium just as they do in the normal person. Only with a further increase in water intake and further acute expansion of body fluid volume does the sodium balance become negative again and then only until a new steady state is established. When vaso-

Fig. 10-3 Mechanism of increased sodium excretion in the development of hyponatremia with a normal circulation.

Hyponatremia with Normal Circulation

(Syndrome of Inappropriate ADH Secretion)

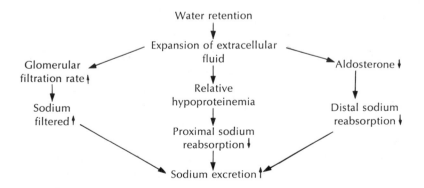

Hyponatremia with Normal Circulation

(Syndrome of Inappropriate ADH Secretion)

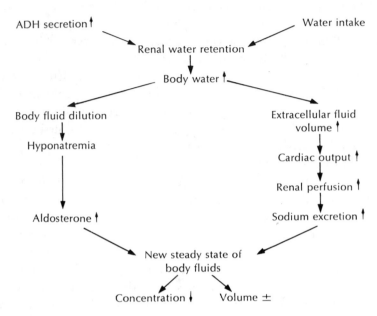

Fig. 10-4 Pathophysiology of the persistent state of hyponatremia with normal circulation.

pressin is withdrawn, water diuresis occurs, and a phase of intense sodium retention follows until the deficits of sodium are replaced (17). During this stage the urine may become essentially free of sodium. The pathophysiology of this persistent state of hyponatremia is summarized in Figure 10-4.

The state produced by prolonged administration of antidiuretic hormone, therefore, manifests hyponatremia resulting primarily from retention of water, with dilution of body fluids, and secondarily from a transient stage of sodium diuresis; and absence of the signs of volume deficiency. Since the primary event is water retention, the volume of body fluids is normal or slightly expanded. Thus, the hyponatremia in this condition is not associated with clinical evidence of a contracted extracellular volume. There is no hypotension, loss of skin turgor, hemoconcentration, or depression of glomerular filtration rate with rising blood urea levels. The volume and sodium content of the urine are unremarkable except during the acute induction of or release from this state. The presence or absence of thirst is not distinctive, and established habits of fluid ingestion are such that several subjects who were allowed an ad lib fluid intake during the period of vasopressin administration drank themselves into a state of hyponatremia (17) (see Table 10-1). Unless symptoms of water intoxication develop during the acute onset of hyponatremia, this type of hyponatremia has justifiably been called "asymptomatic hyponatremia." Of therapeutic importance is the fact that the hyponatremia results from the water retention induced by the hormone rather than from any direct action of the hormone itself. Restriction of water intake can, therefore, prevent the entire sequence from developing, despite the administration of vasopression (17).

The occurrence of this type of hyponatremia was first recognized as a clinical entity by Schwartz and his associates (23), who described two patients with bronchogenic neoplasms and hyponatremia who exhibited all the features of the state that may follow prolonged administration of vasopressin. Since antidiuretic hormone obviously was not being administered to these patients, these workers postulated that the condition developed secondarily to an inappropriate endogenous release of the hormone. Since recognition of this syndrome clinically, it has been described in association with a number of different states. Most of the patients have had either intrathoracic or intracranial disease. Pneumonia and tuberculosis as well as pulmonary neoplasms

TABLE 10-1 *Clinical Features of Hyponatremia with Normal Circulation*
(Syndrome of Inappropriate ADH Secretion)

---

1. Normal cardiovascular function
   Blood pressure normal
   Skin turgor normal
   No orthostatic hypotension
   No edema

2. Normal renal function
   Blood urea nitrogen and serum creatinine normal
   Creatinine clearance normal

3. Hyponatremia and hypochloremia

4. Urinary sodium reflecting dietary sodium

5. Urine concentration $\sim$ 300 to 700 mOsm/kg water

---

have been incriminated. Meningitis, brain tumors, and just "cerebral dysrhythmia" recognized by electroencephalography have been associated with the syndrome of inappropriate antidiuretic hormone secretion. But neoplasms elsewhere, for example, of the pancreas, and a variety of seemingly unrelated conditions, for example, myxedema and acute intermittent porphyria, have been reported in association with this syndrome.

Several studies have shown that bronchogenic tumors and fibrosing tuberculosis lung lesions contain large amounts of assayable antidiuretic activity and may themselves produce substances, presumably peptides, possessing antidiuretic hormone-like activity (24, 25), which is the likely cause of persistent antidiuresis. In the case of intracranial pathology it is thought that hormone is being released from the subject's neurohypophysis. In some of these latter cases successful control of the syndrome has been reported from the use of diphenylhydantoin, which apparently suppresses the irritative focus (Table 10-2).

Increasingly prominent as causes of this syndrome have been a variety of drugs and medications. It has been known that many medi-

TABLE 10-2 *Causes of Hyponatremia with Normal Circulation*

1. Tumors
    Lung—oat cells
    Other—pancreatic

2. Central nervous system disorders
    Head injury
    Brain tumors
    Meningitis

3. Lung disease
    Tuberculosis
    Pneumonia

4. Drugs
    Chlorpropamide
    Clofibrate
    Vincristine
    Cyclophosphamide
    Tricyclic compounds—carbamazepine

5. Miscellaneous
    Acute intermittent porphyria
    Myxedema

cations can cause antidiuresis by stimulating release of antidiuretic hormone from the neurohypophysis. Thus, morphine, other opiates, codeine, barbiturates, nicotine, acetylcholine, several anesthetics, and beta-adrenergic stimulation, act to release vasopressin and hence to provoke antidiuresis. Emotional states of fright and pain may also elicit antidiuresis by release of antidiuretic hormone. Neither these medications nor emotional states are, however, likely to be sufficiently prolonged to induce the sustained water retention associated with the syndrome. By contrast, the hypoglycemic agent chlorpropamide (16), and the anticholesterolemic drug clofibrate (26), are generally prescribed for chronic usage. Both may cause hyponatremia; and seem to act by potentiating the effect of small amounts of circulating antidiuretic hormone. Enough residual hormone seems to circulate, even during mild water diuresis, so that these compounds promote antidiuresis, water retention, and the syndrome.

As one might anticipate from the physiologic basis of this syndrome the hyponatremia is very resistant to correction by administration of sodium. The expanded state of extracellular fluid volume apparently makes the subject quite sensitive to additional sodium, which is promptly excreted in the urine. Even with hypertonic saline solution administered intravenously, only a transient correction of hyponatremia can be achieved because of the rapidity of the renal excretion of the sodium. I once attempted to prevent the development of hyponatremia in a dog during the period of vasopressin administration by giving all liquids as isotonic saline solution rather than water. At the end of 3 days the animal's serum sodium concentration had fallen to 99 mEq/liter, just as would have been expected in the absence of added sodium. The administered sodium was all excreted in the urine, but the water was nevertheless retained in response to the action of vasopressin.

Hyponatremia with circulatory insufficiency and contracted extracellular fluid volume

The existence of this kind of hyponatremia seemed until recently to contradict our understanding of the normal regulation of the serum sodium and total solute concentrations, although its pathogenesis had been suggested years ago (43). Figure 10-5 demonstrates from studies of McCance (27) the development of this state experimentally in a normal subject during forced sodium depletion. The subject was

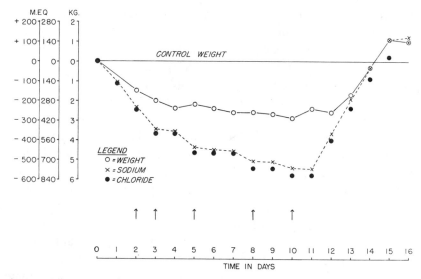

Fig. 10-5 Effect of salt depletion on sodium and chloride balance in man.

maintained on a diet containing very little sodium, with water as desired. On the occasions indicated by the small vertical arrows he was made to lose further sodium by sweating. On the ordinate are plotted body weight and cumulative sodium and chloride balances. The scales are adjusted so that a loss of 140 mEq of sodium or 100 mEq of chloride would correspond to a weight reduction of 1 kg, the relation to be expected if water losses accompanying sodium and chloride depletion were in fact isotonic.

Initially, the weight loss and sodium balance coincided, but after the first 2 or 3 days, body weight stabilized, despite continued losses of sodium. Since caloric intake was maintained and the study was of short duration, this could mean only that water was being retained in spite of the depletion of sodium. The fall in serum sodium concentration, from an initial level of 148 to 131 mEq/liter at the conclusion of the period of sodium depletion, was a necessary consequence of sodium loss without concomitant water loss.

Normal kidneys respond to sodium depletion by excreting a urine that is almost free of sodium; however, the sodium losses in the sweat, which also decrease as depletion progresses (28), were sufficient to increase the net body loss to 760 mEq in McCance's study. This is the amount of sodium in 5.1 liters of extracellular fluid, which is the volume of water that would have been lost if isotonicity of the extracellular fluids had been maintained. It is also about a third of the volume of the extracellular fluids in an adult of average size. A reduction in plasma volume of the magnitude that would have accompanied such a loss of extracellular volume would have led to serious circulatory disturbances. The response avoided this catastrophe by retention of water. The total loss of water was only about 2.4 liters. The resultant dilution of the plasma (fall in concentration of sodium in this study from 148 to 131 mEq/liter) is evidently the lesser of the two evils.

These changes in tonicity of the extracellular fluids are not without effect on the state of hydration of the cells. The normal adult weighing approximately 75 kg contains about 2100 mEq of sodium distributed evenly in some 15 liters of extracellular water. Removal of 760 mEq in the study cited leaves 1340 mEq. At normal concentration, this would require only about 10 liters of water. But since 2.5 liters of water were lost, some 12.5 liters remained. If all 12.5 liters of water had remained in the extracellular space, the concentration of sodium would have fallen to 107 instead of the actual 131 mEq/liter. The observed higher concentration results from net transfers of water into cells as the concentration of the extracellular fluids falls, until osmotic equilibrium between the two compartments is reestablished.

This type of hyponatremia is often encountered clinically in conditions associated with net deficits of body sodium and contracted extracellular fluid volume. Losses of fluid via the gastrointestinal tract by severe diarrhea or vomiting, overuse of diuretics, excessive diaphoresis, adrenal insufficiency, uncontrolled diabetes, and salt-wasting renal lesions may all induce this form of hyponatremia.

In a consideration of the cause of this relative retention of water, one of two different points of view is usually adopted. One view is that vasopressin may be released in response to stimuli from volume depletion as well as to the established osmotic regulation discussed above. The other explanation is that intrinsic renal factors, not involving release of antidiuretic hormone, are responsible. It now seems most likely from the evidence that both mechanisms are involved.

Strauss and his associates (29) produced water diuresis by infusing isotonic solutions into normal subjects, which suggested that expansion of intravascular volume may inhibit secretion of antidiuretic hormone. Diuresis or antidiuresis dependent on recumbent or upright position, respectively, of the experimental subject has been so interpreted (30). Weinstein, Berne, and Sachs (31) demonstrated increased vasopressin in the blood of dogs after acute hemorrhage. Using the same method for partial isolation of antidiuretic hormone from blood and its bioassay, Share (32) reported an increased titer of antidiuretic hormone in jugular vein blood after an acute isotonic reduction of plasma volume in the dog. More recent studies by Robertson, who used a sensitive radioimmunoassay for vasopressin, support the presence of circulating antidiuretic hormone in chronic states of extracellular volume depletion even with reduced osmolality of plasma (33, 62).

Much has been written on the sensing and effector systems that promote water diuresis when the effective vascular volume expands and antidiuresis when the critical volume contracts. There is evidence for the existence of receptors that are involved in the regulation of vasopressin release in response to changes in volume rather than concentration. Henry and his co-workers (34, 63) demonstrated stretch receptors in the left atrium, stimulation of which produced a water diuresis similar to that resulting from inhibition of antidiuretic hormone secretion. That this diuretic response to left atrial distention can be abolished by cervical vagotomy (35) implicates parasympathetic afferent pathways in the suppression of vasopressin release. Moreover, the antidiuresis associated with cervical vagotomy has been found to occur in the absence of changes in renal hemodynamics or solute excretion and to be abolished by hypophysectomy in the dog, suggesting that it is mediated by vasopressin (36). Attempts to show concomitant changes in plasma levels of antidiuretic hormone have led to conflicting results (37), but methods of measuring the very low circulating levels of antidiuretic hormones are still generally unsatisfactory.

In addition to the stretch receptors of the left atrium, there are receptors on the arterial or high-pressure side of the circulation that appear to regulate the release of vasopressin, also in accord with volume rather than osmolar changes. Berl and associates (38) tested the effect of bilateral reduction in carotid perfusion pressure by 25 mm Hg, either above or below the carotid sinus in dogs undergoing water diuresis. When the carotid was constricted below the carotid sinus, antidiuresis occurred. The same degree of constriction distal to the carotid sinus did not alter water excretion. Since the antidiuresis associated with carotid compression has been found to be associated with increased bioassayable titers of antidiuretic hormone activity in plasma, the carotid sinus seems implicated in mediating these changes in vasopressin secretion.

It is apparent, however, that the absence of circulating antidiuretic hormone is only one of the prerequisites for the elaboration of a copious dilute urine. In the absence of this hormone, the permeability of the renal tubular epithelium to water in the distal portions of the nephron is reduced, allowing the hypotonic fluid formed in the ascending limb of the loop of Henle to be excreted as dilute urine. For a hypotonic fluid to be formed, however, a sufficient volume of fluid containing sodium and chloride must reach the ascending limb of the loop of Henle. Reabsorption of sodium chloride at this site leaves the tubular fluid hypotonic as it enters the distal convoluted tubules, and it is the "free water" remaining in the tubules after removal of the sodium that is excreted during a water diuresis. Failure of delivery of sufficient sodium-containing fluid to the distal nephron blunts or prevents a water diuresis and thus promotes water retention and hyponatremia (39). A reduction of glomerular filtration rate, which is likely to accompany the sodium-depleted state, is one of the conditions that might be expected to reduce the volume of sodium-containing fluid reaching the distal nephron, where "free water" is created (see Fig. 10-6). In fact, Berliner and Davidson (40) demonstrated that a reduction in glomerular filtration rate in the absence of antidiuretic hormone can reduce urine flow and increase urine concentration. When glomerular filtration in one kidney was acutely reduced by arterial compression during water diuresis, the urine became slightly more concentrated than the plasma. One surmises that such a reduction in the glomerular filtration rate interferes with the formation of "free water," as stated, and that the subsequent reabsorption of even small amounts of water as the fluid passes finally down the collecting ducts through the surrounding hypertonic medullary interstitial fluid concentrates the urine.

Pursuing this explanation of the impaired water diuresis, Schedl and Bartter (41) infused sodium-depleted normal subjects with mannitol or saline solution and succeeded in increasing the "free-water" excretion thereby. They suggested that the mannitol and the saline solution in the infusates act by "delivering" proximal fluid to distal sites where "free water" is generated. These workers found that the defect in water excretion can occur during sodium depletion in normal subjects without a measurable decrease in glomerular filtration

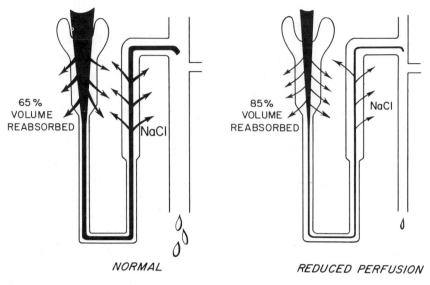

65%
VOLUME
REABSORBED

NaCl

85%
VOLUME
REABSORBED

NaCl

NORMAL   *REDUCED PERFUSION*

Fig. 10-6 The effect of reduced renal perfusion and glomerular filtration rate per nephron on urine flow and "free-water" clearance. With reduced perfusion an increased percentage of the filtered fluid is reabsorbed in the proximal tubule leaving a smaller volume of fluid to reach the thick ascending limb of Henle's loop. Even with further reabsorption of sodium and chloride at this site a smaller volume of "free water" will be formed. During hydropenia the reduced filtration rate per nephron will decrease the amount of sodium and chloride pumped out of the thick ascending limb of Henle's loop. The hypertonicity of the medullary interstitium will be decreased as will the maximal urine concentrating ability. Thus both water excretion and water conservation are impaired.

rate. They suggested that tubular reabsorption of sodium may occur in such circumstances, largely in the proximal tubules as isosmotic fluid, leaving only small volumes of filtrate for distal "free-water" production (see Fig. 10-6).

This concept would account for the impaired ability of the sodium-depleted subject to excrete a water load. Both the rate of urine flow and the maximal dilution of the urine would be less than that achieved by the normal subject. But a hypertonic urine, which occurs in the presence of antidiuretic hormone, would not be expected until the hyponatremia and dilution of body fluids were corrected. The sodium-depleted dog may show a persistent hyponatremia so long as sodium is withheld (42). The urine concentration during such periods may return to levels suggesting the presence of circulating antidiuretic hormone (43). The sodium-depleted rat, on the other hand, excretes a dilute urine, contracting its body water content until normal levels of serum sodium concentration are attained (44). Regulation in man seems to be more like that in the dog than the rat in this regard (see Fig. 10-7).

It now appears that the interaction among left atrial stretch receptors, carotid sinus baroreceptors, intrarenal factors, and hypothalamic osmoreceptors helps to maintain both the tonicity of body fluids and the adequacy of the intravascular fluid volume. Under physiologic conditions the osmoreceptors may be expected to dominate regulation of the release of vasopressin. When intravascular volume—or its effective perfusion pressure—is threatened, vasopressin release may be controlled by volume or pressure. Changes of 1–2% in plasma osmolality normally effect significant changes in secretion of vasopressin (45), whereas assays of plasma vasopressin levels suggest that as much as 7–10% depletion of vascular volume may be needed to alter vasopressin secretion significantly (33). In sheep, findings suggest that the suppressive effect on the release of vasopressin of a decrease in plasma

Fig. 10-7 Pathophysiologic mechanisms in hyponatremia with circulatory insufficiency, the sodium-depletion states.

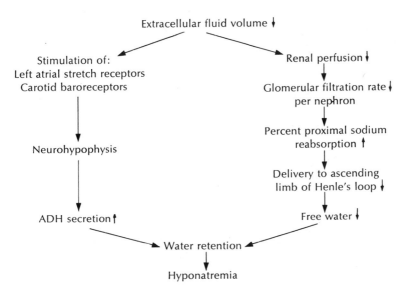

Hyponatremia with Circulatory Insufficiency

(Sodium-Depletion Syndromes)

osmolality of 3.5 mOsm/kg of water may be obscured by a fall in blood volume of 10% (46).

In the hyponatremia with circulatory insufficiency and contracted extracellular fluid volume we have just been discussing, the reduction in left atrial volume, the decreased arterial pressure at the carotid sinus, and intrarenal factors would all combine to promote antidiuresis, water retention, and hyponatremia, overriding the effect of plasma dilution to suppress secretion of vasopressin. Such an interpretation is consistent with our present stage of understanding.

Clinically this form of hyponatremia is the expected response to sodium depletion, regardless of cause. Sodium depletion is encountered clinically when renal sodium losses are excessive, as may be the case with overuse of diuretics, adrenal insufficiency, or renal diseases associated with salt wasting. If the kidneys have induced the negative sodium balance, the expectation is that urinary sodium losses will exceed 10 mEq/liter. On the other hand, sodium depletion may result from extrarenal losses, as with excessive sweating or with gastrointestinal losses. Under these conditions the kidneys will conserve sodium and concentration of sodium in the urine may be expected to be less than 10 mEq/liter.

The clinical features of this syndrome are dominated by the consequences of circulatory insufficiency and when sodium depletion is profound, shock may ensue. The clinical features are summarized in Table 10-3.

TABLE 10-3   *Clinical Features of Hyponatremia with Circulatory Insufficiency, Sodium Depletion*

---

1. Extracellular fluid volume contraction
   hypotension
   rapid pulse
   orthostatic hypotension
   skin turgor decreased
   dry mucous membranes

2. Hemoconcentration
   blood urea nitrogen and serum creatinine increased

3. Hyponatremia and hypochloremia

4. Urine concentration unremarkable
   urine sodium
       <10 mEq/liter—nonrenal Na loss
       >10 mEq/liter—renal Na loss

Hyponatremia with circulatory insufficiency and overexpanded extracellular fluid volume

A variant of the hyponatremia just discussed is commonly seen in edematous patients. The same antidiuretic pattern may be demonstrated in these patients as has been described in the sodium-depleted subject (43). This suggests that the severe heart failure, nephrotic syndrome, or liver disease seen in these patients triggers the same mechanism leading to water retention and expansion of body fluid volume that is active in the normal individual who suffers an absolute reduction in the volume of extracellular or intravascular fluid. Weston and associates (47) have observed water retention with resultant dilution of body fluids in patients during periods of cardiac decompensation and excretion of the water with recovery of compensation. Walker and associates (48) studied water balance in cardiac patients requiring pacemakers because of heart block; slowing the heart rate was associated with water retention, whereas increasing heart rate and cardiac output enhanced water excretion. Figure 10-10 presents a case of corrected hyponatremia in which cardiac function was improved by digitalization. I have come to regard the occurrence of marked hyponatremia in an edematous subject as an ominous prognostic sign that can be relieved permanently only by improvement in function of the failing heart or liver.

The pathophysiology of this type of hyponatremia also remains a topic of debate. The difficulty seems to lie in the spectrum of responses exhibited by these patients. Those presumably with the mildest degree of circulatory insufficiency may have only slight hyponatremia and excrete a water load normally. With more advanced circulatory embarrassment, further hyponatremia, blunting of a water diuresis, and an inability to produce urine of normal dilution following a water load may occur. Finally, one may encounter severe hyponatremia, with complete absence of diuretic response, as shown in Figures 10-8 and 10-9, and no further increase in urine concentration on administration of vasopressin, as in Figure 10-9. By selecting subjects for study at one level in this functional continuum, an investigator may correctly conclude that one factor is of greater importance than others in causing the hyponatremia. Another investigator, studying patients in a different phase, may with equal correctness come to the opposite conclusion regarding the etiology of the hyponatremia. When the entire

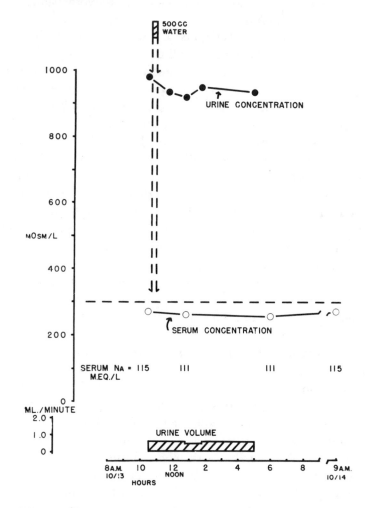

Fig. 10-8 Serum sodium concentration, and serum and urine osmolality in a patient with severe congestive heart failure. Reproduced from (43) with permission of the *Journal of Clinical Investigation.*

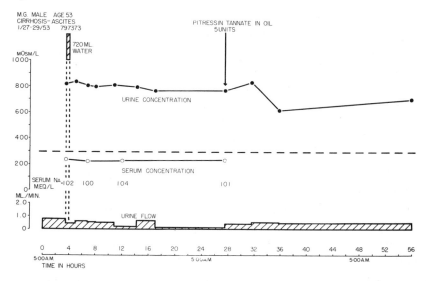

Fig. 10-9 Serum sodium concentration, and serum and urine osmolality in a patient with cirrhosis of liver. Reproduced from (60) with permission of the *New England Journal of Medicine.*

functional continuum is analyzed, at least three factors must be considered: intrinsic renal factors, as considered above in the discussion of contracted extracellular fluid volume; the release of antidiuretic hormone in response to deficits in "effective" circulatory volume; and the resetting of the "osmostat" to preserve a less than normal serum sodium concentration (49)—the rarest and least documented factor. At different stages of circulatory incompetence the relative importance of each factor may change.

It should be stressed that, though the antidiuretic hormone may be related to water retention in cases of severe derangement in body fluid volume, primary retention of water does not produce edematous states. Studies of normal subjects have demonstrated that primary water retention induced by injections of long-acting preparations of vasopressin results in only initial expansion of volume, which in turn produces large renal losses of sodium and hyponatremia. Death from water intoxication would ensue before a clinically significant edema developed. Thus, some factor causing sodium retention would appear necessary for the development of the edematous state, and overproduction of antidiuretic hormone cannot be implicated as a primary cause of edema.

DISTRIBUTION OF SODIUM AND WATER
IN HYPONATREMIA

It was mentioned in the introductory paragraphs of this chapter that cell membranes do not constitute absolute barriers to penetration by water and that the concentration or activity of water is essentially the same inside and outside cells.

In spite of this fact, frequent attempts are made to account for hyponatremia on the basis of the movements of extracellular sodium into cells that may occur in states of illness. Unless such sodium became osmotically inactive within the cells, it would obligate as much water intracellularly as it did extracellularly. The result would, therefore, be shrinkage of extracellular volume by translocation to the intracellular compartments, but no decrease in sodium concentration of the extracellular fluids. Bone is the one tissue known to contain considerable quantities of sodium in a "bound," osmotically inactive form (50, 51). The evidence indicates, however, that this sodium is not available to bolster the volume or regulate the tonicity of body fluids in acute sodium depletion (52).

There is a further serious obstacle to explaining dilution of the extracellular fluids by a decrease in the osmotic activity of sodium or potassium within cells. If such large decreases could occur, intracellular water presumably would be free to move into the extracellular fluid, diluting it. But dilution of the extracellular fluids, as stated previously, normally inhibits secretion of antidiuretic hormone, allowing the kidneys to excrete a dilute urine and thus to correct the tonicity of the body fluids. Why the water transferred from the intracellular to the extracellular compartment would not be excreted promptly with correction of the serum sodium concentration to normal requires explanation. The end result of osmotic inactivation of intracellular solute would thus be only a reduction in intracellular fluid volume. The same difficulty applies to the suggestion (53, 54) that hyponatremia results from depletion of intracellular potassium. Since extracellular fluids are in equilibrium with intracellular fluids, but only the former are directly regulated by the kidneys, changes within cells can have a sustained effect on extracellular fluid composition only by virtue of alterations that they may induce in the normal functions of the kidney and its neural and hormonal regulators. Even if intracellular osmotic deficits can have a primary role in producing hyponatremia, one still must seek some explanation of alterations in regulation of extracellular tonicity to account for the way intracellular osmotic deficits can influence the sodium concentration of the serum. One is thus left with the problem of accounting for hyponatremia in terms of aberrations in regulation of extracellular fluid composition, as discussed above in the sections on hyponatremia with circulatory insufficiency.

One way to reconcile this requirement that hyponatremia can result only from an alteration in the normal regulation of tonicity of the extracellular fluids, and still postulate that intracellular changes play an important part in the development of the hyponatremia, may be to consider the osmoreceptors as cells also sharing the intracellular osmotic deficit. Differences between the tonicity of extracellular and intracellular fluid of the osmoreceptors causing shrinkage or swelling of the latter might serve as the afferent impulse for regulating release of antidiuretic hormone (45). A loss of intracellular potassium or osmotic inactivation of intracellular solute that affects the osmoreceptor cells, as well as other body cells, might serve to reset the osmoregulatory mechanism to preserve some total solute concentration of body fluids below the normal range, to produce hyponatremia. Although there is evidence that some changes in the "setting of the osmostat" may occur (49, 55), one would expect administered water to result in prompt diuresis of dilute urine in hyponatremia if regulation were simply readjusted at some new level of osmotic activity of body fluids. As mentioned, however, water diuresis is usually blunted in hyponatremic subjects and in some induces no diuresis or dilution of the urine, even though serum tonicity and sodium concentrations are further diluted. Such cases are shown in Figures 10-8 and 10-9. Thus, a resetting of the normal regulatory mechanisms to preserve a lower level of tonicity of body fluids does not appear to be an adequate explanation for the development of hyponatremia, except very rarely.

Miscellaneous hyponatremias
Excessive water drinking by a person with normal cardiovascular and renal systems will not cause hyponatremia—only a copious urine flow. There must be some impairment of the kidneys' ability to excrete free water: extracellular or plasma volume depletion, disturbed cardiac function, or renal dysfunction from reduced perfusion, intrinsic disease, or circulating antidiuretic activity. I once tried to drink myself into a state of hyponatremia, but 3 hours later after 4 liters of water I was slightly nauseated and 150 ml in negative water balance!

Rarely, however, there has been described a patient with hyponatremia attributed to a resetting of the "osmostat" to preserve a low level of serum sodium concentration (49, 55, 64). To establish this etiology the following conditions should be rigorously demonstrated: (1) The patient should be able to excrete a water load normally. When a standard water load (20 ml/kg body weight) is administered orally, 80% of the ingested water should be excreted within 4 hours, and the osmolality of urine passed during this period should drop to 100 mOsm/ kg water or less. (2) The patient should be in sodium balance and should not correct the hyponatremia with a high sodium intake. (3) The patient should excrete a concentrated urine with water restriction before serum osmolalties increase to normal levels. Thus the patient should, in fact, protect a hyponatremic state just as a normal person protects a normonatremic state.

Hyponatremia from a reset "osmostat," which has been described in cachectic patients (64), can be relieved by improvement in general nutrition. If one adheres to the above etiologic criteria, the condition must be very rare, as I have only seen two such patients despite a special interest in clinical hyponatremic syndromes.

One should be aware of two further clinical conditions associated with a low serum sodium concentration, which may be referred to as "spurious" hyponatremias. The first occurs when some solute that penetrates cell membranes poorly accumulates in the extracellular fluids and, therefore, draws water osmotically from the cells. This shift of water from the intracellular to the extracellular compartment will lower the sodium concentration in the latter. This occurs in diabetic patients with marked hyperglycemia. In this situation the serum osmolality will be elevated despite the hyponatremia. An elevated blood urea or ethanol level will also increase the serum osmolality, but because urea and ethanol readily penetrate cell membranes their acccumulation does not dislocate body fluid compartments and the serum sodium concentration is unaffected.

The second condition of "spurious" hyponatremia results from the method of determining serum sodium concentration. If a patient has a very marked hyperlipidemia, as may occur in diabetic ketoacidosis, or a marked hyperproteinemia, as may occur in multiple myeloma, a significant proportion of the volume of the serum sample may be the nonaqueous lipid or protein, respectively. Since sodium salts are dissolved only in the aqueous portion of the serum, a low serum sodium value will be reported; and since the sodium concentration may be quite normal in the aqueous phase of the serum, the serum osmolality will be normal here.

TREATMENT OF HYPONATREMIA

The treatment of hyponatremia depends upon its etiology and is based simply on the physiologic principles discussed.

1. *Hyponatremia with adequate circulation,* the syndrome of inappropriate secretion of antidiuretic hormone, is corrected by simple restriction of water. If water intake is sufficiently restricted, then despite persistent antidiuretic hormone activity, no positive water balance or dilution of body fluids can occur. If hyponatremia has developed, then water intake must be reduced to produce a negative water balance via the insensible loss of water from skin and lungs, together with the minimal urinary losses. Only if coma or seizure occur is it useful to administer hypertonic saline intravenously, and there must be concurrent water restriction or hyponatremia will promptly recur. Fluid intake must be restricted as long as the abnormal or inappropriate antidiuretic activity persists. Demeclocycline, which produces a nephrogenic diabetes insipidus, has proven useful in improving water excretion in these patients (65).

2. *Hyponatremia with circulatory insufficiency and contracted extracellular fluid volume,* sodium depletion, is corrected by administration of sodium salts in amounts sufficient to correct the deficit. As extracellular volume returns to normal, the excess water is excreted and the hyponatremia is corrected. Correction of concomitant acidosis, alkalosis, or potassium depletion should be incorporated into the replacement therapy.

3. *Hyponatremia with circulatory insufficiency and edema,* as observed in congestive heart failure or cirrhosis of the liver, is the most difficult form of hyponatremia to treat. Administration of sodium is usually irrational in the presence of the excesses of that ion already sequestered in the edema fluid. Further edema, without a rise in serum sodium concentration, is the usual result of salt administration to these patients. Administration of hypertonic

saline solution to cardiac subjects with hyponatremia raises the serum sodium concentration in a predictable manner, but frequently results in death from pulmonary edema. Hypertonic sodium chloride solutions should be given to these patients only when the degree of hyponatremia is so marked that symptoms of water intoxication interfere with the treatment of the patient. In such cases only enough salt should be given to raise the serum sodium concentrations to levels that do not in themselves pose a threat to the patient—that is, usually up to about 120 mEq/liter. Fluid intake must simultaneously be stringently curtailed; otherwise, the serum sodium is likely to be promptly diluted to its prior low levels. Administration of the salt by mouth is safer than by the parenteral route. The only safe and rational means of raising the serum sodium in these patients is to reduce the daily fluid intake to a level below the obligatory water losses. This usually means curtailing fluid intake to about 500 ml daily. On this fluid restriction the serum sodium concentration gradually rises; however, the patients may complain bitterly of thirst. It is a well-documented but unexplained observation that intense thirst develops seemingly paradoxically in these patients in spite of the existing dilution of the body fluids. This stimulation of thirst is analogous to the assumed stimulation of antidiuretic hormone that would also participate to produce and maintain the hyponatremia.

Hyponatremia in the edematous subject is an ominous prognostic sign. Only if the function of the heart or liver can be improved can lasting relief of hyponatremia be expected. The physician's primary effort should, therefore, be directed toward treatment of the underlying heart or liver disease while the hyponatremia, if severe is arrested or reversed by careful restriction of fluids. Figure 10-10 shows the correction of hyponatremia that can be achieved in this group if the underlying organ failure can be corrected.

"DEHYDRATION"

In conclusion I should like to refer to an unfortunate instance of confusing terminology. Two conditions that have a different pathologic physiology, a different clinical picture, and a different specific treat-

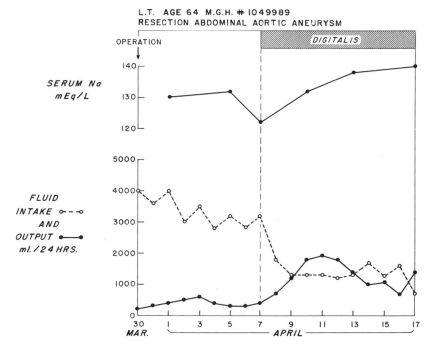

Fig. 10-10 Correction of hyponatremia by improvement in cardiac function. Reproduced from (60) with permission of the *New England Journal of Medicine*.

ment are both frequently referred to as *dehydration*. These two pure types can be readily distinguished, and each has been produced experimentally.

Loss of sodium and chloride with contraction of extracellular volume

As discussed above, McCance (27) produced this state by causing his subjects to sweat excessively and by simultaneously restricting salt intake. Kerpel-Fronius (56) and Darrow and Yannet (57) obtained similar results in animals by injecting isotonic glucose solutions into the peritoneal cavity. After several hours the same amount of fluid was removed from the peritoneal cavity. The glucose had disappeared, and the fluid contained much sodium and chloride. The removal of the peritoneal fluid brought the body content of water back to its original volume and at the same time reduced the amount of extracellular ions. As the extracellular fluid became hypotonic, the osmolality of the intracellular fluids was similarly reduced by passage of water from the extracellular space to the cells. This caused swelling of the cells. The reduction of the extracellular volume resulted in increased concentration of plasma proteins and blood cells. The functional disturbances rest upon the interference with the circulation due to decreased volume and increased vicosity. Nadal and associates (58) obtained analogous sodium depletion in man by removal of intestinal secretions.

Primary loss of water
This is the second condition to which the term *dehydration* is applied. It can be produced simply by drastic limitation of water. The following is an account of the disturbance experienced by a medical student (59). His diet was so arranged that caloric balance was maintained. The water present in the food plus the water produced by oxidation amounted to about 700 ml daily. On the fourth day the subject's mouth was so dry that he could not swallow the food, and it was necessary to terminate the study. At the end of the 4 days the deficit of water incurred was approximately 4 liters. On the fourth day the urine concentration rose to a specific gravity of 1.037, and protein, casts, and red blood cells appeared in the urine, indicating some renal irritation from water lack. Since only a slight increase in concentration of plasma protein and blood cells developed, the extracellular volume did not shrink much. Evidently, as water left the extracellular space and the concentration of the extracellular fluid increased, water was drawn osmotically from the intracellular fluids, and the extracellular volume was largely sustained. The consequent dehydration of the cells may have interfered with their activities sufficiently to account for the student's mental confusion, vomiting, unsteady gait, and general incapacity.

The clinical differences between these two pure types are summarized in Table 10-4; an equal loss of body weight is assumed for each condition. A simple calculation will explain the differences. A 75-kg man has a total body water content of approximately 45 liters, of which some 15 liters is extracellular. If sodium depletion results in a weight loss of 3 kg, the loss of body fluid is all sustained from the extracellular fluid. Serious disturbances in vascular volume may be expected. If simple water lack causes an equal weight loss, the water loss is distributed over total body water, and the extracellular volume is

TABLE 10-4 *"Dehydration"*[a]

CLINICAL FEATURES	SALT DEPLETION	WATER LACK
Thirst	Not remarkable	Intense
Skin turgor	Decreased	Normal
Pulse	Rapid	Normal
Blood pressure	Low	Normal
LABORATORY FINDINGS		
Urine volume	Not remarkable	300–500 ml/day
Urine concentration	Not remarkable	Maximal
Serum proteins	Increased	Normal
Hemoglobin & hematocrit	Increased	Normal
Blood urea nitrogen	Elevated	High normal
Plasma sodium & chloride	Reduced	Elevated
TREATMENT	Salt	Water

[a] An equal weight loss 3–5% of body weight is assumed for both conditions. Reproduced from (60) with permission of the New Eng. J. Med.

compromised by only 1 liter, a loss that can be borne without serious manifestations of vascular insufficiency.

References

1. Edelman, I. S., Leibman, J., O'Meara, M. P., and Birkenfeld, L. W. Interrelations between serum sodium concentration, serum osmolarity and total exchangeable sodium, total exchangeable potassium and total body water. J. Clin. Invest. 37:1236–1256, 1958.
2. Relman, A. S. and Schwartz, W. B. Kidney in potassium depletion. Am. J. Med. 24:764–773, 1958.
3. Levitt, M. F., Halpern, M. H., Polimeros, D. P., Sweet, A. Y., and Gribetz, D. Effects of abrupt changes in plasma calcium concentrations on renal function and electrolyte excretion in man and monkey. J. Clin. Invest. 37:294–305, 1958.
4. Epstein, F. H., Rivera, M. J., and Carone, F. A. Effect of hypercalcemia induced by calciferol upon renal concentrating ability. J. Clin. Invest. 37:1702–1709, 1958.
5. Singer, I., Rotenberg, D., and Puschett, J. B. Lithium-induced nephrogenic diabetes insipidus: *in vivo* and *in vitro* studies. J. Clin. Invest. 51:1081–1091, 1972.
6. Singer, I. and Rotenberg, D. Demeclocycline-induced nephrogenic diabetes insipidus. Ann. Int. Med. 79:679–683, 1973.
7. de Graeff, J. and Lips, J. B. Hypernatremia in diabetes mellitus. Acta med. Scandinav. 157:72–75, 1957.
8. Williams, R. H. and Henry, C. Nephrogenic diabetes insipidus: transmitted by females and appearing during infancy in males. Ann. Int. Med. 27:84–95, 1947.

9. McQuarrie, I., Johnson, R. M., and Ziegler, M. R. Plasma electrolyte disturbance in patient with hypercorticoadrenal syndrome contrasted with that
   found in Addison's disease. Endocrinology 21:762–772, 1937.

10. Conn, J. W. Presidential address: painting background: primary aldosteronism,
    new clinical syndrome. J. Lab. & Clin. Med. 45:3–17, 1955.

11. Kleeman, C. R., Maxwell, M. H., and Rockney, R. Mechanism of impaired
    water excretion in adrenal and pituitary insufficiency. I. Role of altered glo-
    merular filtration rate and solute excretion. J. Clin. Invest. 37:1799–1808, 1958.

12. Peters, J. P. Role of sodium in production of edema. New Eng. J. Med. 239:
    353–362, 1948.

13. Bartter, F. C., Liddle, G. W., Duncan, L. E., Jr., Barber, H. K., and Delea, C.
    Regulation of aldosterone secretion in man: role of fluid volume. J. Clin. In-
    vest. 35:1306–1315, 1956.

14. Leaf, A. Diabetes Insipidus. In P. B. Beeson and W. McDermott, eds. Textbook
    of medicine W. B. Saunders, Philadelphia, 14th ed., 1975, pp. 1700–1701.

15. Crawford, J. D., Kennedy, G. C., and Hill, L. E. Clinical results of treatment
    of diabetes insipidus with drugs of chlorothiazide series. New Eng. J. Med.
    262:737–743, 1960.

16. Miller, M. and Moses, A. M. Mechanism of chlorpropamide action in diabetes
    insipidus. J. Clin. Endocrinol. Metab. 30:488–496, 1970.

17. Leaf, A., Bartter, F. C., Santos, R. F., and Wrong, O. Evidence in man that
    urinary electrolyte loss induced by pitressin is function of water retention. J.
    Clin. Invest. 32:868–878, 1953.

18. Leaf, A., Chatillon, J. Y., Wrong, O., and Tuttle, E. P., Jr. Mechanism of
    osmotic adjustment of body cells as determined in vivo by volume of distribu-
    tion of large water load. J. Clin. Invest. 33:1261–1268, 1954.

19. Yannet, H. Changes in brain resulting from depletion of extracellular electro-
    lytes. Am. J. Physiol. 128:683–689, 1940.

20. Müller, A. F., Riondel, A. M., and Mach, R. S. Control of aldosterone excre-
    tion by change in volume of body fluids. Lancet 1:831, 1956.

21. Levinsky, N. G., Davidson, D. G., and Berliner, R. W. Changes in urine con-
    centration during prolonged administration of vasopressin and water. Am. J.
    Physiol. 196:451–456, 1959.

22. Hays, R. H. and Leaf, A. Problem of clinical vasopressin resistance: in vitro
    studies. Ann. Int. Med. 54:700–709, 1961.

23. Schwartz, W. B., Bennett, W., Curelop, S., and Bartter, F. C. Syndrome of renal
    sodium loss and hyponatremia probably resulting from inappropriate secretion
    of antidiuretic hormone. Am. J. Med. 23:529–532, 1957.

24. Bowers, B. F., Mason, D. M., and Forsham, P. H. Bronchogenic carcinoma with
    inappropriate antidiuretic activity in plasma and tumor. New Eng. J. Med.
    271:934–938, 1964.

25. Vorherr, H., Massry, S. G., Fallet, R., Kaplan, L., and Kleeman, C. R. Anti-
    diuretic principle in tuberculosis lung tissue of a patient with pulmonary tu-
    berculosis and hyponatremia. Ann. Int. Med. 72:383–387, 1970.

26. Moses, A. M., Howanitz, J., van Gemert, M., and Miller, M. Clofibrate-induced
    antidiuresis. J. Clin. Invest. 52:535–542, 1973.

27. McCance, R. A. Experimental sodium chloride deficiency in man. Proc. Roy.
    Soc., London, s. B. 119:245–268, 1936.

28. Conn, J. W. Mechanism of acclimatization to heat. Advances in Int. Med. 3:
    373–393, 1949.

29. Strauss, M. B., Davis, R. K., Rosenbaum, J. D., and Rossmeisl, E. C. "Water

diuresis" produced during recumbency by intravenous infusion of isotonic saline solution. J. Clin. Invest. 30:862–868, 1951.

30. Brun, C., Knudsen, E. O. E., and Raaschow, F. Influence of posture on kidney function. I. Fall of diuresis in erect posture. Acta med. Scandinav. 122:315–331, 1945.

31. Weinstein, H., Berne, R. M., and Sachs, H. Vasopressin in blood: effect of hemorrhage. Endocrinology 66:712–718, 1960.

32. Share, L. Acute reduction in extracellular fluid volume and concentration of antidiuretic hormone in blood. Endocrinology 69:925–933, 1961.

33. Dunn, F. L., Brennan, J. J., Nelson, A. E., and Robertson, G. L. The role of blood osmolality and volume in regulating vasopressin secretion in the rat. J. Clin. Invest. 52:3212–3219, 1973.

34. Henry, J. P., Gauer, O. H., and Reeves, J. L. Evidence of atrial location of receptors influencing urine flow. Circulation Research 4:85–90, 1956.

35. Henry, J. P. and Pearce, J. W. The possible role of cardiac atrial stretch receptors in the induction of changes in urine flow. J. Physiol. (Lond.) 131:572–585, 1956.

36. Schrier, R. W. and Berl, T. Mechanism of the antidiuretic effect associated with interruption of parasympathetic pathways. J. Clin. Invest. 51:2613–2620, 1972.

37. Schrier, R. W. and Berl, T. Nonosmolar factors affecting renal water excretion. New Eng. J. Med. 292:81–88 and 141–146, 1975.

38. Berl, T., Cadnapaphornchai, P., Harbottle, J. A., and Schrier, R. W. Mechanism of stimulation of vasopressin release during beta-adrenergic stimulation with isoproterenol. J. Clin. Invest. 53:857–867, 1974.

39. Berliner, R. W., Levinsky, N. G., Davidson, D. G., and Eden, M. Dilution and concentration of urine and action of antidiuretic hormone. Am. J. Med. 24:730–744, 1958.

40. Berliner, R. W. and Davidson, D. G. Production of hypertonic urine in absence of pituitary antidiuretic hormone. J. Clin. Invest. 36:1416–1427, 1957.

41. Schedl, H. P. and Bartter, F. C. An explanation for and experimental correction of the abnormal water diuresis in cirrhosis. J. Clin. Invest. 39:248–261, 1960.

42. Darrow, D. C. and Yannet, H. Metabolic studies of changes in body electrolyte and distribution of body water induced experimentally by deficit of extracellular electrolyte. J. Clin. Invest. 15:419–427, 1936.

43. Leaf, A. and Mamby, A. R. An antidiuretic mechanism not regulated by extracellular fluid tonicity. J. Clin. Invest. 31:60–71, 1952.

44. Baker, G. P., Levitin, H., and Epstein, F. H. Sodium depletion and renal conservation of water. J. Clin. Invest. 40:867–873, 1961.

45. Verney, E. B. Croonian Lecture: antidiuretic hormone and factors which determine its release. Proc. Roy. Soc., London, s. B. 135:25–106, 1947.

46. Johnson, J. A., Zehr, J. E., and Moore, W. W. Effects of separate and concurrent osmotic and volume stimuli on plasma ADH in sheep. Am. J. Physiol. 218:1273–1280, 1970.

47. Weston, R. E., Grossman, J., Boron, E. R., and Hanenson, I. B. Pathogenesis and treatment of hyponatremia in congestive heart failure. Am. J. Med. 25:558–572, 1958.

48. Humphries, J. O., Hinman, E. W., Bernstein, L., and Walker, W. G. Effect of artificial pacing of the heart on cardiac and renal function. Circulation 36:717–723, 1967.

49. Orloff, J., Walser, M., Kennedy, T. J., and Bartter, F. C. Hyponatremia. Circulation 19:284–299, 1959.

50. Neuman, W. F. and Neuman, M. W. Nature of mineral phase of bone. Chem. Rev. 53:1–45, 1953.

51. Forbes, G. B. and Lewis, A. M. Total sodium, potassium and chloride in adult man. J. Clin. Invest. 35:596–600, 1956.

52. Winters, R., Whitlock, R. T., DeWalt, J. L., and Welt, L. G. Effect of alterations of sodium concentration of serum upon content of sodium in bone. Am. J. Physiol. 195:697–701, 1958.

53. Edelman, I. S. Symposium: water and electrolytes: pathogenesis of hyponatremia: physiologic and therapeutic implications. Metabolism 5:500–507, 1956.

54. Maffly, R. H. and Edelman, I. S. Role of sodium, potassium and water in hypoosmotic states of heart failure. Progr. Cardiovas. Dis. 4:88–104, 1961.

55. Earley, L. E. and Sanders, C. A. Effect of changing serum osmolality on release of antidiuretic hormone in certain patients with decompensated cirrhosis of liver and low serum osmolality. J. Clin. Invest. 38:545–550, 1959.

56. Kerpel-Fronius, E. Uber die Beziehungen zwischen Salz- und Wasserhaushalt bei experimentellen Wasservelusten. Ztschr. f. Kinderh. 57:489–504, 1935.

57. Darrow, D. C. and Yannet, H. Changes in distribution of body water accompanying increase and decrease in extracellular electrolyte. J. Clin. Invest. 14:266–275, 1935.

58. Nadal, J., Peterson, S., and Maddock, W. Comparison between dehydration from salt loss and from water deprivation. J. Clin. Invest. 20:691–703, 1941.

59. Leaf, A. and Newburgh, L. H. Significance of the body fluids in clinical medicine, 2nd ed. Charles C Thomas, Springfield, Illinois, 1955, pp. 1–72.

60. Leaf, A. The clinical and physiologic significance of the serum sodium concentration. New Eng. J. Med. 267:24–30, 77–83, 1962.

61. Cohen, J. J., Hulter, H. N., Smithline, N., Melby, J. C., and Schwartz, W. B. The critical role of the adrenal gland in the renal regulation of acid-base equilibrium during chronic hypotonic expansion. J. Clin. Invest. 58:1201–1208, 1972.

62. Robertson, G. L., Shelton, R. L., and Athar, S. The osmoregulation of vasopressin. Kidney Int. 10:25–37, 1976.

63. Gauer, O. H. and Henry, J. Neurohormonal control of plasma volume. Int. Rev. Physiol. 9:145–190, 1976.

64. DeFronzo, R. A., Goldberg, M., and Agus, Z. S. Normal diluting capacity in hyponatremic patients. Ann. Int. Med. 84:538–542, 1976.

65. Forrest, Jr., J. N., Cox, M., Hong, C., Morrison, G., Bia, M., and Singer, I. Superiority of demeclocycline over lithium in the treatment of chronic syndrome of inappropriate secretion of antidiuretic hormone. N. Eng. J. Med. 298:173–177, 1978.

11

Calcium, Magnesium, and Phosphate

About 99% of the calcium, 85% of the phosphate, and 50% of the magnesium in the body are in bone. Because of their prevalence in bone, calcium and phosphorus comprise 1.9% and 1.0% of total body weight, respectively. The magnesium content of the body is only about 0.05% of body weight. The purpose of this chapter is to deal, not with bone formation and metabolism, but rather with the distribution of the nonosseous portion of these ions and their excretion by the kidneys.

CALCIUM IN BODY FLUIDS

In man the concentration of ionized calcium is normally about 5 mg/dl of extracellular fluid or 1.25 mM. Normal serum total calcium concentration in man is 10 mg/dl plasma (8.5 to 10.5 mg/dl or 2.0 to 2.5 mM are the usual accepted normal range). Of this concentration about 50% is ionized, 40% is bound to serum proteins, chiefly albumin, and 5–10% is complexed with citrate and other organic anions so that it is nonionized, but ultrafiltrable. This is shown in Table 11-1 (1). The most constant moiety is the ionized calcium, whose level is normally precisely controlled and expresses the chemical activity of

247

TABLE 11-1   *The State of Calcium in 100 ml of Normal Serum (in mg)*

TOTAL CALCIUM				10.0
I. Nonfiltrable			3.5	
A. Albumin		2.8		
B. Globulin		0.7		
II. Filtrable			6.5	
A. Calcium ion		5.3		
B. Complexes		1.2		
1. Bicarbonate	0.6			
2. Citrate	0.3			
3. Phosphate	0.2			
4. Others	?			

Reproduced from (1) with permission of *American Journal of Medicine*.

calcium. It is this chemical activity of calcium in the body fluids on which many vital bodily functions depend. The ionized calcium is thus the physiologically important and carefully controlled fraction of total serum calcium concentration.

By contrast, the portion that is protein bound may vary greatly, depending on the concentration of serum proteins. Normally, the largest amount is bound to albumin. In diseases such as multiple myeloma that are often characterized by elevated levels of serum protein, the total serum calcium concentration may be elevated while ionized calcium levels are maintained normally. Perhaps the extreme example of protein-bound calcium occurs in the hen. To transport the large quantities of calcium necessary for the egg shell, an estrogen-induced, calcium-binding protein, phosvitin, is added to the serum of the hen as she deposits the shell around the egg she is about to lay. Very high total serum calcium levels are attained while the ionized moiety still retains a normal concentration.

Because of the presence of citrate, amino acids, and other organic anions in the extracellular fluids a small portion of circulating calcium is complexed, nonionized but soluble, and ultrafiltrable.

Because calcium is a strongly positive ion, it binds tightly to anions, and being divalent, it has the ability to cross-link two separate negative charges. Because of these chemical properties it serves as an important molecular "glue" holding molecules, cell membranes, and cells together. In the absence of Ca^{++} cell membranes become leaky;

tight intercellular junctures come undone. By linking together negative phosphate groups in adjacent phospholipid molecules, calcium stabilizes lipid membranes and reduces their permeability (2); presumably the same occurs in cell membranes. It competes with sodium for entry sites in nerve membranes and controls the gating of sodium fluxes across the nerve cell membranes that constitute the conduction of the nerve impulse (3). Thus the integrity of neuromuscular function is critically dependent on the concentration of ionized calcium in the extracellular fluids and accounts for the need to regulate this concentration precisely. The concentration of calcium ions seems to determine the threshold potential of excitable tissues (see Figure 5-2, page 119). A high ionized calcium concentration in the serum reduces neuromuscular irritability, whereas a low calcium concentration in the serum has the opposite effect.

An elevated level of ionized calcium (as may occur in hyperparathyroidism, or with malignancy metastatic to bone) affects neuromuscular irritability and also affects autonomic functions, causing constipation and later dulling of the sensorium with coma at very high concentrations. Clinically more common and more dramatic are the signs of low concentrations of ionized calcium. Annoying spontaneous muscle cramps may accompany minor reductions; tetany and generalized tonic and clonic seizures develop with more severe reductions in concentration of this ion.

Evidence of hypocalcemia may be elicited by simple bedside tests. Tapping with a finger over the supramandibular portion of the parotid gland causes spasm in the muscles innervated by the 7th, or facial, nerve. The examiner carefully observes the upper lip of the patient. In the presence of low ionized calcium, such tapping provokes twitches in the upper lip on the side of the stimulation. This is the so-called Chvostek's sign. Some normal persons without hypocalcemia, however, exhibit a positive response, and many persons with hypocalcemia have negative responses.

Another, somewhat more specific, test is that of Trousseau. In this test a blood pressure cuff is inflated around the upper arm of the subject and maintained until carpopedal spasm develops (flexion contraction of wrist and metacarpophalangeal joints with fingers held straight and grouped with tips together, the so-called *main d'accoucheur*). If no carpopedal spasm develops in 3 minutes of ischemia, the test is regarded as negative. If no carpopedal spasm occurs, the cuff is removed and the subject asked to take about 30 deep breaths in a minute. The resulting slight respiratory alkalosis is likely to elicit carpopedal spasm in the hypocalcemic individual when the Trousseau test alone was negative.

Both alkalosis and hypocalcemia may give a positive Trousseau test. The effect of the tourniquet or blood pressure cuff is not to cause ischemia to the arm as was once assumed, but directly to irritate the underlying motor nerve by pressure. This can be simply shown by using two cuffs or tourniquets, one above the other on the upper arm. If the upper cuff is inflated first and pressure maintained until carpopedal spasm occurs, inflation of the lower cuff and removal of the more proximal one results in relaxation of the muscle of the arm and hand, even though ischemia is sustained.

Erb's test examines the electrical excitability of peripheral motor nerves by measuring the twitch threshold for galvanic stimulation; in hypocalcemia stimulation is elicited by a weaker current than is required in the normal person.

Tetany may be life threatening if the laryngeal or respiratory muscles are affected. Biliary colic and broncospasm are occasional visceral manifestations of hypocalcemia. In the presence of hypocalcemia many seemingly unrelated factors may elicit tetany. Pressure on nerves, which can occur on crossing the legs, excitement, or activity that may be associated with respiratory alkalosis as well as an elevated serum potassium may evoke tetany in the hypocalcemic subject.

The role of potassium has been mentioned. Occasionally a patient with a malabsorption syndrome presents with very low serum concentrations of both calcium and potassium but without neuromuscular symptoms. Replacement of potassium without correction of the associated hypocalcemia is likely to cause tetany. Conversely, administration of calcium to a hyperkalemic subject ameliorates the disturbance in the neuromuscular system due to the high serum potassium concentration, and potassium administered in the presence of hypercalcemia is likewise beneficial, especially to the critical conduction system in the heart. Thus a low calcium ion concentration in extracellular fluid increases the excitability of motor nerve fibers and lowers the threshold of sensory nerve receptors to excitation—an effect that is antagonized by low potassium, but also by high magnesium.

Calcium is inhibitory to adenylate cyclase and thus opposes the actions of various peptide hormones when its concentration is elevated. Hypercalcemia is, however, itself a stimulus for gastric acid secretion and thus may be associated with peptic ulcer disease. This raises questions regarding the use of calcium carbonate or other antacids containing calcium in the treatment of hyperchlorhydria.

Hypercalcemia, especially in the presence of normal or elevated concentrations of phosphates, entails the likelihood of metastatic calcification's affecting the extraosseous soft tissue. Calcification occurs earliest in the more alkaline areas of the body. There are alkaline sites on the contraluminal side of acid-secreting epithelia: gastric mucosa, renal tubules, alveoli of lung. In these tissues metastatic calcification may quickly develop, but periarticular soft tissues are also the site of amorphous deposits of calcium salts—true bone formation does not occur, and the calcium deposits are gradually reabsorbed from such deposits once the hypercalcemia is corrected.

The cornea of the eye is another place where metastatic calcification occurs in hypercalcemia. Usually, the calcium crystals deposited in the cornea are visible only by examination with the slit lamp. If extensive, however, the deposits may be visible to the naked eye as a band keratopathy. This consists of semilunar whitish bands, forming "parentheses" at the lateral margins of the cornea that do not extend over the upper and lower poles of the cornea, which are normally covered by the eyelids. Since the cornea is avascular, solutes diffuse into it from the circumferential limbal blood vessels. But the cornea is covered by a moist mucous membrane through which carbon dioxide readily escapes, leaving a slightly alkaline interstitial fluid in the cornea. Calcium diffuses into this alkaline interstitium and is precipitated in the characteristic limbal arc of band keratopathy. The eyelids prevent loss of carbon dioxide from the upper and lower margins of the cornea, which they normally cover, and no calcium salts deposit there (4).

Cells are held together in tissues by calcium. Most methods of separating cells in tissues depend on reducing the concentration of extracellular calcium ions either by incubating the tissue in a calcium-free medium or by adding ethylene diamine tetraacetic acid (EDTA) or some other chelating agent that reacts with calcium to lower its ionic concentration drastically. Calcium is important in the electrical coupling of adjacent cells via the intercellular junctions (5). Within cells calcium ions are very toxic because of their ability to bind to negative sites. They interfere with the action of many enzymes, bind nucleic acids, and uncouple oxidative metabolism. Nevertheless, at the appropriate low concentration maintained within the cells, calcium is not only tolerated but also necessary for vital activities. Intracellular calcium is essential to the coupling of electrical or chemical excitation to electrical, contractile, or secretory responses.

The intracellular concentration of calcium is of the order of 10^{-5} to 10^{-7} M (10 to 0.1 μM), as compared with its concentration in extracellular fluids of some 10^{-3} M (1.0 mM). The details of how cells maintain such low intracellular concentrations of calcium are not understood. The mechanism for the active transport of calcium out of the cell is unknown, but calcium must be transported up large electrical and chemical gradients from cell interior to extracellular fluids. In red blood cells there is evidence for a Ca-sensitive Mg-ATPase involved in the active extrusion of cellular calcium. There is also evidence that such a transport ATPase exists in kidney cells (49). Some excitable tissues have been found to possess a Ca/Na exchange mechanism by which sodium entering the cell is coupled to extrusion of calcium (37). This mechanism has been suggested for other cells also.

The major regulation of intracellular calcium concentration, however, is most likely the intracellular organelles, especially the mitochondria (38). Calcium is actively transported from the cytosol to the mitochondrial matrix, and roughly half of the intracellular calcium is found in the mitochondria. Isolated mitochondria can lower the free calcium concentration of their bathing medium to 10^{-6} to 10^{-7} M. Calcium transport into the matrix of the mitochondria is probably driven by the active ejection of protons from the mitochondria. In the presence of permeable anions, isolated kidney mitochondria can accumulate calcium at rates that greatly exceed the rate of calcium transport across the plasma membranes. A further large pool of intracellular calcium is bound to other cellular components: proteins, nuclei, membranes, and endoplasmic reticulum. It is the release and uptake of calcium by intracellular organelles, rather than the traffic of calcium across plasma membranes, that determine the concentration of free calcium in the cytosol.

Calcium effects muscular contraction. Movement of calcium from specific binding sites in the sarcoplasmic reticulum to actinomyosin is believed to initiate muscular contraction; removal of the calcium from the actinomyosin and its reaccumulation in the sarcoplasmic reticulum result in relaxation (6). There is a calcium-activated adenosine triphosphatase in muscle that is believed to play a role in the excitation–contraction coupling mediated by calcium. Calcium is required for the appropriate response to excitation in many tissues. A rise in free calcium ion concentration within cells inhibits intercellular electrical coupling (5).

INTESTINAL ABSORPTION OF CALCIUM

The concentration of calcium ions in the extracellular fluids depends on the delicate balance maintained by uptake of calcium from the gut and deposition in bone or excretion via kidneys or gut.

The usual American diet includes close to 1 gm of calcium each day—the amount in a quart of milk. Exclusion of dairy products from the diet lowers the daily intake of calcium to about 200 mg. The major portion—about 75–85%—of ingested calcium is excreted in the feces; the remainder appears in the urine if the subject is in calcium balance. Intestinal absorption is not linearly proportional to calcium intake but shows "saturation" kinetics, that is, it rises steeply at low levels of intake but the rate of increase diminishes as the amount ingested increases. This is shown in Figure 11-1 (1) in which the urinary excretion reflects the kinetics of calcium absorption from the intestine. Note that there is a large variation in the individual absorption (urinary excretion) rates. Urinary excretion is less than 300 mg of calcium per day in 85–90% of normal adults. Furthermore, within the same individual the absorption can be modified according to physiologic states. Calcium deprivation results in a more efficient absorption of ingested calcium. This is a slow adaptation, dependent on the presence of vitamin D.

Calcium absorption takes place in the proximal regions of the small intestine, largely in the duodenum. Calcium secretion as well as absorption has been demonstrated. The absorption of calcium is dependent on the presence of vitamin D, which is now known to possess the characteristics of a hormone rather than a dietary constituent (7, 8, 9). Under the influence of ultraviolet light, 7-dehydrocholesterol in the skin is converted first to precholecalciferol that in turn is thermally converted slowly to cholecalciferol (vitamin D_3), or the latter may be ingested as vitamin D. In the liver microsomes and mitochondria the cholecalciferol is enzymatically hydroxylated to form 25-hydroxycholecalciferol ($25\text{-}(OH)D_3$). This 25-hydroxylase reaction in

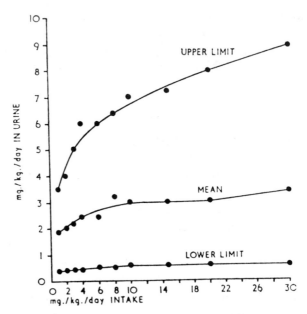

Fig. 11-1 Relation between urinary and dietary calcium in normal subjects, from data of Knapp (19). Note the minimal further increase of urinary calcium with increase of dietary intake levels of calcium. Reproduced from (1) with permission of the *American Journal of Medicine.*

the liver is not influenced by concentrations of calcium or phosphate in body fluids.

The 25-(OH)D₃ has very little physiologic activity until it undergoes a further hydroxylation. This is accomplished by a 1α-hydroxylase, a mitochondrial enzyme restricted to the kidney. The resultant 1α,25-dihydroxycholecalciferol (1,25-(OH)₂D₃) is the active form of the hormone. Details of the control of its synthesis are under investigation.

It seems that parathyroid hormone (PTH) turns on production of the 1,25-(OH)₂D₃ so that with hypocalcemia 1,25-(OH)₂D₃ is synthesized in the kidney. But 1,25-(OH)₂D₃ in turn activates a 24-hydroxylase, also in the kidney, to produce an alternative product, 24,25-dihydroxycholecalciferol. Production of the 24,25-(OH)₂D₃ occurs at serum calcium concentrations above 9.5 mg/dl in the presence of adequate amounts of phosphate and vitamin D₃. There is controversy regarding a possible role for the 24,25-(OH)₂D₃ in the expression of vitamin D action. The same may be said for another product, 1α,24,25-(OH)₃D₃, which arises from the introduction of the 24-hydroxyl into the $1\alpha,25$-$(OH)_2D_3$.

Thus the correction of hypocalcemia by $1,25$-$(OH)_2D_3$ and PTH shuts off PTH and switches further hydroxylation of 25-$(OH)_2D_3$ from the 1α-position to the 24-position. Conversely, a fall in the serum calcium concentration turns on PTH, which restores activity of the 1α-hydroxylase in the kidney and turns off the 24-hydroxylase.

A low serum phosphate concentration produced by PTH excess or by phosphate deprivation stimulates the production of $1,25$-$(OH)_2D_3$ by enhancing the activity of 1α-hydroxylase of the kidney. It may be the level of phosphate in renal tubule cells that controls the activity of 1α-hydroxylase. Both phosphate depletion and parathyroid hormone excess may act through a common pathway, low renal cellular phosphate levels, to stimulate production of $1,25$-$(OH)_2D_3$. Low serum calcium concentrations also stimulate formation of $1,25$-$(OH)_2D_3$, but this effect is thought to be secondary to its stimulation of PTH secretion.

The adaptation of intestinal absorption of calcium to a low calcium intake mentioned earlier, probably occurs as a result of the increased synthesis of $1,25$-$(OH)_2D_3$ stimulated by the low calcium intake. Administering excess $1,25$-$(OH)_2D_3$ increases calcium absorption from a low calcium dietary intake and abolishes further adaptation.

In summary, low serum phosphate, or phosphate depletion, increases activity of the 1α-hydroxylase of the kidney directly. Hypocalcemia has a similar, but indirect, effect on the renal enzyme. By its well know action of stimulating PTH secretion, hypocalcemia also increases the renal 1α-hydroxylase. The resulting increase of $1,25$-$(OH)_2D_3$ enhances intestinal absorption of calcium and phosphate and, with PTH, mobilizes these ions from bone. The overall effect is to raise serum calcium and phosphate levels which in turn shut down PTH and $1,25$-$(OH)D_3$ production. It is this feedback regulation of its metabolism that justifies the application of the term "hormone" to vitamin D (39). Whether $1,25$-$(OH)_2D_3$ has direct effects on renal handling of calcium or phosphate independent of PTH or of the changes in serum calcium and phosphate induced by its action on the intestines, has not yet been established. The full effects of PTH on bone and on the kidney, however, require the presence of adequate levels of $1,25$-$(OH)_2D_3$. It is the failure of the 1α-hydroxylation in severe renal disease that causes the vitamin D-resistant malabsorption of calcium from the intestine and bones, long recognized as a feature of chronic renal failure.

Renal disease can alter the metabolism of vitamin D by a second mechanism in the nephrotic syndrome. When proteinuria in this condition is massive, urinary losses of the vitamin D binding protein, which normally transports the vitamin in the circulation, can deplete 25-(OH)D_3 and thus produce a state of hypovitaminosis D (40).

How vitamin D acts to promote intestinal absorption of calcium remains unclear. It has been demonstrated that rachitic chicks given small amounts of vitamin D synthesize large amounts of a calcium-binding protein that Wasserman has isolated from their intestinal mucosa (10). But there have been aspects of calcium absorption that are difficult to explain solely on the basis of the induction of a calcium-binding protein that acts as a carrier for transepithelial transport of calcium in the duodenum. There is a calcium-activated adenosine triphosphatase in the intestinal mucosa, whose activity appears to be enhanced by vitamin D (11, 12), and by analogy with the Na, K-dependent ATPase, may be involved in intestinal transport, since this transport can occur "uphill" from intestinal lumen to body fluids and thus be an active, energy-requiring process.

Adrenal corticosteroids are able to antagonize the action of vitamin D on calcium absorption from the intestine. A curious excessive intestinal absorption of calcium occurs in sarcoidosis, which may be linked to increased 1,25-(OH)$_2$D$_3$ (41). Adrenal glucocorticosteroids inhibit this vitamin D activity in sarcoidosis.

Parathyroid hormone probably does not exert direct effects on intestinal absorption of calcium. In man hypoparathyroidism reduces the fraction of ingested calcium that is absorbed and hyperparathyroidism increases it. This is the opposite effect from what might have been anticipated purely on the serum calcium concentrations in the two states—low in hypoparathyroidism and elevated in hyperparathyroidism. Furthermore, low dietary calcium stimulates parathyroid hormone secretion, and high calcium intake reduces parathyroid activity. It is likely that parathyroid hormone exerts these effects on intestinal absorption via its known role in the production of 1,25-(OH)$_2$D$_3$ in the kidneys.

The deposition and resorption of calcium from bone depend on many factors. The ionic composition of the interstitial fluid bathing the surface of bone is important, particularly the concentrations of calcium and phosphate, but hydrogen ions and probably other ions have an influence. Parathyroid hormone increases the turnover rate of calcium in bone and, with $1,25-(OH)_2D_3$, facilitates release of calcium, whereas calcitonin has as its major action an inhibition of bone resorption. Physical stress plays a role in maintaining mineralization. Adrenal corticosteroids demineralize bone, and sex hormones may have the opposite effect. The purpose of this chapter is not to consider the very complex regulation of bone mineralization but only to indicate that bone constitutes a major reservoir of calcium that is available to buffer the concentration of ionized calcium in body fluids; the release from bone to, or removal from, extracellular fluids is subject to numerous controls.

URINARY EXCRETION OF CALCIUM

Renal handling of calcium is also subject to several interrelated controls. One factor determining urinary excretion is the quantity of calcium filtered through the glomeruli. Only ionized and soluble-complexed calcium is filtered. If the serum calcium concentration falls to 7.5 mg/dl or less with normal serum proteins, calcium virtually disappears from the urine. Reductions in glomerular filtration rate, both acute and chronic, diminish renal calcium clearance. Urinary calcium falls with progressive loss of renal tissue in hyperparathyroidism or the milk–alkali syndrome in spite of persistent high serum levels of ionized calcium in these conditions.

Of the approximately 10 gm of calcium filtered through the glomeruli daily about 98% is reabsorbed. Most of the calcium (65 to 75%), like sodium, is reabsorbed in the proximal tubule, 20–25% is reabsorbed in the loop of Henle, 10% in the distal convolution, and most of the remainder in the collecting duct, as determined by micropuncture studies in the rat (13). The concentration of calcium in luminal fluid of the proximal tubule remains unchanged from the ultrafiltrate of plasma, indicating that, again like sodium, calcium is absorbed with water in the same proportion that exists in the glomerular filtrate. With the poorly reabsorbable solute, mannitol, retarding water reabsorption in the proximal tubule, the concentration of calcium may fall to 20–30% of its ionic concentration in plasma, implying an active transport mechanism for calcium reabsorption in the proximal tubule. Further active reabsorption of calcium occurs in the distal nephron. There is a gradient of calcium concentration increasing from cortex to medulla, presumably consequent to active reabsorption of calcium by the ascending limb of Henle's loop and trapping of calcium in the medullary interstitium by the countercurrent system there. This reabsorption of calcium in the ascending limb of the loop of Henle reduces its concentration in the distal tubule to approximately 60% of the ionized calcium of plasma, again mimicking the handling of sodium.

The striking similarities in the handling of calcium and sodium in the nephron suggest that they may share a common transport pathway. Little is known, however, regarding the mechanism of calcium transport in the kidney. The sodium, potassium-activated adenosine triphosphatase, which is believed to be an integral part of the active transport mechanism, is actually inhibited by calcium ions, so that calcium does not share this step in active sodium transport. Under usual circumstances calcium excretion follows sodium excretion: high rates of sodium excretion are associated with high rates of calcium, and low rates of sodium excretion reduce calcium excretion (14). It is in the proximal tubule that sodium and calcium are most closely linked. An acute expansion of extracellular fluid volume with saline reduces fractional calcium as well as sodium reabsorption in the proximal tubule, leading to a large excretion of both ions (15).

Administration of most diuretics results initially in an increased excretion of both sodium and calcium. Continued administration of a diuretic such as chlorothiazide results in a state of mild salt depletion and slightly reduced extracellular volume. This results in nearly total reabsorption of calcium while the diuretic sustains blockage of sufficient sodium reabsorption to maintain sodium balance in the mildly salt-depleted state. Hypercalcemia may ensue from chronic thiazide diuretic usage. It is probably in the proximal tubule that changes in extracellular fluid volume affect parallel alterations in sodium and calcium excretion.

Dissociation of rates of sodium and calcium excretion have also been achieved by manipulating distal reabsorption with mineralocorticoids that affect sodium but not calcium reabsorption (16). Acute administration of desoxycorticosterone causes an abrupt decrease in sodium excretion, owing to the stimulation of distal sodium reabsorption, but without affecting calcium excretion. With the expansion of extracellular fluid volume that ensues as salt intake and desoxycorticosterone administration are continued, proximal tubular reabsorption is inhibited by hemodynamic influences (17). Sodium excretion rises to control levels as a result of diminished proximal and enhanced distal absorption to achieve a new steady state. Calcium excretion remains markedly elevated, however, since the decreased proximal reabsorption is not counterbalanced by increased distal reabsorption, as is the case for sodium.

Hypercalciuria is the expected finding in primary hyperparathyroidism despite the action of the hormone to increase tubular reabsorption of calcium. The consequence of continued excessive parathyroid hormone (PTH) activity on bone is to elevate serum calcium and this ultimately increases urinary calcium excretion despite the continued stimulus for calcium reabsorption. Enhancing calcium reabsorption by PTH in experimental animals apparently occurs both prior to and beyond the distal tubule (42). The effects of parathyroid hormone on responsive kidney tubular cells may be summarized as follows (42): (1) the total calcium content of the cells is increased; (2) calcium influx into the cells and the total cellular calcium exchangeable pool is increased; (3) both cytosolic and mitochondrial pools and their rates of exchange are increased, but the effects are much larger on the mitochondrial pool. These effects can all be replicated by cyclic AMP, which also stimulates efflux of calcium from the cells. The increased efflux of calcium induced by cyclic AMP will occur even in the absence of extracellular calcium. Thus, it seems that PTH, via cyclic AMP, increases the release of calcium from mitochondria, thus elevating cytosolic calcium. In turn, the increased cytosolic concentration of calcium stimulates influx and efflux in and out of the tubular cell. The rate of calcium transport across the plasma membrane appears generally to be regulated by the level of cytosolic calcium; the two increase together. Metabolic and respiratory acidosis and alkalosis affect calcium excretion via effects on intracellular pH, which in turn alters cytosolic calcium concentrations. Alkalosis increases cytosolic calcium levels and enhances tubular reabsorption of calcium, while acidosis increases calcium excretion (38). The fall in serum concentration in hypoparathyroidism likewise decreases urinary calcium excretion, despite absence of the PTH-dependent stimulus for calcium reabsorption. Generally, calcium disappears from the urine at serum concentrations less than 7.5 mg/dl.

Many other factors affect calcium excretion. Reduced urinary calcium excretion is of no clinical significance except that it may indicate underlying pathology. Any reduction of glomerular filtration rate or of serum calcium concentration reduces urinary calcium excretion. The latter accompanies vitamin D deficiency, inadequate calcium intake, malabsorption syndromes, and hypoparathyroidism—all conditions that reduce gastrointestinal absorption of calcium or mobilization of calcium from bone. Acute binding of serum calcium by free fatty acids may occur in acute pancreatitis as lipases hydrolyze depot triglycerides. Some snake venoms have similar effects.

Factors causing hypercalciuria are listed in Table 11-2 (1). Hypercalciuria is important in its own right, in addition to indicating often serious underlying pathology. Hypercalciuria increases the risk of renal calculi; at least 90% of all renal stones in man contain calcium as a major constituent. Calcium oxalate stones are the most common, but calcium phosphate and stones of mixed composition occur. Hypercalciuria is not a requirement for stone formation; it occurs only in about one-third of patients who are stone formers, but the majority of these have "idiopathic hypercalciuria." In this condition more than 300 mg of calcium are excreted in the urine daily when the subjects are ingesting usual levels of calcium—from 800–1000 mg.

Although the term "idiopathic hypercalciuria" was originally coined by Albright to describe patients with normocalcemic hypercalciuria

TABLE 11-2   *Causes of Hypercalciuria*

DISSOLUTION OF BONE

Hyperparathyroidism
Metastatic cancer
Multiple myeloma
Excess adrenal glucocorticoids
Immobilization
Hyperthyroidism
Renal tubular acidosis
Phosphate depletion

EXCESSIVE ABSORPTION OF CALCIUM

High calcium intake
Vitamin D intoxication
Sarcoidosis and berylliosis
"Idiopathic" hypercalciuria*

---

* This category may also include some individuals with defective tubular reabsorption of calcium. Adapted from (1) with permission of the *American Journal of Medicine.*

and a tendency to hypophosphatemia, three pathogenic mechanisms are now recognized to cause this condition (43). These are: (1) a primary intestinal hyperabsorption of calcium, (2) a primary renal loss or "leak" of calcium, and (3) a subtle primary hyperparathyroidism with normocalcemia or only intermittent hypercalcemia.

"Absorptive" hypercalciuria is associated with increased intestinal absorption of calcium, with at least postprandial suppression of parathyroid function and spillage of the absorbed load of calcium into the urine. Some of these patients have a primary renal "leak" of phosphate, the resulting hypophosphatemia or phosphate depletion enhances $1,25\text{-}(OH)_2D_3$ synthesis which then accounts for the increased intestinal absorption of calcium.

"Renal" hypercalciuria is associated with a defect in renal tubular calcium reabsorption. The resulting decreased serum calcium concentration results in secondary hyperparathyroidism. This in turn promotes hypophosphatemia which, with increased PTH, stimulates $1,25\text{-}(OH)_2D_3$ synthesis and calcium absorption.

"Subtle hyperparathyroidism" is a primary hyperparathyroidism. The increased PTH results in hypophosphatemia and increases in $1,25\text{-}(OH)_2D_3$ synthesis. The latter enhances calcium absorption and the mobilization of calcium from bone so that mild hypercalcemia or at least intermittent hypercalcemia may be expected.

A calcium tolerance test has been proposed to distinguish between these three main causes of idiopathic hypercalciuria (43). Following a 7 to 10 day period of a low calcium intake (~400 mg per day), the response to a standard oral dose of calcium (1000 mg) is observed. The resulting calciuric response provides an index of calcium tolerance, and the parathyroidal response an index of parathyroid suppressibility. All three groups will show hypercalciuria in response to the calcium load (> 0.2 mg/dl of GFR). The "absorptive" hypercalciuric subjects will exhibit only a modest increase in serum calcium within the normal range (< 10.5 mg/dl) and suppress PTH secretion. Subjects with "renal" hypercalciuria will have the lowest serum calcium concentrations before and after the calcium challenge and will minimally but appropriately suppress PTH. Subjects with subtle hyperparathyroidism will exhibit intolerance to the high calcium intake, exhibiting elevation of serum calcium concentrations above 10.5 mg/dl without significant suppression of PTH despite the hypercalcemia.

Other causes of hypercalciuria most frequently found in patients with kidney stones include frank hyperparathyroidism, renal tubular acidosis, and excessive ingestion of calcium especially if combined with low fluid intake and an alkaline urine.

There is a diurnal variation in calcium excretion; more is excreted during the day. This is fortunate, since the urine is more concentrated during the night. The increased calcium excretion during the day seems to be caused by the effects of glucose and protein in the diet (18, 19). Metabolic acidosis increases urinary calcium, probably by bone dissolution (20). The hypercalciuria, associated with hyperparathyroidism and hyperadrenocorticism, is also secondary to bone dissolution. Very high rates of urinary calcium excretion may accompany thyrotoxicosis (21), but only rarely is this a cause of hypercalcemia. Calcium excretion tends to vary inversely with phosphate intake. This effect is due to enhanced deposition of calcium in bone and not to reduced calcium absorption in the intestines. In addition, excessive calcium intake increases urinary calcium, probably through a slight increase in serum calcium with reduced secretion of parathyroid hormone. The response is not striking, as shown in Figure 11-1, for the increment in calcium excretion decreases progressively as dietary calcium increases.

Other factors besides urinary calcium concentration are important in stone formation. Normally, urine contains citrate and other chelators of calcium that inhibit precipitation of calcium salts, even in urines supersaturated with respect to calcium salts. There may be factors in normal urine, as yet undetermined, that inhibit crystal formation and growth. Absence or decreases in such factors, which may occur with urinary tract infections or stasis, allow deposition of calcium salts, even in the absence of hypercalciuria. Increased urinary oxalate due to dietary intake or endogenous production may be responsible for stone formation. The extreme of this condition is primary hyperoxaluria, a genetic inborn error of metabolism, in which renal failure from calcium oxalate deposits in the kidney occurs at an early age (22). But pyridoxine (vitamin B_6) deficiency and inflammatory bowel disease with excessive bacterial conversion of bile salt glycine to oxalate may also increase oxalate excretion or enhance intestinal absorption of ingested oxalate.

CALCIUM NEPHROPATHY

Experimental hypercalcemia decreases sodium reabsorption from both the proximal and distal tubules and impairs renal concentrating ability. Thus polyuria and sodium depletion may accompany hypercalcemia irrespective of cause. These functional effects of calcium are the result of the general action of calcium to tighten membranes and reduce their permeability and of its inhibitory effect on vasopressin-responsive adenylate cyclase. But calcium is inhibitory to several key enzymes involved in energy metabolism: phosphofructokinase, pyruvic kinase, and pyruvic carboxylase (23), as well as to the Na,K-adenosine triphosphatase essential for active sodium transport (24). The loss of concentrating ability with calcium excess is most likely the result of failure of the kidney to produce a hypertonic medullary interstitium, owing to interference with sodium transport rather than to inhibition of the action of antidiuretic hormone on its adenylate cyclase (25, 26). The latter probably requires higher calcium ion concentrations than even those attained in most instances of hypercalcemia.

With excessive passage of calcium through the nephrons, deposition of calcium occurs. This occurs earliest and is most pronounced in the medulla and collecting ducts, where the urine is most concentrated and calcium attains its highest concentration. But thickening of the basement membranes of proximal tubules occurs, and later all zones of the kidneys are affected.

Deposits of calcified cellular debris originally obstruct the lumen of the collecting duct, producing intrarenal hydronephrosis, dilatation of tubules, and reduction in renal function. Such calcification, which was initially extracellular or intratubular, may gradually erode through the tubular epithelium or be covered by regenerating epithelium and become interstitial. Within the renal interstitium these deposits are often treated as foreign bodies evoking inflammatory reactions with fibrosis, scar formation, and distortion of renal architecture extending the impairment of function to neighboring nephrons. Frequently infection occurs in these areas of medullary scarring, and hypertension, with its adverse effects on renal vasculature, contributes to the impairment of renal function.

Though hypercalcemia may produce a nephropathy in which intrarenal calcification may be visible radiologically as discrete calculi or as stippled flecks of radiopaque material within the medulla, usually the deposits are too fine to be visualized radiographically, although the calcium content of the kidneys is markedly increased, and at a postmortem the prosector may note a gritty sensation when the kidneys are cut.

Loss of distal nephron functions from such nephrocalcinosis, in addition to compromising concentrating ability, may produce renal tubular acidosis of the distal variety. Primary distal renal tubular acidosis can also produce nephrocalcinosis. In time, renal failure ensues because of reduced glomerular filtration rate. With moderate, longstanding hypercalcemia and hypercalciuria, azotemic renal failure may be the first manifestation of the disturbance in calcium metabolism.

How reversible the renal lesions of calcium nephropathy are after correction of the hypercalcemia depends on the degree of scarring in the interstitium of the kidneys. If irreversible scars have not become too prevalent, then gradual improvement in renal function may be expected. If general distortion of renal architecture is present, improvement may not appear or progression of renal failure may even continue after the disorder of calcium metabolism is corrected.

When the serum calcium becomes very elevated, as may occur in severe hyperparathyroidism, vitamin D intoxication, metastatic bone disease, or Paget's disease of bone with immobilization, acute hypercalcemic crisis may supervene. This occurs only at serum calcium concentrations above 15 mg/dl. This condition is characterized by a rapid progression from polyuria to dehydration, oliguria, and azotemia; death from renal failure may supervene, or coma and cardiac arrhythmias may be terminal events. Such high serum calcium concentrations thus constitute medical emergencies. Correction of dehydration with saline is the initial need, usually accomplished together with increasing urinary excretion of calcium with calcium-binding agents such as sodium citrate or with diuretics that increase sodium and calcium excretion. Finally, correction of the specific defect responsible for the hypercalcemia, such as vitamin D intoxication or hyperparathyroidism, is mandatory. Adrenal steroids counteract the effects of vitamin D on intestinal absorption and of most metastatic lesions on bone resorption but generally are ineffective in hyperparathyroidism. Administration of inorganic phosphate may help reduce serum calcium levels but should not be used if the serum phosphate is normal or elevated, since it increases metastatic calcium deposits and hastens loss of renal function.

MAGNESIUM

Much less magnesium than calcium is present in bone and much more is intracellular, where it plays an important role as cofactor in many enzyme systems. All adenosine triphosphatases require magnesium. Magnesium is, moreover, required for the synthesis of proteins and nucleic acids. Next to potassium it is the major intracellular cation. It can be taken up by mitochondria by an energy-requiring process, and cell membranes presumably can take up magneisum from its low concentrations in extracellular fluids by similar active transport processes. But the intracellular concentration of free magneisum ions is not known, and intracellularly, much of this divalent cation must be bound electrostatically to polyanions. Muscle contains some 26 mEq of magnesium per liter of intracellular water.

The concentration of magnesium in serum is some 1.5–2.5 mEq/ liter and is not as rigorously regulated as is the case with calcium. During magnesium depletion the serum concentration may be reduced to one-half or even less at a time when only a small portion of total body magnesium has been lost (27). Normally, about 25–35% of plasma magnesium is bound to protein, largely albumin. The remainder is ionized except for a small soluble fraction that is complexed to anions such as citrate, phosphate, and sulfate (28).

Low concentrations of plasma magnesium may occur with starvation or with increased gastrointestinal losses from malabsorption or diarrhea. Magnesium deficiency should be anticipated following extensive intestinal resection (44). Because renal conservation of magnesium is effective, depletion is difficult to produce experimentally in human subjects. Alcohol ingestion is said to increase magnesium excretion in the urine, and chronic alcoholism may lead to magnesium depletion from this effect plus poor intake and increased gastrointestinal losses (29).

Symptoms resulting from magnesium deficiency are referable to neural dysfunction. In man, neuromuscular hyperexcitability with muscular weakness, tremors, athetoid movements, and fasciculations may be seen. Tetany, generalized tonic-clonic or focal seizures, and a positive Chvostek's sign also may be present. Some patients develop irritability, depression, and even psychotic behavior. The peripheral effects of magnesium are to decrease liberation of acetylcholine at the neuromuscular junction and sympathetic ganglia. Thus deficiency of magnesium is associated with an increased neuronal excitability and neuromuscular transmission.

An important consequence of severe hypomagnesemia (< 1.0 mEq/ liter) is hypocalcemia which is resistant to correction so long as the magnesium depletion persists. Positive Chvostek's and Trousseau signs may be present, but the patient may exhibit more prominent clinical evidence of hypocalcemia with carpopedal spasms, tetany, and even seizures. Marked hypocalcemia is found, which is only transiently relieved with supplementary calcium, even when the supplementation is administered intravenously. Correcting the magnesium deficiency returns serum calcium levels to normal. The resistant hypocalcemia in this condition is attributable to deficient parathyroid hormone activity. Hypomagnesemia has been shown to impair secretion of PTH (45), but it may also blunt the peripheral actions of PTH on bone and kidney. The resulting functional PTH deficiency accounts for the resistant hypocalcemia.

Hypermagnesemia is not uncommon in chronic renal failure. It has been found that the concentration of total magnesium was elevated in one-half, and that of ionic magnesium increased in one-third of uremic patients studied in one series (30). Thus, most but not all of the increase is attributable to binding to the retained anions in the serum of uremic subjects.

Symptoms of magnesium excess include retardation of neuromuscular transmission, central nervous system depression with somnolence and coma, peripheral vasodilation with hypotension, and disturbances in cardiac conduction. High magnesium levels block neuromuscular transmission by decreasing the liberation of acetylcholine at neuromuscular junctions. Reflex activity, such as the patellar reflex, is suppressed early, and respiratory failure and coma occur at very high levels, greater than 10 mEq/liter. At these levels direct effects on the heart may also occur with bradycardia, prolonged PR intervals, widening of QRS complexes, and finally, cardiac arrest in diastole (31). These toxic effects of magnesium excess may be reversed by the administration of large amounts of calcium.

Such severe degrees of magnesium intoxication are rarely encountered clinically, but can supervene in patients with severe renal failure who receive antacids or laxatives containing magnesium. Such medications should, therefore, be avoided in markedly azotemic subjects.

Little is known about the mechanisms by which serum levels of magnesium are maintained. The serum magnesium concentration has an effect similar to that of calcium on the secretion of parathyroid hormone, but an efficient feedback control does not exist. Parathyroid hormone is only moderately effective in restoring low magnesium concentrations to normal. It seems that intracellular levels of magnesium are protected at the expense of considerable fluctuations in extracellular fluid concentrations.

Magnesium reabsorption, like that of calcium, is closely linked to sodium reabsorption in the proximal tubule. As described, chronic mineralocorticoid secretion or administration can expand extracellular fluid volume with reduction of proximal tubular reabsorption of magnesium, as well as of calcium, and increased urinary losses of these ions (32). This mechanism probably accounts for the renal magnesium wasting and hypomagnesemia noted in primary aldosteronism.

In magnesium deficiency lesions are seen in the distal tubular epithelium somewhat similar to those found with potassium deficiency and thought to be characterized by an increase in lysosomes (27). Since its salts are generally much more soluble than those of calcium, magnesium does not occur as a constituent of intrarenal deposits or kidney stones except as the complex salt magnesium ammonium phosphate. This crystal occurs only in the presence of highly alkaline urine produced by infection with urea-splitting organisms.

PHOSPHATE

Phosphate, like calcium, is predominantly in bone, but, even more than magnesium, it plays an important role within cells. Phosphate covalently linked to diverse organic compounds constitutes the machinery of life. It is incorporated into labile sugar molecules in energy-producing, intracellular reactions—the final steps of which involve the transfer of phosphate group and energy to nucleotides. The phosphonucleotides are the energy currency of life. But they may also be linked together in sequence to code genetic information into DNA and RNA. Phosphoproteins and phospholipids are also essential intracellular molecules. Phosphorylated compounds within cells are so labile that values for the concentration of free intracellular inorganic phosphate are not reliable.

In the serum, phosphate values in man range from 3.0–4.5 mg of phosphorus*/dl in normal man (1.0–1.5 mM). This value is not regulated precisely, as is ionized calcium, but varies in the same individual with age and with functional state. In growing children values up to

---

* It is conventional to measure inorganic phosphate in serum, but to report the results as milligrams of inorganic phosphorus.

6.0 or 7.0 mg/dl of serum are normal. In any species there is a positive correlation between serum phosphate levels and growth. But a recent meal, glucose, insulin, muscular activity, hyperventilation, and other functional states lower the serum phosphate by increasing cellular uptake of phosphate as sugar phosphates are formed.

High levels of serum inorganic phosphate are deleterious because they promote precipitation of calcium in nonosseous sites. Sustained high levels of serum phosphate as occur in chronic renal failure may depress the serum calcium level to the point at which muscle cramps, tetany, and even seizures occur when the concomitant acidosis is treated.

On the other hand, very low levels of serum phosphate are associated with muscle weakness. This may occur in malabsorption syndromes, rickets, or osteomalacia and dramatically in parenteral hyperalimentation if supplementary phosphate is not supplied to a depleted individual. Knochel (46) emphasized the consequences of severe hypophosphatemia that may occur following acute and chronic alcoholism. During the third to fifth day of hospitalization malnourished, chronic alcoholics given parenteral glucose may have reductions of serum phosphate to less than 1.0 mg/dl. This is associated with weakness; elevation in the serum of muscle enzymes, creatinine phosphokinase, and aldolase; and rhabdomyolysis. The release of myoglobin may be associated with acute renal failure. In the dog, experimental dietary deficiency of phosphate has been shown to depress myocardial performance (47). Depletion of intracellular stores of high-energy phosphate compounds is the probable common feature of the widespread dysfunction associated with phosphate depletion.

Aside from the regulation of serum phosphate that results from uptake and release of phosphate from bone, cells, and gut, the kidneys have an important role in regulating its concentration. Inorganic phosphate is freely filtered at the glomerulus, and a variable amount is then reabsorbed in the proximal tubule. This is an active process, and, as with phosphate uptake in the gut and elsewhere, depends on the presence of sodium. This transport mechanism appears to be subject to saturation, though the limits of reabsorption are not as constant as once believed (33).

Of great importance is that parathyroid hormone inhibits this proximal reabsorption of phosphate. The hormone affects this process by stimulating production of cyclic adenosine monophosphate in cells of the proximal nephron (34). The phosphaturic action of parathyroid hormone occurs within minutes after its administration and results in an increased excretion of phosphate with a rise in renal phosphate clearance as the serum phosphate falls. It is now apparent that parathyroid hormone reduces phosphate reabsorption in the loop of Henle and distal convoluted tubule as well as in the proximal tubule (48).

In hypoparathyroidism serum phosphate rises above normal as its renal clearance falls associated with a reciprocal fall in serum calcium concentration. In hyperparathyroidism, either primary or secondary, the serum phosphate is depressed (less than 3.0 mg/dl) and renal clearance of phosphate is high so long as kidney function is normal. But a large reduction in glomerular filtration rate interferes with the phosphaturic action of parathyroid hormone in regulating the serum phosphate concentration. Thus a normal adult excretes some 500–800 mg of phosphate daily in the urine, depending on the dietary intake. With a normal serum phosphate of 3.5 mg/dl and a glomerular filtration rate of 180 liters/24 hours, he filters some 6000 mg of phosphate/day. Thus, by reabsorbing 90% of filtered phosphate, he can excrete 600 mg, the daily intake. If glomerular filtration rate should fall to only 17 liters/24 hours in our hypothetical subject, then he could excrete the daily intake of 600 mg of phosphate without elevating serum phosphate concentration only by suppressing tubular reabsorption completely. Any further fall in glomerular filtration rate would prevent the excretion of the 600-mg intake in the urine unless an increase in serum phosphate concentration occurs. As serum phosphate rises, serum calcium falls with stimulation of more parathyroid secretion, but the low glomerular filtration rate prevents the physiologic action of the hormone to increase phosphate clearance. In such secondary hyperparathyroidism of renal failure, the hormone continues to have some effects on bone metabolism, although its renal effects are severely blunted or abolished. Even its effects on bone are reduced because of the associated deficiency of $1,25\text{-}(OH)_2D_3$, the active form of vitamin D.

Thus, in practice, reductions of glomerular filtration rate to one-tenth or less of normal cause a fall in the renal clearance of phosphate and a rise in its serum concentration despite maximal effects of parathyroid hormone to depress tubular reabsorption of phosphate. In fact, serum phosphate levels may rise before the glomerular filtration rate is so profoundly depressed; the actual level is, of course, modified by the quantities of phosphate absorbed from the gut. When glomerular filtration rate falls much below 10% of normal, all tubular reabsorption of phosphate stops and the clearance of phosphate becomes equal to that of inulin. The osmotic diuresis, as well as other mechanical factors, and the high concentrations of circulating parathyroid hormone in the uremic subject are together responsible for the cessation of phosphate reabsorption by the renal tubule. When the ingested load of phosphate exceeds the ability of the failing kidney to excrete it, some is excreted into the bowel (35) and some may be precipitated in bone and soft tissues. Total renal phosphate excretion in severe renal failure may drop to one-tenth of the amounts usually excreted. Administration of aluminum hydroxide gels binds intestinal phosphate as insoluble aluminum phosphate and is helpful in reducing serum phosphate levels when the kidneys fail. Overadministration of aluminum hydroxide or carbonate can deplete the body of phosphate, lower serum phosphate below normal, and actually demineralize the skeleton (36), but huge quantities of aluminum gels are required to cause such depletion.

In contrast to the common renal failure in which reduction in glomerular filtration rate dominates the clinical picture, producing the syndrome of azotemic renal failure, there is a group of nephropathies characterized by loss of tubular functions while glomerular filtration is relatively well sustained. The prototype of such conditions is the Fanconi syndrome, in which a variety of pathologic disturbances can result in loss of all proximal tubular functions—cystinosis, heavy metal poisoning, and other proximal tubular toxins. Phosphate wasting is a common feature of such tubular nephropathies, owing to loss of the proximal tubular reabsorptive mechanism. But glucosuria, aminoaciduria, enhanced uric acid clearance, proteinuria of tubular origin, impaired bicarbonate reabsorption, and potassium depletion are also features of this generalized proximal tubular nephropathy. The excessive loss of phosphate in the urine lowers serum phosphate, with interference in mineralization of bone. Rickets develop in childhood and osteomalacia in the adult.

In contrast to the general loss of proximal tubular functions, which characterizes the Fanconi syndrome, there are isolated disturbances as well. An isolated defect in proximal tubular reabsorption results in excessive losses of phosphate analogous to another isolated proximal reabsorptive defect that causes renal glycosuria. Rickets or osteomalacia results that is vitamin D resistant. The pathogenesis of this disturbance has been confusing. It would seem that at least three quite different etiologies might produce a similar clinical picture:

1. Loss of the proximal tubular phosphate reabsorptive mechanism, or congenital failure or absence of some critical component of it, would result in excessive renal clearance of phosphate.

2. A primary, vitamin D-resistant, intestinal defect in the mechanism for intestinal calcium reabsorption would tend to lower the concentration of calcium in serum, which would in turn stimulate parathyroid hormone secretion. A depression in the tubular reabsorption of phosphate would occur and cause a high phosphate clearance.

3. A primary failure or congenital defect of the α-hydroxylase system in the kidney or of the 25-hydroxylase of liver would result in a vitamin D-resistant defect in intestinal absorption of calcium with consequences similar to those indicated.

It is likely that "vitamin D-resistant rickets" includes these and other pathogenic mechanisms. With improved techniques available to measure parathyroid hormone and the various vitamin D metabolities in body fluids this confusing group of hypophosphatemic, hyperphosphaturic disorders is subject to clarification.

References

1. Epstein, F. H. Calcium and the kidney. Am. J .Med. 45:700–714, 1968.
2. Tobias, J. M., Agin, D. P., and Pawlowski, R. Phospholipid-cholesterol membrane model: Control of resistance by ions or current flow. J. Gen. Physiol. 45:989–1001, 1962.
3. Hodgkin, A. L. The Croonian Lecture: Ionic movements and electrical activity in giant nerve fibres. Proc. Royal Soc. (Biol) ser. B. 148:1–37, 1958.
4. Newman, E. V. and Lawrence, A. Respiration, acid secretion and calcium deposition; the eye as a clinical and experimental example. Trans. Assoc. Amer. Physicians 71:85–92, 1958.
5. Loewenstein, W. R. Cell surface membranes in close contact. Role of calcium and magnesium ions. J. Colloid and Interface Sci. 25:34–46, 1967.
6. Davies, R. E. A molecular theory of muscle contraction: calcium-dependent contractions with hydrogen bond formation plus ATP-dependent extensions of part of the myosin-actin cross-bridges. Nature 199:1068–1074, 1963.
7. Omdahl, J. L. and DeLuca, H. F. Regulation of vitamin D metabolism and function. Physiol. Revs. 53:327–372, 1973.
8. DeLuca, H. F. Vitamin D—1973. Am. J. Med. 52:1–12, 1974.
9. Kodicek, E. The story of vitamin D from vitamin to hormone. Lancet 1:325–329, 1974.
10. Wasserman, R. H., Corradino, R. A., and Taylor, A. N. Vitamin D-dependent calcium-binding protein. J. Biol. Chem. 243:3978–3986 and 3987–3993, 1968.

11. Mellancon, M. J. and DeLuca, H. F. Vitamin D stimulation of calcium-dependent adenosine triphosphatase in chicken intestinal brush borders. Biochem. 9:1658–1664, 1970.

12. Hausseler, M. R., Nagode, L. A., and Rasmussen, H. Induction of intestinal brush border alkaline phosphates by vitamin D and identity with calcium-ATP'ase. Nature 228:1199–1201, 1970.

13. Lassiter, W. E., Gottschalk, C. W., and Mylle, M. Micropuncture study of renal tubular reabsorption of calcium in normal rodents. Am. J. Physiol. 204:771–775, 1963.

14. Walser, M. Calcium clearance as a function of sodium clearance in the dog. Am. J. Physiol. 203:1099–1104, 1961.

15. Massry, S. G., Coburn, J. W., Chapman, L. W., and Kleeman, C. R. Effect of NaCl infusion on urinary Ca^{++} and Mg^{++} during reduction in their filtered loads. Am. J. Physiol. 213:1218–1224, 1967.

16. Massry, S. G., Coburn, J. W., Chapman, L. W., and Kleeman, C. R. The acute effect of adrenal steroids on the interrelationship between the renal excretion of sodium, calcium and magnesium. J. Lab. and Clin. Med. 70:563–570, 1967.

17. Earley, L. E. Influence of hemodynamic factors on sodium reabsorption. Ann. N.Y. Acad. Sci. 139:312–327, 1966.

18. Lennon, E. J. and Piering, W. F. A. comparison of the effects of glucose ingestion and NH_4Cl acidosis on urinary calcium and magnesium excretion in man. J. Clin. Invest. 49:1458–1465, 1970.

19. Knapp, E. L. Factors influencing the urinary excretion of calcium: I. In normal persons. J. Clin. Invest. 26:182–200, 1946.

20. Lemann, J., Jr., Litzow, J. R., and Lennon, E. J. Studies of the mechanism by which chronic metabolic acidosis augments urinary calcium excretion in man. J. Clin. Invest. 46:1318–1328, 1967.

21. Krane, S. M., Brownell, G. L., Stanbury, J. B., and Corrigan, H. Effect of thyroid disease on calcium metabolism in man. J. Clin. Invest. 35:874–887, 1956.

22. Smith, L. H., Jr., and Williams, H. E. Kidney stones. In M. B. Strauss and L. G. Welt, eds. Diseases of the kidney, vol. II, 2nd ed. Little Brown and Co., Boston 1971, Chap. 26, pp. 973–996.

23. Bygrave, F. L. The ionic environment and metabolic control. Nature (London) 214:667–671, 1967.

24. Epstein, F. H. and Whittam, R. The mode of inhibition by calcium of cell-membrane adenosine-triphosphatase activity. Biochem. J. 99:232–238, 1966.

25. Manitius, A., Levitin, H., Beck, D., and Epstein, F. H. The mechanism of impairment of renal concentrating ability in hypercalcemia. J. Clin. Invest. 39:693–697, 1960.

26. Bank, N. and Aynedjian, H. S. On the mechanism of hyposthanuria in hypercalcemia. J. Clin. Invest. 44:681–693, 1965.

27. Gitelman, H. J. and Welt, L. G. Magnesium deficiency. Ann Rev. Med. 20:233–242, 1962.

28. Elkinton, J. R. The role of magnesium in the body fluids. Clin. Chem. 3:319–331, 1957.

29. Vallee, B. L., Wacker, W. E. C., and Ulmer, D. D. The magnesium-deficiency tetany syndrome in man. New Eng. J. Med. 262:155–161, 1960.

30. Walser, M. The separate effects of hyperparathyroidism, hypercalcemia of malignancy, renal failure and acidosis on the state of calcium, phosphate and other ions in plasma. J. Clin. Invest. 41:1454–1471, 1962.

31. Smith, P. K., Winkler, A. W., and Hoff, H. E. The pharmacological actions of parenterally administered magnesium salts. Anesthesiology 3:323–329, 1942.

32. Massry, S. G., Coburn, J. W., Chapman, L. W., and Kleeman, C. R. The effect of long-term desoxycorticosterone acetate administration on the renal excretion of calcium and magnesium. J. Lab. Clin. Med. 71:212–219, 1968.

33. Massry, S. C., Coburn, J. W., and Kleeman, C. R. The influence of extracellular volume expansion on renal phosphate reabsorption in the dog. J. Clin. Invest. 48:1237–1245, 1969.

34. Chase, L. R. and Aurbach, G. D. Renal adenyl cyclase: anatomically separate sites for parathyroid hormone and vasopressin. Science 159:545–547, 1968.

35. Liu, S. H., Su, C. C., Chou, S. K., Chu, H. I., Wang, C. W., and Chang, K. P. Calcium and phosphorus metabolism in osteomalacia: V. The effect of varying levels and ratios of calcium to phosphorus intake on their serum levels, paths of excretion and balances, in the presence of continuous vitamin D therapy. J. Clin. Invest. 16:603–611, 1937.

36. Dent, C. E., Harper, C. M., and Philpot, G. R. The treatment of renal-glomerular osteodystrophy. Quart. J. Med. 30:1–32, 1961.

37. Blaustein, M. P. The interrelationship between sodium and calcium fluxes across cell membranes. Rev. Physiol. Biochem. Pharmacol. 70:33–82, 1974.

38. Borle, A. B. A cybernetic view of cell calcium metabolism. In Calcium in Biological Systems, C. J. Duncan, ed. Cambridge: Cambridge University Press. 1976, p. 141–160.

39. Haussler, M. R. and McCain, T. A. Basic and clinical concepts related to vitamin D metabolism and action. N. Eng. J. Med. 297:974–983 and 1041-1050, 1977.

40. Massry, S. G. and Goldstein, D. A. Calcium metabolism in patients with nephrotic syndrome. A state with vitamin D deficiency. Am. J. Clin. Nutr. 31:1572–80, 1978.

41. Papapoulos, S. E., Fraher, L. J., Sandler, L. M., Clemens, T. L., Lewin, I. G., and O'Riordan, J. L. H. 1,25-Dihydroxycholecalciferol in the pathogenesis of the hypercalcemia of sarcoidosis. Lancet 1:627–630, 1979.

42. Sutton, R. A. L. and Dirks, J. H. Renal handling of calcium. Fed. Prod. 37: 2112–2119, 1978.

43. Broadus, A. E. and Thier, S. O. Metabolic basis of renal-stone disease. N. Eng. J. Med. 300:839–845, 1979.

44. Hamed. I. A. and Lindeman, R. D. Dysphagia and vertical nystagmus in magnesium deficiency. Ann. Int. Med. 89:222–223, 1978.

45. Mennes, P., Rosenbaum, R., Martin, K., and Slatopolsky, E. Hypomagnesemia and impaired parathyroid secretion in chronic renal disease. Ann. Int. Med. 88:296–209, 1978.

46. Knochel, J. P. The pathophysiology and clinical characteristics of severe hypophosphatemia. Arch. Intern. Med. 137:203–220, 1977.

47. Fuller, T. J., Nichols, W. W., Brenner, B. J., and Peterson, J. C. Reversible depression in myocardial performance in dogs with experimental phosphorus deficiency. J. Clin. Invest. 62:1194–1200, 1978.

48. Pastoriza-Munoz, E., Colindres, R. E., Lassiter, W. E., and Lechene, C. Effect of parathyroid hormone on phosphate reabsorption in rat distal convolution. Am. J. Physiol. 235:F321–F330, 1978.

49. Kinne-Saffran, E. and Kinne, R. Localization of a calcium-stimulated ATPase in the basal-lateral plasma membranes of the proximal tubule of rat kidney cortex. J. Membr. Biol. 17:263–274, 1974.

12

Glomerulonephritis

In the kidney diseases known collectively as glomerulonephritis (GN) the primary injury is to the glomeruli. Because the renal glomerulus plays such a central role in the anatomy and physiology of the kidney, glomerular injury often affects a variety of renal functions, and in the advanced stages of glomerular disease there is always structural damage to the tubules, blood vessels, and interstitial tissue. Chronic glomerulonephritis is the most common cause of chronic renal failure requiring chronic dialysis or renal transplantation in man.

In the past two decades, remarkable insights into the various forms of glomerulonephritis have been gained. In particular, advances in immunobiology, the development of experimental and spontaneous animal models, and the use of renal biopsy in early stages of the disease have increased our understanding of the pathogenesis of these diseases and have improved our ability to differentiate among the types of glomerulonephritis and perhaps to predict ways of interfering with their natural history.

There are several types of glomerulonephritis, but no entirely satisfactory classification is available. Table 12-1 lists the forms that have reasonably well-defined morphologic and clinical characteristics.

It can be seen that the glomerulonephritides may be primary, in which the kidney is the only or predominant organ involved; or a

TABLE 12-1   *Glomerular Diseases*

Primary Glomerulonephritis
Acute Diffuse Proliferative Glomerulonephritis (GN)
  Poststreptococcal
  Nonpoststreptococcal
Rapidly Progressive (Crescentic) Glomerulonephritis
Membranous Glomerulonephritis
Lipoid Nephrosis (Minimal change disease)
  Focal and Segmental Glomerulosclerosis
Membranoproliferative Glomerulonephritis
Focal Glomerulonephritis
  IgA Nephropathy
Chronic Glomerulonephritis

Systemic Diseases
Systemic Lupus Erythematosus
Goodpasture's Syndrome
Polyarteritis Nodosa
Wegener's Granulomatosis
Henoch-Schönlein Purpura
Bacterial Endocarditis
Diabetes Mellitus
Amyloidosis

Hereditary Disorders
e.g., Alport's Syndrome, Fabry's Disease

---

manifestation of a variety of systemic diseases; or a component of some hereditary disorders. In this chapter we will discuss the various types of primary GN and only briefly touch on the glomerular alterations in some systemic diseases.

In reviewing the specific types of GN, it is useful to consider each in terms of (1) *morphology* of the glomerular lesion, (2) *etiology* and *pathogenesis,* and (3) the *clinical presentation.* There are remarkably limited ways by which glomerular injury can be manifested either histologically or clinically, and only a small number of known pathogenetic mechanisms, and these will be summarized before specific types are discussed.

TISSUE REACTIONS IN GLOMERULONEPHRITIS

The number of histological changes that occur in the glomerulus is limited, and the various glomerulonephritides are characterized by one or more of four basic tissue reactions:

1. *Cellular proliferation* is seen histologically as an increase in the number of cells in the glomerular tuft. This is a common response, and detailed histological studies have shown that endothelial, mesangial, and epithelial cells undergo proliferation. In certain diseases, there is a florid proliferation of the parietal epithelial cells of the glomerulus that takes the form of a crescent—this histological feature is characteristic of diseases that present clinically with rapidly progressive glomerulonephritis.

2. *Leukocytic exudation.* Infiltration of the glomerulus by leukocytes, both neutrophils and monocytes, sometimes occurs in association with cellular proliferation.

3. *Basement membrane thickening.* The normal glomerular basement membrane (GBM), especially as visualized with the periodic acid Schiff (PAS) stain, is a thin sinewy structure that increases in thickness slightly with age. Distinct thickening of the basement membrane seen by light microscopy is a component of some of the glomerulonephritides, such as membranous nephropathy. By electron microscopy this thickening is found to be due to one or combinations of four events: (a) thickening of the basement membrane proper, as occurs in diabetic glomerular disease; (b) deposition of amorphous electron-dense material on the endothelial side of the basement membrane (subendothelial), as in the glomerulonephritis associated with lupus erythematosus; (c) deposition of abnormal materials within the GBM proper, as in dense deposit disease (p. 309); or (d) most commonly, the deposition of electron-dense material on the epithelial side of the basement membrane (subepithelial). In most instances, these deposits are thought to be immune complexes (see below).

4. *Sclerosis or hyalinization.* This represents the deposition of mildly eosinophilic, homogeneous acellular material in the glomerulus, with resulting obliteration of the structural detail of the glomerular tuft. It usually denotes glomerular obsolescence and irreversible injury and is the end result of various forms of glomerular damage.

Because many of the glomerulonephritides are of unknown etiology, they are often classified by their histological characteristics, which include the four terms listed above. The histological changes can be either diffuse, that is, involving the entire glomerulus and all glomeruli; or focal and segmental, that is, involving only a few glomeruli or segments of each glomerulus; or mesangial, affecting predominantly the mesangial region. Thus, the terms *diffuse, focal, segmental* and *mesangial* are sometimes appended to the histological classifications, as seen in Table 12-1.

PATHOGENESIS OF GLOMERULONEPHRITIS

One of the most impressive advances in nephrology in the past twenty years has been the elucidation of pathogenetic mechanisms that operate in glomerulonephritis. It is now widely accepted that most forms of glomerulonephritis in man are caused by immunological processes (1, 2, 3). Support for these views comes from clinical observations and from the resemblance of various forms of glomerulonephritis to experimental models in which immunological mechanisms have been well worked out.

Table 12-2 lists the various types of immunologically induced glomerular injury. Two of these, *circulating immune complex nephritis* and *antiglomerular basement membrane (anti-GBM) antibody nephritis,* have been well established for years; the third, *in situ immune complex nephritis* has only recently been recognized but is being rapidly delineated by experimental work (3). *Activation of the alternate complement pathway* plays a role in some types of GN (e.g.,

TABLE 12-2   *Immunological Mechanisms in Glomerulonephritis*

A. Immune Complex Deposition
   1. Circulating immune complexes
        Exogenous antigens (e.g., serum sickness; postinfectious GN)
        Endogenous antigens (e.g., DNA in lupus nephritis; tumor
          antigens)
   2. *In-situ* immune complexes
        Endogenous fixed antigens (e.g., Heymann nephritis)
        Endogenous planted antigens (e.g., DNA)

B. Antiglomerular Basement Membrane Antibody (Anti-GBM) nephritis
   (e.g., Goodpasture's syndrome)

C. Activation of the Alternate Complement Pathway (e.g., membranoproliferative GN)

D. (?) Cell-Mediated Immune Mechanisms

---

membranoproliferative GN or MPGN), and will be referred to in the discussion of MPGN. In some experimental models and human diseases, more than one mechanism may operate simultaneously. Finally, there is early, but as yet inconclusive, evidence that *cell-mediated immune reactions* may induce glomerular damage, and these are briefly discussed later. Immunopathologic studies of a large series of patients (2) suggest that about 70% of cases of glomerulonephritis are immune-complex mediated (circulating or *in situ*), and 5% anti-GBM mediated. Unknown, possibly nonimmunogenic mechanisms account for the rest, and these are referred to in the discussion of specific types of glomerulonephritis.

Circulating immune-complex nephritis

Circulating immune-complex nephritis is defined as the condition resulting from glomerular deposition of circulating antigen–antibody complexes that do not bear any antigenic relationship to the glomerulus. Immune-complex nephritis can be subdivided further on the basis of whether the antigens involved are *exogenous* or *endogenous:*

1. *Exogenous antigens* are foreign proteins or microbial agents. Acute serum sickness nephritis, Hepatitis B associated nephritis, and poststreptococcal glomerulonephritis in man are exogenous immune-complex diseases.

2. *Endogenous antigens* are antigens derived from the patient's own tissues. Examples of endogenous immune-complex diseases include systemic lupus erythematosus in man, where the complexes have been shown to represent, in the main, DNA–anti-DNA complexes, and immune-complex disease occurring in New Zealand mice.

The pathogenesis of glomerular injury by circulating immune complexes can best be understood by briefly reviewing the experimental model of acute serum sickness (4). To produce serum sickness, a rabbit is injected with a large dose of foreign protein, for example, bovine serum albumin (BSA). Between 8 and 14 days after injection, a number of rabbits develop inflammatory lesions in the hearts, joints, and kidneys. The glomerular lesions, virtually identical to those seen in some forms of human glomerulonephritis, consist of cellular proliferation and leukocytic infiltration in the glomeruli. If the serum level of antigen is determined, one finds that it diminishes first gradually,

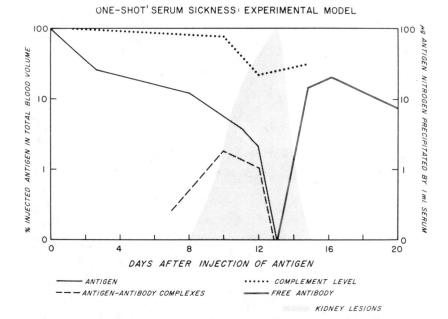

Fig. 12-1 Serum levels of antigen–antibody complexes and complement in acute one-shot serum sickness nephritis.

then precipitously, disappearing after about 2 weeks (Fig. 12-1). Just at the time that the BSA disappears, free antibody to BSA is detectable in the serum; the antibody level rises rapidly, reaching a maximum between 14 and 18 days after the initial injection of antigen. Circulating immune complexes appear in the serum about the sixth day, rising rapidly as the lesions appear and reaching a maximum as the lesions become fully developed. This suggests that the complexes in some way cause the development of the lesions, and a number of experimental studies have shown that an important prerequisite for the development of the lesion is the development of _soluble antigen–antibody complexes_ formed in antigen excess (1, 5).

In several experimental models of serum sickness, components of the immune complexes can be shown to localize in the glomerulus by immunofluorescence microscopy, a technique in which tissue sections are treated with fluorescein-labeled specific antibody. Immunoglobulin representing antibody, antigens, and complement can be seen in the glomerulus in the form of discrete granules in the mesangium

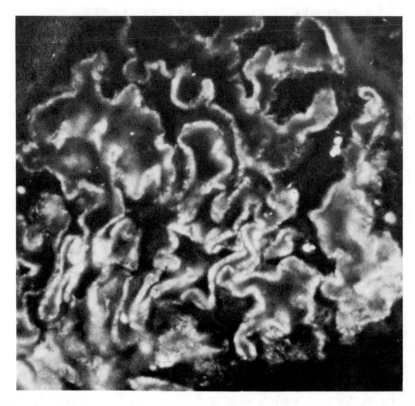

Fig. 12-2 Glomerulus, showing immunofluorescent pattern of *granular* deposits along the basement membrane, characteristic of immune-complex nephritis.

and along the basement membrane. The fluorescence pattern is distinctly *granular* or lumpy and is characteristic of immune-complex disease, both in experimental animals and man, Fig. 12-2 (1). By electron microscopy these graular deposits appear as electron-dense, amorphous precipitates on the subendothelial surface of the basement membrane, in the mesangium, or along the epithelial side of the basement membrane; in the latter location they often have the shape of a camel's "hump." The light, fluorescent, and electron microscopic features of acute serum sickness nephritis are similar to those seen in acute post-streptococcal glomerulonephritis in man. Serum complement activity falls during the formation of immune complexes because complement is bound to the complexes.

If, instead of a large amount of foreign protein in a single injection, smaller doses are given repeatedly, some rabbits produce just enough antibody so that circulating soluble complexes are present in the circulation for long periods of time, and chronic serum sickness develops. This experimental model, developed in the classic experiments of Dixon, Feldman, and Vasquez (6) results in glomerular histological lesions that are more chronic and resemble those seen in membranous glomerulonephritis in man. In this model, immunoglobulins, antigen, and complement are also seen by immunofluorescence microscopy as granular deposits along the basement membrane; by electron microscopy, chronic serum sickness and membranous glomerulonephritis are characterized by numerous electron-dense deposits present virtually exclusively along the epithelial side of the basement membrane (epimembranous). However, as will be discussed later, this pattern of localization is now thought to occur also as a result of *in situ* (rather than circulating) immune complex deposition (3).

Other forms of experimental circulating immune-complex disease include:

1. *Viral-induced immune-complex diseases.* Many animals with circulating viral complexes develop glomerular lesions. This has been established in animals with persistent lymphocytic choriomeningitis virus, equine infectious anemia virus, Gross or Raucher leukemia virus, and Aleutian disease of mink (1, 7). In man, cases of glomerulonephritis associated with hepatitis B virus, vaccinia, and measles, have been reported (2).

2. *Immune-complex nephritis associated with parasitic disease.* A variety of experimental or human acute and chronic parasitic infections, such as schistosomiasis, malaria, and toxoplasmosis are associated with glomerulonephritis and the deposition of immune complexes containing parasite antigen (10, 11).

3. *Immune-complex disease in New Zealand mice.* The development of a spontaneous syndrome resembling systemic lupus erythematosus was observed in inbred New Zealand black mice (8). The black and white NZB/W hybrids develop glomerular renal lesions similar to those of lupus nephritis in man. It has been shown that the renal lesions are induced by immune complexes and that at least two antibodies can be eluted from the nephritic kidneys: (a) antibodies against nuclear antigens (b) antibodies directed

against antigens of the Gross virus, which infects these animals naturally (9). Thus, both viral and autologous immune complexes are involved.

Factors affecting glomerular localization of circulating complexes in any of these models are, unfortunately, not well understood (12). As mentioned above, the lesions develop when *soluble* antigen–antibody complexes are formed in *antigen excess.* Size, shape, charge, and chemical composition of the antigen may affect the capacity of the complexes to localize in the glomeruli, but these determinants have not been studied in great detail. Cochrane and Hawkins (13) found that, in *acute* serum sickness in rabbits, very small complexes were nonpathogenic while those over 19S induced glomerulonephritis. In a series of studies on rabbits immunized with bovine serum albumin (reviewed in 14), Germuth found *diffuse* glomerulonephritis in animals with complexes ranging from 300,000 to 500,000 in molecular weight; complexes with a molecular weight of more than 1 million developed *focal* lesions localized to mesangial areas, suggesting that physical characteristics of the complexes may affect the distribution of renal lesions. Because of the importance of molecular charge in glomerular permeability (see Chapter 2), the charge of antigen or complexes may be relevant (3a). In addition, active host factors may also play a role in the localization of complexes. For example, it has been shown that the immunologically mediated release of vasoactive amines (such as histamine and serotonin) from platelets increases the glomerular accumulation of complexes. Experimentally, antagonists of serotonin and histamine largely prevent glomerular deposition of complexes in acute serum sickness in rabbits (15).

Finally, the pattern of localization of complexes in the glomerulus (mesangial, subendothelial, or subepithelial) is influenced not only by the physicochemical characteristics of the complexes but by the local properties of the glomerulus itself. Experimental studies suggest that alterations in glomerular hemodynamics, mesangial function, and charge-selective properties of the glomerulus (reviewed in refs. 3, 3a) may affect the intraglomerular distribution of immune complexes and the resultant glomerular morphological alterations.

In summary, circulating *immune-complex deposition* is an established pathogenetic mechanism in human and experimental glomerulonephritis. A variety of exogenous (foreign protein, bacterial, parasitic, or viral antigen) and endogenous (DNA) antigens can induce circulating immune-complex nephritis; the resulting glomerular lesions can be either acute or chronic, proliferative or membranous, and are characterized by a pattern of granular deposition of immunoglobulins and complement when examined by immunofluorescence microscopy.

In situ immune complex nephritis

Until recently it was believed that a granular pattern of localization of immune complexes in the glomerulus was almost always caused by preformed *circulating* immune complexes, distinct from the linear pattern characteristic of anti-GBM disease described below. Current evidence, however, indicates that this was an oversimplified view of these pathogenic mechanisms. Several pieces of data suggest that at least one form of immune complex glomerulonephritis with granular fluorescence, membranous GN, may be caused by reaction of antigen with antibody, *in situ*, within the glomerulus. In the first place, a variable but large (31–100%) proportion of patients with membranous glomerulonephritis (exhibiting diffuse granular deposits by fluorescence microscopy, and subepithelial deposits by EM) fail to exhibit immune complexes in their serum when studied by a variety of newly developed techniques (3, 16, 17). Secondly, it has been difficult to induce membranous glomerulonephritis in experimental animals by injections of preformed immune complexes. In the vast majority of such experiments preformed complexes deposit in the mesangium or subendothelial space (reviewed in ref. 3) with no subepithelial localization whatsoever.

The critical experiments documenting the occurrence of *in situ* complex GN were performed using an experimental model called *Heymann nephritis*. In this model rats immunized with an antigen derived from the brush border of proximal tubular cells develop granular immune deposits indistinguishable from those of human membranous GN (18, 19). Earlier studies showed that Heymann nephritis was caused by the formation of antibodies to an antigen normally largely sequestered from the circulation, followed by glomerular deposition of small circulating immune complexes containing the brush border antigen—a form of *autologous* circulating immune complex disease. Recently, however, two groups have shown that immune deposits are formed in the glomerulus after 10 minutes to 1 hour of passive perfusion of antibody to brush border antigens in bloodless rat kidneys (20), or in an isolated perfused rat kidney system (21) in which the presence of circulating complexes could be excluded. Presumably the antibody reacted with a fixed antigenic component in the glomerulus that cross reacted with the immunizing brush border antigen. The granular pattern of the fluorescent deposits could conceivably be caused by particulate distribution of the antigen in the glomerular capillary wall.

In situ immune complex formation can theoretically result from the following circumstances:

1. Circulating autoantibodies can react to a fixed endogenous glomerular antigen, as suggested by the experiments on passive Heymann nephritis described above.

2. Circulating antibodies can react with antigens that had been previously "planted" in the glomerulus. Such planted antigens may be exogenous (e.g., viral or bacterial products) and may deposit in the glomerulus because of their size or because of some chemical affinity to glomerular constituents. While no direct proof for this sequence is known, Golbus and Wilson (22) showed that administration of the glycoprotein-binding plant lectin Con A (which binds to the glomerular capillary wall), followed by anti-Con A, results in the local formation of immune complexes and the development of glomerulonephritis. The planted antigens may also be endogenous. Izui et al. (23) have shown that free DNA will bind avidly *in vitro* to collagen and collagenlike structures in the glomerulus; addition of anti-DNA antibody results in *in situ* DNA–anti-DNA immune complex formation on the GBM.

Before leaving the subject of immune complex nephritis, it must be stressed that although both circulating and *in situ* immune complex deposition are plausible pathogenetic mechanisms in glomerulonephritis, the nature of the antigens involved in the vast majority of cases of immunologically mediated glomerulonephritis in humans is unknown.

Anti-GBM nephritis

In this type of immunological injury, antibodies are directed against a component of the glomerulus proper—in fact, the basement membrane. The earliest experimental model was so-called nephrotoxic or Masugi nephritis. In a typical model, homogenates of rat kidney or, better still, preparations of rat glomerular basement membrane, are injected into a rabbit (1, 2, 24). The rabbit then develops antibodies to the basement membrane. Serum from this rabbit, containing circulating antibodies to rat kidney, is injected back into a rat; the antibodies react with the rat glomerular basement membrane, and a glomerulonephritis develops. In this case, immunofluorescence localization of immunoglobulin and complement takes a distinctly *linear* diffuse pattern (Fig. 12-3), in contrast with the granular pattern seen in immune-complex disease.

To come back to the nephrotoxic model, the deposited rabbit IgG is itself foreign to the host and thus acts as an antigen, eliciting antibodies in the rat, the latter reacting with the rabbit IgG on the GBM and leading to further glomerular damage. A similar disease can also be produced by injection of heterologous or homologous glomerular basement membrane preparations, usually with Freund's adjuvant (25).

Anti-GBM nephritis is much less common that immune-complex nephritis in man accounting for less than 5% of cases of GN. It is well established as the mechanism of nephritis associated with Goodpasture's syndrome. In this syndrome, pulmonary hemorrhage and glomerulonephritis occur, and it is thought that lung and renal basement membrane have antigenic similarities. Some cases of rapidly progressive glomerulonephritis, discussed later, appear to be of this type.

Mediators of immunologic glomerular injury

Once complexes or antibody to basement membrane have localized in the glomerulus, how does glomerular damage ensue? A well-established sequence of events in immune injury involves activation of the complement sequence by fixation of complement to immune complexes. In this sequence, activation of C3 to C9 components is initiated with generation of biologically active compounds, principally C3 and C5 fragments, which act as chemotactic stimuli for the localization of polymorphonuclear leukocytes (25). Leukocytes that contain a number of destructive enzymes can then act on the glomerular basement membrane to cause damage. Acid proteases from neutrophils have been shown to damage the GBM directly, and Cochrane and his associates have shown that animals depleted of polymorphonuclear leukocytes by antineutrophilic sera or by nitrogen mustard are protected from

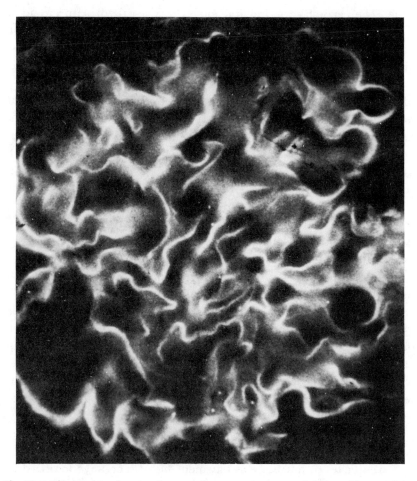

Fig. 12-3 Glomerulus, showing immunofluorescent pattern of diffuse *linear* staining, characteristic of anti-GBM nephritis. Compare with Fig. 12-2.

the development of glomerulonephritis in some experimental models. In addition, this glomerular injury can be inhibited by decomplementing animals before induction of nephritis (25). This *complement–leukocyte-dependent mechanism* has, however, been shown to apply to a limited number of experimental models; many human glomerulonephritides do not exhibit neutrophilic infiltration in the glomerulus, and in some human and experimental forms complement is not present in the basement membrane as seen by fluorescence microscopy.

For these reasons, it is assumed that there are other mechanisms of glomerular damage that do not involve neutrophils or the complement cascade. Antigen–antibody complexes may directly activate the kinin-forming system, which could result in increased permeability without neutrophilic emigration, but the role for such a mechanism in nephritis has not been established (25). Alterations in charge selectivity of the glomerular filter may well be involved. Kreisberg et al. have shown rapid focal loss of negative charge early in nephrotoxic serum nephritis, associated with mononuclear infiltration (25a).

The *coagulation system* may also be a mediator of glomerular damage. Fibrin and fibrin degradation products are frequently present in the glomeruli in GN, and fibrinogen may leak into Bowman's space, serving as a stimulus to cell proliferation. Pretreatment of animals with anticoagulants (26) or defibrinating agents (27) prevents the development of proliferative glomerular lesions in some experimental models of GN. Although the beneficial effect is by no means uniform, the balance of evidence indicates that intraglomerular coagulation plays a role in progressive renal damage in GN.

Recently, prominent *monocytic infiltration* of the glomerulus has been shown in some forms of human and experimental proliferative GN (28). Depletion of monocytes by irradiation prevented the proteinuria and histologic alterations in experimental nephritis, suggesting a role for monocytes in the induction of renal damage (29). Further, the histologic lesions in two experimental models of nephritis could be transferred with lymphocytes (30, 31). In humans, cell-mediated immunity to altered GBM has been found in some patients with progressive GN (32). These studies are still preliminary but have opened up the possibility that *cell-mediated hypersensitivity* reactions may be involved in immunologic glomerular damage.

CLINICAL MANIFESTATIONS OF GLOMERULAR DISEASE
The principal clinical features that reflect glomerular injury are:

1. *Hematuria,* which denotes the presence of blood in the urine and reflects damage to the glomerular capillary wall.

2. *Proteinuria.* Mild or moderate proteinuria is common to most of the glomerular diseases, but severe, persistent proteinuria amount-

ing to more than 3.5 gm of protein per day is characteristic of the nephrotic syndrome.

3. *Oliguria,* the production of decreased amounts of urine, usually less than 600 ml/day.

4. *Azotemia* or the accumulation in the blood of nitrogenous substances.

5. *Edema.* Mild to moderate edema can be present in most types of glomerulonephritis, but severe edema is usually associated with heavy proteinuria as a feature of the nephrotic syndrome.

6. *Hypertension.*

These six clinical manifestations often occur in groups or syndromes. The five major syndromes (Table 12-3) include:

1. *Acute nephritis,* which is dominated by the acute onset of hematuria, usually visible, and mild to moderate hypertension. The classical example of an acute nephritic presentation is poststreptococcal glomerulonephritis.

2. *Rapidly progressive glomerulonephritis.* A syndrome with an acute onset dominated by hematuria, but additionally with severe oliguria leading to renal failure within weeks.

3. The *nephrotic syndrome* is characterized by heavy proteinuria (more than 3.5 gm/24 hours), hypoalbuminemia, edema, hyperlipemia, lipiduria.

4. *Chronic renal failure* (Chapter 9).

5. Asymptomatic urinary abnormalities such as *hematuria, proteinuria,* or both.

TABLE 12-3 *Clinical Syndromes in Glomerulonephritis*

Acute Nephritic Syndrome
Rapidly Progressive Nephritis
Nephrotic Syndrome
Chronic Renal Failure
Asymptomatic Hematuria and/or Proteinuria
A. Primary
B. As part of systemic disease

These signs of glomerular injury can occur either as a manifestation of a systemic disorder or as primary glomerulonephritis, which denotes a disease that involves the kidney exclusively. The systemic diseases that most frequently affect the glomeruli are diabetes mellitus, lupus erythematosus, amyloidosis, subacute bacterial endocarditis, and the vasculitides.

SPECIFIC TYPES OF GLOMERULONEPHRITIS

Acute poststreptococcal (proliferative) glomerulonephritis
This is a fairly common glomerular disease, which occurs most often in children but also affects adults of any age. In a typical case, signs and symptoms of glomerular disease appear 1 or 2 weeks after a streptococcal infection of the throat or, occasionally, of the skin. The onset is usually abrupt and is manifested by the appearance of smoky-colored urine, representing hematuria; edema, usually limited to swelling around the eyes; mild proteinuria, rarely exceeding 2 gm of protein per day; oliguria; and mild to moderate hypertension. This constellation of clinical manifestations is typical of the acute nephritic syndrome outlined above. Unusual cases may present with only gross or microscopic hematuria, and severe forms of the disease can develop into the rapidly progressive form discussed below.

ETIOLOGY AND PATHOGENESIS
The association of beta-hemolytic streptococcal infection and glomerulonephritis has long been known, and the following specific features are relevant to the etiology and pathogenesis of the disease:

1. Not all types of Group A streptococci can cause glomerulonephritis; 90% of cases can be ascribed to Types 12, 4, and 1, but other types have occasionally been implicated, for example, the Red-Lake strain responsible for an epidemic of glomerulonephritis on an Indian reservation in Minnesota. Skin infections are responsible for many cases in certain geographical areas, and there have been elegant studies on the characteristics of glomerulonephritis associated with skin infections in Trinidad.

2. Even within a certain *nephritogenic* type, the incidence of acute glomerulonephritis varies considerably. This suggests that strain

differences within individual types can occur or that host factors may be important determinants for the development of glomerulonephritis.

3. The blood, urine, and kidneys are sterile, and the lesion is clearly not produced by bacterial proliferation in renal tissue.

4. Antibodies to the extracellular antigens of the hemolytic streptococcus are frequently identified in the serum during the development of acute glomerulonephritis. Although antibodies confer little or no immunity on the patient infected with these organisms, serum antibody levels are useful diagnostically in implicating streptococcal infection as the cause of the glomerulonephritis; for example, the antistreptolysin O (ASO) titer is a frequently used clinical test.

It is now accepted that poststreptococcal glomerulonephritis is immunologically mediated (33). The latent period between the streptococcal infections and nephritis, and the elevated antistreptococcal antibody titers in the serum have always pointed to hypersensitivity reaction. Serum complement levels are usually low in acute glomerulonephritis; this reflects the utilization of complement in the antigen–antibody reaction, rather than loss of complement components in the urine. The most convincing evidence comes from the immunofluorescent and electron microscopic findings. By fluorescence microscopy, there is granular deposition of IgG and C3 in the diseased glomeruli, and by electron microscopy, there are subepithelial electron–dense deposits—these features are similar to those seen in acute experimental serum sickness nephritis described above, suggesting a circulating immune complex mechanism. To date, however, it has not been possible to determine the type of streptococcal antigen responsible for the immune complexes, and except for scattered reports, it has not been possible to reproduce a glomerular lesion in experimental animals with streptococcal infection.

Further, although circulating immune complexes are found regularly in the serum of these patients, they are equally prevalent in streptococcal sequelae not associated with GN (34). Additional or alternative mechanisms of immunological injury are being explored. The absence in some cases of C1 and C4, the early components of complements in glomeruli, suggests activation of the alternate complement pathway (35). Cross-reactivity between group A streptococcal antigens and glycosidase-treated GBM has suggested that while streptococci initiate antibody formation, the antibody reacts with GBM components, not streptococci. There is also evidence of cell-mediated reactivity to such altered GBM membranes (30). Whatever the precise mechanism, the evidence is substantial that this is a form of immunologically mediated nephritis triggered by an antecedent streptococcal infection.

PATHOLOGIC CHANGES

The *light microscopic* changes in the glomeruli are characteristic and, in the typical case, easy to recognize (Fig. 12-4). The glomeruli appear enlarged and hypercellular, the hypercellularity being caused by *proliferation* of endothelial, mesangial, and often epithelial cells. The proliferation is diffuse, that is, involving all lobules of all glomeruli, and there is frequently *infiltration with leukocytes,* both neutrophils and monocytes. There is also swelling of endothelial cells, and the combination of proliferation, swelling, and leukocyte infiltration obliterates the capillary lumina. The tubules often contain red cell casts and may show evidence of degeneration; there is frequently edema in the interstitium. Deposits of fibrin in the lumina and mesangium are present in many cases.

By *fluorescence microscopy,* there are granular deposits of IgG and complement in the mesangium and along the basement membrane. Although present, they are often focal and sparse.

The *electron microscopic* features in poststreptococcal glomerulonephritis are also characteristic. Discrete amorphous electron-dense deposits are seen on the epithelial side of the basement membrane (Fig. 12-5). Such deposits have the appearance of a "hump" and are present in most patients biopsied in the first 6 weeks of illness. They presumably represent antigen–antibody complexes trapped at the epithelial surface. Subendothelial and intramembranous deposits are sometimes seen. Other electron microscopic findings include swelling of endothelial and mesangial cells, occasional discontinuities in the basement membrane, and fibrin deposits.

PATHOPHYSIOLOGY AND CLINICAL COURSE

Patients with acute glomerulonephritis exhibit a distinctive pattern of abnormalities in renal function. Glomerular filtration rate is mod-

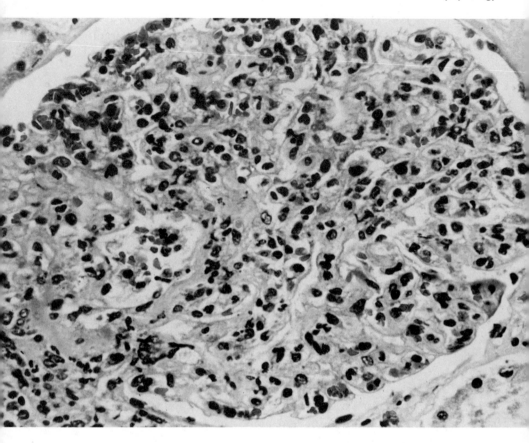

Fig. 12-4 Glomerulus, showing diffuse hypercellularity and infiltration by leukocytes, characteristic of acute proliferative poststreptococcal GN.

erately or markedly depressed, this almost certainly being due to the obstruction of glomerular capillary lumina by endothelial proliferation and swelling. Renal blood flow, however, is slightly reduced or normal, and thus the filtration fraction is low. Although tubular function is also impaired, as measured by PAH clearance, it is less severely impaired than glomerular function.

The *course* of poststreptococcal glomerulonephritis is favorable, especially in children. In childhood, more than 95% of patients heal either spontaneously or with conservative therapy aimed at maintaining sodium and water balance. Signs of recovery appear within days or weeks, beginning with diuresis, loss of edema, and return of the blood pressure to normal. In a biopsy specimen, the proliferation sub-sides, the neutrophils disappear, and the capillary lumina open up. The electron-dense humps and immunoglobulin usually disappear within 6 weeks. A small minority of patients do not undergo diuresis, become severely oliguric, and develop a rapidly progressive form of glomerulonephritis. Other rare patients, less than 1–2% of children, may undergo slow progression to chronic glomerulonephritis, with or without recurrences of an active nephritic sediment. A biopsy in such patients shows persistent hypercellularity, predominantly in the mes-angium, and with time, increasing sclerosis of individual glomeruli.

There is some controversy over the clinical course in adults. In one

Fig. 12-5 Electron micrograph from patient with poststreptococcal GN. There is a characteristic subepithelial electron-dense deposit (hump—arrow), as well as de-posits in the basement membrane.
CAP: capillary; BM: basement membrane; Ep: epithelial cell

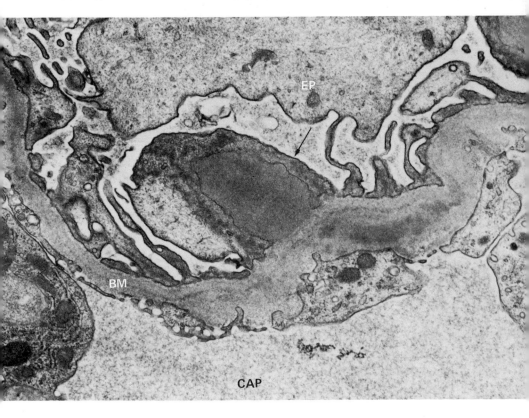

study, as many as 40% of patients failed to resolve completely either histologically or clinically and about one-third of patients developed progressive renal damage (36). Other investigators have questioned these rather grim statistics (37). Factors leading to progression in some patients are unclear, but cell-mediated immunologic reactions directed to GBM cross-reacting with or altered by streptococci have been implicated (30).

Although most patients with acute glomerulonephritis have post-streptococcal disease, a similar form has been reported sporadically which is associated with staphylococcal infection, especially endocarditis, and a number of viral diseases, such as mumps, varicella, infectious mononucleosis, and hepatitis B (1, 38). The best studied cases have been those with staphylococcal endocarditis, and hepatitis B antigenemia. In both of these granular immunofluorescent deposits and subepithelial humps characteristic of immune complex nephritis have been documented (39, 40).

Rapidly progressive glomerulonephritis (RPGN)

This type of glomerulonephritis represents a clinical–pathological syndrome in which glomerular injury is accompanied by rapid and progressive decline in renal function, frequently with severe oliguria, or anuria, usually resulting in irreversible renal failure in weeks or months. The disease is characterized histologically by widespread proliferation of cells in Bowman's space, with conspicuous *"crescent"* formation (Fig. 12-6). Hematuria is a common finding, but proteinuria is variable, and hypertension and edema may or may not be present.

The syndrome of rapidly progressive glomerulonephritis may occur in the course of several diseases that can affect the glomerulus (27) (Table 12-4). In this chapter, only three of these are discussed.

POSTSTREPTOCOCCAL RAPIDLY PROGRESSIVE NEPHRITIS

In some cases of RPGN, there is a history of poststreptococcal glomerulonephritis that either does not resolve or progresses rapidly to anuria and renal failure. This type of complication of poststreptococcal glomerulonephritis is rare in children but somewhat more common in adults. The initial clinical manifestations and pathogenetic mechanisms are similar to those of diffuse proliferative glomerulonephritis: the antistreptolysin serum titers are usually elevated, serum complement levels are reduced, and there is granular deposition of IgG and

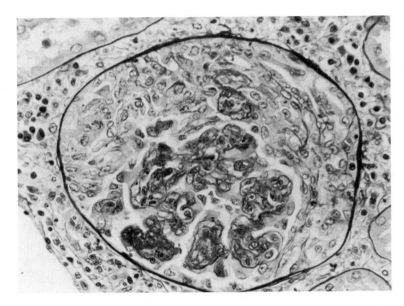

Fig. 12-6 Glomerulus from patient with RPGN, showing typical "crescent" in Bowman's space.

C3 in the glomeruli. Histologically, in addition to the diffuse proliferation, there is abundant crescent formation.

GOODPASTURE'S SYNDROME
This condition is characterized by rapidly developing renal insufficiency and recurrent lung hemorrhages, the latter manifested by hemoptysis and radiologically visible pulmonary infiltrates (42).

TABLE 12-4 *Diseases Associated with Rapidly Progressive Glomerulonephritis*

Poststreptococcal Rapidly Progressive
Glomerulonephritis
Goodpasture's Syndrome
Wegener's Granulomatosis
Lupus Erythematosus
Polyarteritis Nodosa
Henoch–Schönlein Purpura
Essential Cryoglobulinemia
Idiopathic Rapidly Progressive
Glomerulonephritis

Although rare, the condition is of great interest because the pathogenetic mechanism of glomerular damage has been documented to be the result of antiglomerular basement membrane antibodies. Immunofluorescence studies reveal the characteristic continuous *linear* staining for IgG seen in experimental anti-GBM nephritis (Fig. 12-3). When immunoglobulins are eluted from glomeruli, they can be shown to react *in vitro* with glomerular basement membrane, and when they are injected into monkeys, glomerular disease with typical linear staining is found in glomeruli. Circulating antiglomerular basement membrane antibodies can be detected in the serum of most patients with Gooodpasture's syndrome by using either immunofluorescence or radioimmunoassay techniques (2). Immunoglobulins are also found along the alveolar basement membranes, and materials eluted from lung tissue do react with glomerular basement membrane. It is thus assumed that the pulmonary and renal lesions are due to the deposition of circulating antibodies directed against antigens common to both the pulmonary and glomerular basement membrane. It has been possible, experimentally, to induce renal lesions with antibodies against lung alveolar membranes (43). Whereas the pathogenesis of the glomerular and lung disease has been reasonably well established, the etiological factors that stimulate the formation of the autoantibodies to basement membranes are unknown.

Etiological factors implicated in the initiation of antibody production have included influenza or other viral infections (44), exposure to hydrocarbon solvents found in paints or dyes (45), and penicillamine treatment (46); but in most cases no such factors seem to play a role (47). A high prevalence of DRW2 haplotype in patients with Goodpasture's syndrome suggests a genetic predisposition common to many of the autoimmune diseases (48).

The glomerular lesions of Goodpasture's syndrome may be focal and segmental at first, but subsequently they become widespread and necrotizing and exhibit conspicuous crescent formation. By electron microscopy, there is extensive fibrin deposition, epithelial and endothelial degeneration, and focal discontinuities of the glomerular basement membrane. Electron-dense deposits similar to those in poststreptococcal glomerulonephritis are absent.

In most cases, progressive renal failure eventually necessitates dialysis support, and life-threatening pulmonary hemorrhage may occur, occasionally, with a fatal outcome. Therapy has included immunosuppression and corticosteroids; in some instances, removal of the kidneys has ameliorated the pulmonary lesions. Clear-cut benefits from all these modes of therapy are not well documented.

However, dramatic results have been achieved with intensive plasmapheresis (plasma exchange) combined with steroids and cytotoxic agents (49). This therapy reverses both the pulmonary hemorrhage and renal failure and is particularly beneficial when instituted before the patient's urine output has decreased to 400 ml per day. Plasma exchange presumably removes the anti-GBM antibodies as well as secondary circulating mediators of glomerular injury. Despite therapy, severely oliguric patients will eventually require chronic dialysis or transplantation. Since anti-GBM antibodies usually disappear spontaneously from the circulation, transplantation is successful but is usually delayed for several months to reduce the small but definite risk of recurrence in the transplanted kidney.

IDIOPATHIC RAPIDLY PROGRESSIVE GLOMERULONEPHRITIS

In more than half of the patients presenting with rapidly progressive renal failure, and glomerulonephritis, the conditions outlined in Table 12-4 can be excluded. Such patients probably represent a heterogeneous group with differing etiological agents and pathogenetic mechanisms. Immunofluorescent findings show granular fluorescence (immune complex) in about one-third, linear fluorescence (anti-GBM disease) in another third, and either no fluorescence whatsoever or a nonspecific pattern in at least one-third of patients (50). They have in common rapid progression, a poor prognosis, and extensive crescent formation in the glomeruli. The disease in such patients is not a distinct entity but may follow many types of GN of differing etiologies and pathogenesis; the common feature is severe glomerular damage (51, 52).

THE NATURE OF EPITHELIAL CRESCENTS

Because the pathologic hallmark of rapidly progressive glomerulonephritis is crescent formation, the nature and morphogenesis of epithelial crescents deserve consideration. A variety of studies indicate that crescents are formed both by proliferation of the parietal epithelial cells of Bowman's space, and by infiltration of monocytes which are later converted to macrophages (28, 53). Whether the infiltrating monocytes are attracted nonspecifically as a result of glomerular damage or are called forth by antibody or cell-mediated immune mechanisms within the glomerulus is still open to question (28). The crescents form in relation to focal disruptions of the basement membrane, and foreign proteinaceous material having the staining and immunologic characteristics of fibrin is seen within crescents. In some studies, the severity of crescent formation was reduced by prior treatment of the animals with anticoagulants. This has led to the assumption that crescent formation may be a reaction to severe injury to GBM and to fibrin deposition (26). Whatever their pathogenesis, however, it is agreed that when crescents are present in large numbers they are a poor prognostic sign.

Membranous glomerulonephritis

Membranous glomerulonephritis is characterized morphologically by diffuse, widespread thickening of the capillary walls of the glomeruli and clinically by the nephrotic syndrome. The structural changes are distinctive, and the clinical presentation is sufficiently uniform to consider the condition a clinicopathologic entity.

The patients are usually adults who present with all the manifestations of the nephrotic syndrome: heavy proteinuria of more than 3.5 gm of protein/24 hours, edema, hypoalbuminemia, lipiduria, and often hypercholesterolemia. The onset is insidious. Hematuria and hypertension may occur, but they are not constant or necessary features of the entity. Membranous glomerulonephritis is the most common cause of the nephrotic syndrome in adults but is rare in children.

PATHOGENESIS

Because of the close similarity of the lesions of membranous glomerulonephritis to those seen in chronic serum sickness experimentally, it has been assumed that this is a form of chronic immune-complex disease. In particular, the immunofluorescence findings in the glomeruli are those of diffuse granular deposits of IgG and complement along the basement membrane of all glomeruli.

However, as mentioned earlier, immune complexes are frequently absent from the circulation in these patients. Further, the glomerular alterations also resemble those of Heymann nephritis, which is now thought to be a form of *in situ* immune complex nephritis (3). Whatever the mechanism of deposition of immune complex, there is little information about the etiologic agents (antigen) responsible for the immune reactions. Membranous glomerulonephritis is sometimes associated with certain infections (hepatitis B, syphilis, malaria), drugs (gold, penicillamine), and tumors (bronchogenic carcinoma), but in only a minuscule number of patients has a specific antigen been implicated. These include *P. malariae* antigen, hepatitis B antigen, and tumor-specific antigens in patients with membranous glomerulonephritis associated with carcinomas (54, 55).

PATHOLOGIC CHANGES

By light microscopy, there is diffuse thickening of the capillary wall *without proliferation of cells* (Fig. 12-7). The thickening is especially evident when the sections are stained with the periodic acid-Schiff

Fig. 12-7 Glomerulus with diffuse membranous glomerulonephritis. Note the absence of proliferation.

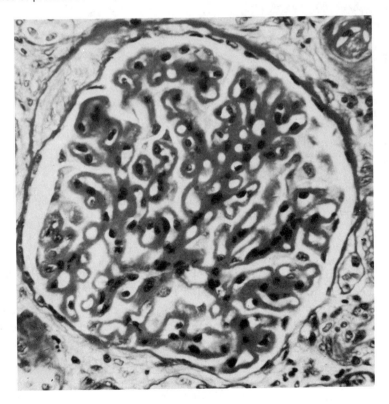

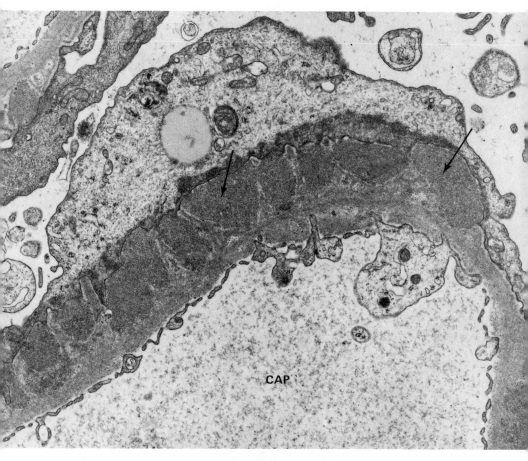

Fig. 12-8 Membranous glomerulonephritis—electron micrograph showing numerous subepithelial deposits (arrows) and obliteration of foot processes overlying the deposits.
CAP: capillary lumen

stain. The characteristic features of membranous glomerulonephritis are seen with the electron microscope: the capillary wall thickening is due mainly to the deposition of numerous, irregular electron-dense deposits between the basement membrane proper and the epithelial cell cytoplasm (Fig. 12-8). The epithelial cells overlying the deposits have lost their foot processes and are somewhat swollen. It is the combination of subepithelial deposits and the altered epithelial cytoplasm that gives the appearance of a diffusely thickened basement membrane by light microscopy. Eventually some of these deposits become incorporated in the basement membrane and, in long-standing disease, the basement membrane itself becomes thickened and acquires a moth-eaten appearance. It is presumed that the electron-dense deposits contain antibody and complement, since by immunofluorescence microscopy there is diffuse granular deposition of these materials along the GBM (Fig. 12-2).

PATHOPHYSIOLOGY AND CLINICAL COURSE

The pathophysiology of membranous glomerulonephritis is that of the nephrotic syndrome, discussed on page 322. The clinical course is variable, but the disease is frequently progressive; the rapidity of the progression is unpredictable, and renal insufficiency may occur from 2–20 years after onset. Spontaneous remissions of proteinuria occur, and in rare cases there appears to be regression of the histological changes and recovery. Progression to renal failure is associated with increasing sclerosis of glomeruli, rising blood urea nitrogen, relative diminution of the amount of proteinuria, and the development of hypertension. The value of corticosteroid therapy in this condition is controversial, but a recent interhospital prospective controlled study has shown significant reduction in progression to renal insufficiency in patients treated with alternate-day corticosteroid therapy as compared to patients given a placebo (56).

Lipoid nephrosis

This term is used to describe a disorder, most common in children, in which the nephrotic syndrome is present but the renal glomeruli show no apparent change by light microscopy. The condition is also known as minimal change or nil change disease. Clinically, it is manifested by the nephrotic syndrome, usually without hematuria, hypertension, or impaired renal function. The peak incidence is in children between 2 and 3 years of age; before age 15 it accounts for more than 85% of cases of the nephrotic syndrome. In adults, it is found in 10% of cases of the nephrotic syndrome. The disease sometimes follows a respiratory infection (25% of cases) or routine prophylactic immunization (9% of cases) (57, 58). Serum complement levels are not usually depressed.

PATHOGENESIS

The etiology and pathogenesis are unknown. The association with respiratory infections and the response to corticosteroid and immunosuppressive therapy suggest an immunological mechanism, but there is no evidence of deposition of immunoglobulins or complement in glomeruli, and by electron microscopy no deposits are seen. For these reasons, it is felt that lipoid nephrosis is not mediated by any of the known mechanisms of immunologic glomerular injury.

However, several features of the disease suggest an immunological basis and these have been thoroughly reviewed and analyzed by Mallik (59). Such factors include: (1) the clinical association with respiratory infections and prophylactic immunizations, (2) the response to corticosteroid and immunosuppressive therapy, (3) the association with other atopic disorders (e.g., eczema, rhinitis), (4) the increased prevalence of HLA-B12 in patients with minimal-change disease associated with atopy (suggesting a possible genetic predisposition), (5) the increased incidence of lipoid nephrosis in patients with Hodgkin's disease (55), in whom defects in T-cell-mediated immunity are well recognized, and (6) the elaboration of lymphokinelike activity by lymphocytes of patients suffering from lipoid nephrosis, when such lymphocytes are cultured with renal tissue. Such findings have led to hypotheses implicating either IgE-mediated reactions, or some dysfunction of T-cell immunity, eventually resulting in the elaboration of a circulating substance that increases the permeability of the glomerular wall.

The molecular basis of protein leakage in this condition and the pathogenesis of the characteristic loss of foot processes have received much attention. An early event in lipoid nephrosis and experimental aminonucleoside nephrosis (a model that mimics lipoid nephrosis) appears to involve loss of the sialic acid-rich glomerular polyanion (Chapter 2). This reduction in negative charge leads to two consequences: (1) enhanced filtration of circulating polyanions, mainly albumin, resulting in proteinuria (60), and (2) decrease of the repulsive forces that normally serve to keep adjacent foot processes separate, leading to the familiar disappearance of these processes (61). Thus, early loss of glomerular fixed negative charges may account for the prime features of the glomerular defect: proteinuria and loss of foot processes. How the glomerular polyanion loss is brought about, however, is still totally unknown.

PATHOLOGIC CHANGES

The glomeruli appear normal by light microscopy: there is no thickening of basement membranes and no cellular proliferation (Fig.

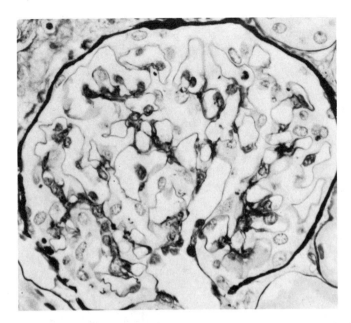

Fig. 12-9 Lipoid nephrosis—glomerulus shows no basement membrane thickening or proliferation.

12-9). By electron microscopy, the basement membrane appears morphologically normal and no electron-dense material is deposited; the principal lesion is in the visceral epithelial cells: the characteristic foot processes of epithelial cells are lost and replaced by a rim of cytoplasm, often showing vacuolization and swelling (Fig. 12-10). This change is often termed "fusion" of foot processes but in fact represents flattening and swelling of foot processes rather than actual fusion of adjacent cells (62). It is characteristic of lipoid nephrosis and other nephrotic states.

PATHOPHYSIOLOGY AND CLINICAL COURSE

The term *lipoid nephrosis* was initially coined because of the presence of lipid in tubules and fat bodies in the urine in the absence or glomerular histologic changes by light microscopy. It is now established, however, that increased glomerular permeability to protein is the *cause* of proteinuria and that the lipid reflects loss and reabsorption of lipoprotein. The proximal convoluted tubules show hyalin and fatty droplets that reflect reabsorption of filtered protein and liproprotein.

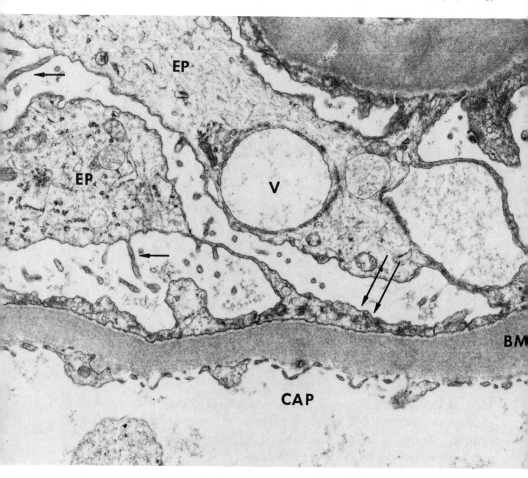

Fig. 12-10 An electron micrograph of glomerulus in lipoid nephrosis. The epithelial cells (EP) show complete obliteration of the foot processes (double arrow), vacuolization (V), and formation of surface microvilli (small arrow). Note that there are no deposits along the basement membrane (BM).

The great majority of patients with lipoid nephrosis exhibit a rapid response to corticosteroid therapy. There is disappearance of the proteinuria, recovery of epithelial foot processes, and restitution of the capillary wall by electron microscopy. Although there are recurrences, they also generally respond to steroid therapy. In a series of 209 patients, followed up to 10 years, it was found that 71% were in complete remission, 10% still exhibited the nephrotic syndrome, and only

3 patients had died of chronic renal insufficiency (57). In adults, relapses after discontinuance of corticosteroids are more frequent, and the prognosis is generally somewhat less favorable.

FOCAL AND SEGMENTAL SCLEROSIS AND HYALINOSIS

In the course of an international study on the effect of corticosteroid therapy in lipoid nephrosis, it was noted that a small proportion of patients responded poorly to steroids (63). In these patients, light microscopic examination of renal biopsies showed that, while most glomeruli were normal, an occasional glomerulus exhibited an area of sclerosis confined to only a segment of the glomerulus (Fig. 12-11). Thus, the lesions were focal in that they involved some glomeruli and segmental in that they involved a segment of the affected glomerulus. Hyaline masses were frequently present in the sclerotic areas (thus focal hyalinosis). Although this is almost certainly a variant of lipoid nephrosis, the entity has now been separated from lipoid nephrosis and termed *focal* sclerosis or focal sclerosing glomerulonephritis (64, 65, 66). Patients with this lesion have the nephrotic syndrome but differ from the usual patients with lipoid nephrosis in the following respects: (1) They have a higher incidence of hematuria and hyperten-

Fig. 12-11 Focal sclerosis—while most of the glomerulus is normal, there is a segment which is obliterated by noncellular hyalin material.

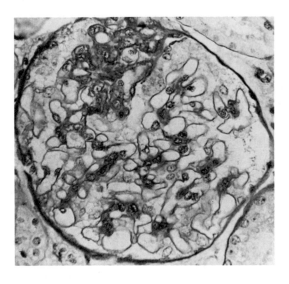

sion, (2) they respond poorly to corticosteroid therapy, (3) many progress to chronic glomerulonephritis, about 50% dying within 10 years of diagnosis, (4) immunofluorescence microscopy shows deposition of IgM and complement in the sclerotic areas of the glomeruli, and (5) there is a high incidence of recurrence in patients with focal sclerosis who receive renal transplants (about two-thirds of cases).

As seen by light microscopy, the segmental lesions may involve only a minority of the glomeruli and initially the juxtamedullary glomeruli, although they subsequently become more generalized. In the sclerotic segments there is collapse of basement membranes, increase in mesangial matrix, and deposition of hyaline masses (hyalinosis), often with lipoid droplets. Glomeruli without segmental sclerosis appear either normal (as in lipoid nephrosis) or may show increased mesangial proliferation. Electron microscopy shows the loss of foot process in nonsclerotic areas, as in lipoid nephrosis, but in the sclerotic lesions there is also pronounced denudation of the podocytes. Granules are also present within the sclerotic areas. Immunofluorescence reveals nodular deposits of IgM and C3 within the sclerotic areas, but nonsclerotic glomeruli show either no staining or slight staining with IgM and C3.

Clinically there is little tendency for spontaneous remission, and responses to corticosteroid therapy are infrequent. Progression of renal failure occurs at variable rates. Some patients follow an unusually rapid course (malignant focal sclerosis), with intractable proteinuria ending in renal failure within two years (67). Of note is the development of focal sclerosis with heavy proteinuria in heroin addicts (68), in whom the prognosis is very poor.

Membranoproliferative glomerulonephritis (MPGN)

As the term implies, this condition is characterized histologically by both thickening of the basement membrane and proliferation of cells. Because the proliferation is predominantly in the mesangium, a frequently used synonym is mesangio–capillary glomerulonephritis; a number of patients with the histologic lesions exhibit persistent hypocomplementemia, and the disease is also known as chronic hypocomplementemic glomerulonephritis.

The condition was first clearly delineated in 1965 when a form of chronic glomerulonephritis in children and young adults was found to be characterized by persistent low levels of serum complement (69). Most of these patients did not have previous poststreptococcal glomerulonephritis or any other condition such as lupus erythematosus, that would account for the hypocomplementemia. Since these initial studies, it has been shown that many patients with similar histologic lesions may have normal serum complement levels at various times, despite the progression of the glomerular disease. The clinical manifestations are variable; some patients present with hematuria or proteinuria, about two-thirds develop the overt nephrotic syndrome, and hypertension may or may not be present.

It is now customary to divide the disease into two types (I and II) depending on the ultrastructural features (see below).

ETIOLOGY AND PATHOGENESIS

As in most other types of glomerulonephritis, no etiologic agent is evident. In most cases of type I MPGN, there is evidence of immune complexes in the circulation or the kidneys (70). However, many with type II lesions have features which suggest that in some (but by no means all) patients the disease results not from activation of complement by immune complexes, but rather from activation of complement via the *alternate pathway* (the properdin system). The latter pathway is activated by bacterial lipopolysaccharides, aggregated globulins, and IgA.

In the first place, depression of serum complement in many patients is limited to C3–C9 components of the system, C1, C2, and C4 being unaltered. Secondly, properdin, a major protein of the alternate system, is deposited in glomeruli, together with C3 components, but often not with C1 or C4. Thirdly, some patients with MPGN have in their serum a factor, termed *C3 nephritic factor* (C3NeF), which is capable of breaking down C3 *in vitro,* thus activating the complement pathway (Fig. 12-12). It has recently been discovered that C3NeF is an immunoglobulin, which acts at the same step in the alternate complement pathway as *properdin,* helping to stabilize the alternate pathway convertase C3bBb by binding to it (71). It may be that C3NeF is acting as an autoantibody to this convertase, adding MPGN to the list of autoimmune diseases affecting the glomerulus. In addition to increased consumption of C3, there is decreased C3 synthesis by the liver, further contributing to the profound hypocomplementemia.

How these complement defects cause glomerular injury is unclear. It has not been possible to induce glomerulonephritis experimentally by activation of the alternate complement pathway (72). Could it be, instead, that the complement defects—either genetic or acquired—pre-

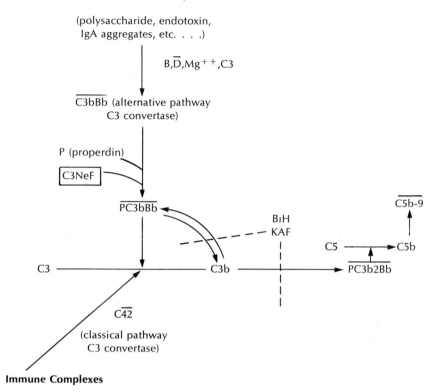

Fig. 12-12 The alternate complement pathway. Note that C3NeF acts at the same site as properdin, serving to stabilize the alternate pathway C3 convertase (C3bBb). Courtesy Dr. A. Arnaout, Children's Hospital Medical Center, Boston.

dispose to GN by limiting the patient's ability to deal with infectious agents or toxins? Could products of complement activation be nephrotoxic only in certain genetically susceptible individuals? A genetic predisposition is suggested by the presence of C3NeF activity in 50% of patients with the genetically determined disease, *partial lipodystrophy* (73), and with the increased frequency of HLA-B7 in patients with type II MPGN (74).

PATHOLOGIC CHANGES

The glomeruli are large and hypercellular, the latter due to a prominent increase in mesangial cells (Fig. 12-13). The GBM is thickened, often focally, particularly in the peripheral capillary loops. The glomerular capillary wall shows a "double contour" or "tram track" appearance in silver of PAS stains. This is caused by "splitting" of the basement membrane because of the inclusion within it of processes of mesangial cells extending into the peripheral capillary loops, so-called *mesangial interposition.*

MPGN is divided into two major types according to the ultrastructural findings (75):

Type I MPGN (two-thirds of cases) is characterized by the presence of *subendothelial* electron-dense deposits. Mesangial and occasional subepithelial deposits may also be present. Immunofluorescence reveals that C3 is deposited in a granular pattern and IgG and early complement components (C1q and C4) are often also present, suggesting an immune complex pathogenesis in the majority of cases.

In the type II lesion, the lamina densa of the GBM is transformed

Fig. 12-13 Membranoproliferative GN–there is both proliferation of mesangial cells and thickening of the capillary wall.

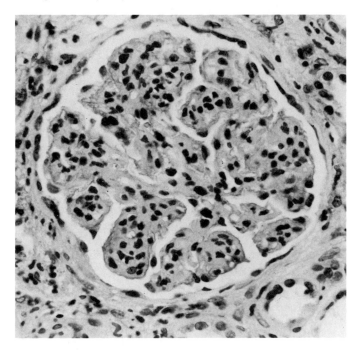

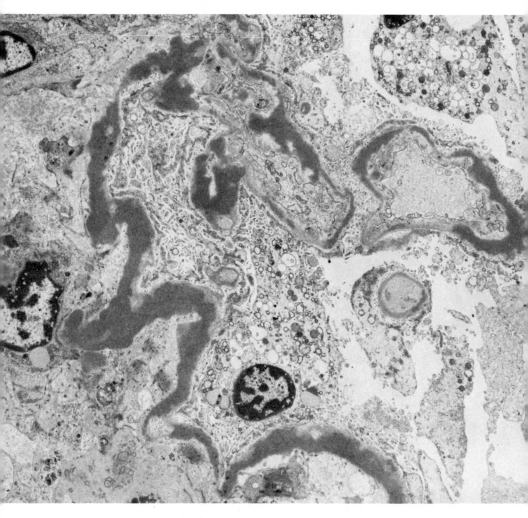

Fig. 12-14 Dense-deposit disease—a variant of membranoproliferative GN. There are dense deposits *within* the basement membrane. (Courtesy of Dr. T. Cavallo)

into an irregular, electron-dense structure, due to the deposition of dense material in the GBM proper, giving rise to the term *dense-deposit disease* (Fig. 12-14). In type II, C3 is present in irregular granular-linear foci within the basement membranes and mesangium, IgG is often absent, and the early acting complement components (C1q and C4) are always absent from the deposits, suggesting activation of the alternate complement pathway.

While most authors (75, 76) agree on this relatively good correlation between the type of MPGN and the complement abnormality described above, others find no distinguishing clinical or laboratory features between the two types (77).

The clinical course of membranoproliferative glomerulonephritis is variable, but many patients in time develop increasing renal insufficiency and chronic glomerulonephritis. If they are transplanted, recurrences in allografts occur with a greater frequency than in diseases such as membranous glomerulonephritis and chronic sclerosing glomerulonephritis. This is especially true with the dense-deposit variety of the condition.

Chronic sclerosing glomerulonephritis

Chronic sclerosing glomerulonephritis is the clinical and pathological expression of many types of protracted, long-standing glomerulonephritis. In its final stages, the syndrome is associated with a series of clinical, biochemical, and metabolic disturbances that are discussed in detail in the chapter on chronic renal failure.

Chronic glomerulonephritis, the most common cause of chronic renal failure in man (78), develops following some of the conditions discussed earlier in this chapter. Poststreptococcal glomerulonephritis is a rare antecedent of chronic glomerulonephritis, except in some adults. Patients with rapidly progressive glomerulonephritis, if successfully dialyzed, invariably end with chronic glomerulonephritis; membranous and membranoproliferative varieties progress more slowly to chronic renal failure; focal sclerosis often develops rather rapidly into chronic glomerulonephritis. Nevertheless, in any series of patients who present with the clinicopathologic syndrome of chronic glomerulonephritis, about one-third give no preceding history of any of the well-recognized forms of early glomerulonephritis. These cases represent the end result of relatively asymptomatic forms of glomerulonephritis, either known or still unrecognized, that progress to uremia.

PATHOLOGIC CHANGES

The kidneys are contracted and have a finely granular external surface. On cut section the cortex is thinned, and there is increase in peripelvic fat. Histologic examination shows replacement of most of the glomeruli by a hyalin material (Fig. 12-15). In early cases, the non-sclerosed glomeruli may show evidence of the primary disease, for example, membranous or membranoproliferative glomerulonephritis. To-

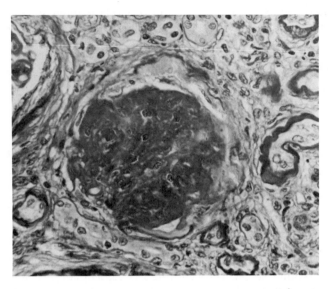

Fig. 12-15 Chronic glomerulonephritis—a totally hyalinized glomerulus is evident.

gether with the glomerular hyalinization, marked atrophy of the associated tubules, irregular interstitial fibrosis, and lymphocytic infiltration occur. Because hypertension is a common accompaniment of chronic glomerulonephritis, arterial and arteriolar sclerosis may be conspicuous. Secondary vascular, tubular, and interstitial changes in end-stage renal failure may make it difficult to determine whether the primary disease affecting the kidney is glomerulonephritis rather than an interstitial or vascular process.

Patients dying with chronic glomerulonephritis exhibit pathological changes outside the kidney that are related to the uremic state and that are also present in other forms of chronic renal failure. Often clinically important, these include uremic pericarditis, uremic gastroenteritis, secondary hyperparathyroidism, left ventricular hypertrophy due to hypertension, and pulmonary changes often ascribed to uremia (uremic pneumonitis).

CLINICAL COURSE

Some patients may go on for years with a relatively stable glomerular filtration rate, whereas others succumb rapidly to uremia or to complications of secondary hypertensive disease. Exacerbations of the active nephritic process with hematuria, oliguria, proteinuria, and on occasion the overt nephrotic syndrome may also occur.

Focal glomerulonephritis (including IgA nehropathy)

Focal glomerulonephritis represents a histologic entity in which glomerular proliferation is restricted to segments of individual glomeruli and commonly involves only a proportion of the glomeruli. The lesions are predominantly proliferative (Fig. 12-16) or necrotizing and should be differentiated from those occurring in focal sclerosis. Defined as such, focal glomerulonephritis occurs under two circumstances:

1. It may be a manifestation of a systemic disease that sometimes involves the entire glomerulus, e.g., systemic lupus erythematosus, polyarteritis nodosa, early Goodpasture's syndrome, Wegener's granulomatosis, Henoch-Schönlein purpura, and subacute bacterial endocarditis.

2. Similar changes can occur in the kidney unrelated to any systemic disease and constitute a form of primary focal glomerulonephritis.

Fig. 12-16 Focal proliferative glomerulonephritis—one segment of the glomerulus shows hypercellularity.

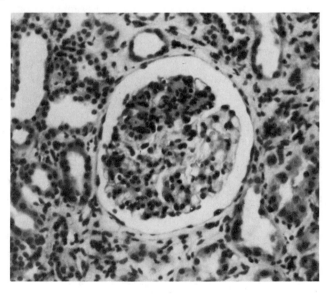

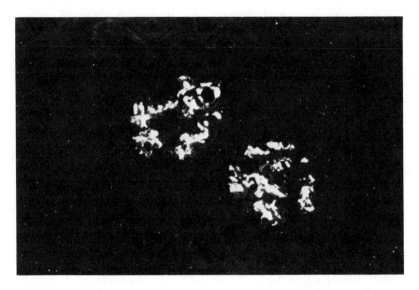

Fig. 12-17 IgA nephropathy. Two glomeruli showing typical immunofluorescent pattern of IgA localization in the mesangium.

In primary focal glomerulonephritis, the clinical manifestations are usually recurrent hematuria, proteinuria, or both.

One type of focal GN, *IgA nephropathy* or Bergers's disease has sufficiently distinctive immunologic features to be described separately. It is characterized by the presence of IgA deposits in the mesangial regions as determined by immunofluorescence microscopy (79) (Fig. 12-17). Clinically there is usually recurrent gross or microscopic hematuria and mild proteinuria. Occasionally the nephrotic syndrome may develop (80). The disease usually affects children and young adults and may arise within a day or two of a nonspecific respiratory infection. Typically, the hematuria lasts for several days, then subsides only to return every few months.

By light microscopy the glomeruli are sometimes normal, but more commonly show mesangial widening and segmental proliferation confined to some glomeruli. The immunofluorescent picture is of mesangial deposition of IgA, often with C3 and properdin and lesser amounts of IgG or IgM. Early complement components are usually absent. Electron microscopy confirms the presence of electron-dense deposits in the mesangium in most cases.

The pathogenesis is unknown. The mesangial deposition of IgA suggests entrapment of large, circulating aggregates or complexes, and the absence of early complement components points to activation of the alternate complement pathway. Up to 50% of patients have elevated IgA serum levels. The hematuria often recurs after a flulike syndrome. Taken together, these findings suggest a peculiar reactivity to some exogenous agent (virus?), resulting in the production of increased levels of IgA, which aggregates or complexes to antigen and becomes entrapped in the mesangium, activating the alternate complement pathway. The peculiar reactivity may be genetically determined as evidenced by familial clustering and by the occurrence of the disease in twins.

Although IgA nephropathy is generally a benign or, at best, a slowly progressive disease, at least 15% of patients progress to renal failure and hypertension over a period of 10 years (79). Insufficient time has elapsed since the discovery of the disease to estimate long-term prognosis.

SUNDRY GLOMERULAR LESIONS ASSOCIATED WITH SYSTEMIC DISEASES

Lupus glomerulonephritis
Glomerulonephritis occurs in up to 70% of patients with systemic lupus erythematosus, but the kidneys of all such patients show some abnormalities when studied by fluorescence or electron microscopy. The pathogenesis of glomerular damage has been well documented as a type of immune-complex nephritis, the lesion being induced by deposition of DNA—anti-DNA complexes in the glomeruli: immunoglobulin, complement, and DNA as antigen can be localized in glomeruli, and antibody eluted from renal tissue has antinuclear activity. The immune reactants may deposit as circulating complexes, but also probably by virtue of an affinity of DNA to collagenlike components of the glomerulus (23), a form of *in situ* immune complex deposition (p. 284). The resulting clinical syndromes are variable and include recurrent gross or microscopic hematuria, acute nephritis, and the nephrotic syndrome. Any of these may progress in time to chronic renal insufficiency, which remains one of the main causes of death in patients with systemic lupus erythematosus.

Four subgroups of lupus nephritis are recognized (81):

Mesangial lupus nephritis is the mildest of the lesions and is seen in those patients who have minimal clinical manifestations such as mild hematuria or proteinuria. There is slight increase in the intercapillary mesangial matrix and the number of mesangial cells. Despite the mild histologic change, mesangial deposits of immunoglobulin and complement are almost always present.

Focal proliferative glomerulonephritis is seen in about one-third of initial biopsies of patients. Typically one or two tufts in an otherwise normal glomerulus exhibit swelling and proliferation of endothelial and mesangial cells, infiltration with neutrophils, and sometimes fibrinoid deposits and intracapillary thrombi. *Hematoxylin bodies* may be present, and fragmentation and breakdown of nuclei produce the degenerative appearance described as "nuclear dust." Focal lesions may be associated with recurrent hematuria and moderate proteinuria, but some patients with focal lesions may have more severe clinical disease progressing to renal failure.

Diffuse proliferative glomerulonephritis is the most serious of the renal lesions in SLE, occurring in 45 to 50% of patients. Most or all glomeruli are involved in both kidneys, and the entire glomerulus is almost always affected. Patients with diffuse lesions are usually symptomatic, showing microscopic or gross hematuria, proteinuria including the nephrotic syndrome, hypertension, and frequently a diminution of glomerular filtration rate. In some patients there is, in addition, membranous thickening; thus the lesion may resemble MPGN.

Membranous glomerulonephritis occurs in 10% of patients. The lesions are very similar to those encountered in idiopathic membranous glomerulonephritis, described more fully earlier. Patients with this histologic change almost always have severe proteinuria or the overt nephrotic syndrome.

All four types are thought to be due to the deposition of DNA–anti-DNA complexes within the glomeruli. Thus deposits of immunoglobulin and complement—sometimes in the mesangium only, sometimes along the entire basement membrane, and sometimes massively throughout the entire glomerulus—are characteristic features. Why this same pathogenetic mechanism produces such different histologic lesions (and clinical manifestations) in different patients is not entirely clear. It is likely that the physical and chemical characteristics of the complexes as well as the state of the glomerular capillary wall play a role in the pattern of deposition of complexes and in the histologic change.

Electron microscopy reveals electron-dense deposits (presumably immune complexes) in three locations within the glomerulus. (1) In the membranous type the deposits are predominantly subepithelial, a location similar to that of deposits in other types of membranous nephropathy. (2) All histologic types show large deposits in the mesangium. (3) *Subendothelial deposits* (between the endothelium and the basement membrane) are particularly characteristic of SLE, since they are present in few other types of glomerulonephritis (Fig. 12-18). When extensive, subendothelial deposits create a peculiar thickening of the capillary wall, which can be seen by means of light microscopy as a "wire loop" lesion. Such "wire loops" are often found in the proliferative types of glomerulonephritis. They usually reflect active disease and are generally a poor prognostic sign.

Although the four types of lupus nephritis have been presented separately, occasionally one type transforms to another in the same patient. Focal proliferative GN transforms fairly frequently to the diffuse type. Of interest is the finding that whereas patients with the diffuse proliferative type of lupus nephritis have large amounts of *precipitating antibody* to native DNA in their serum, those with membranous GN have only low titers of *nonprecipitating antibody* (82). This indicates that the host antibody response may determine the nature of the immune complex and thus the location of its deposition in the glomerulus.

Diabetic glomerulosclerosis

In long-standing diabetes mellitus the kidney rarely escapes damage. Hyaline arteriosclerosis, acute pyelonephritis, necrotizing papillitis, and diabetic glomerulosclerosis are the main forms of diabetic nephropathy. The glomerular involvement takes the form of diffuse or nodular glomerulosclerosis (the latter called Kimmelstiel-Wilson's disease), or, more often, the concurrence of both patterns. The glomerulosclerosis is related to the duration of the disease rather than to its severity, and one or both patterns almost inevitably appear within 15 to 20 years (83).

In the diffuse form the lesions consist of diffuse thickening of the basement membrane proper and increased mesangial cells and mesangial matrix. In the nodular form there is massive deposition of base-

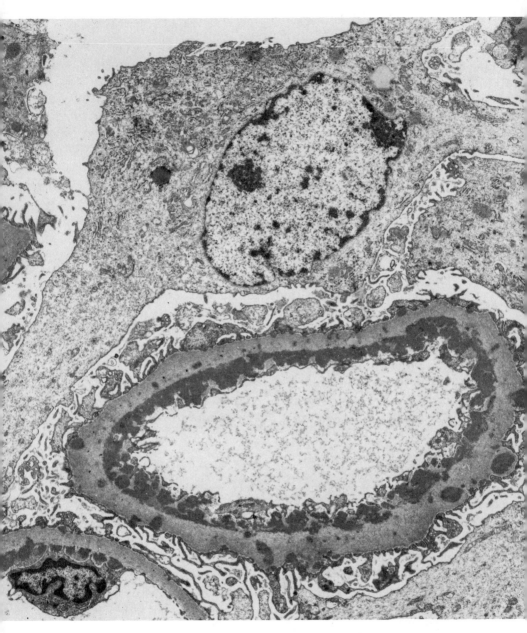

Fig. 12-18 *Subendothelial* deposits seen in lupus nephritis. There are also a few subepithelial deposits.

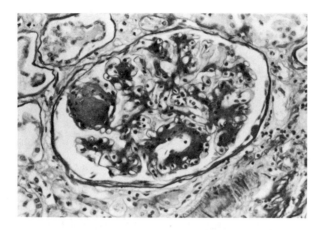

Fig. 12-19 Diabetic glomerulosclerosis. Note the typical acellular nodule and the diffuse thickening of the mesangium. From Robbins and Cotran, Pathologic Basis of Disease (2nd ed.). W. B. Saunders, Philadelphia, 1979.

ment membrane matrix material in the mesangium, producing the typical hyaline mass in the center of a glomerular lobule with capillaries displaced to the periphery (Fig. 12-19). The pathogenesis of these changes is obscure but is clearly related to the pathogenesis of diabetic microangiopathy. Recent studies have shown enhanced glomerular basement membrane synthesis in diabetic rats (84), but decreased degradation of GBM material has not been excluded. The clinical manifestations include recurrent proteinuria often in the nephrotic range, followed by slow progression to chronic renal failure. The ischemic lesions caused by arterial and arteriolar disease almost certainly contribute to the renal insufficiency.

Amyloidosis

Generalized amyloidosis, whether it conforms to the so-called primary or secondary pattern of distribution, may be associated with deposits of amyloid within the glomeruli. The fibrillar deposits of amyloid are present within the mesangium, subendothelium, and occasionally, the subepithelial space. Eventually, they obliterate the glomerulus completely. Deposits of amyloid also appear in blood vessel walls and in the kidney interstitium. Amyloid can be identified by light microscopy with special stains; particularly indicative is the birefringence after staining with Congo red, and the characteristic amyloid fibrillar ultrastructure.

Patients with glomerular amyloid may present with heavy protein-uria or the nephrotic syndrome, and later they succumb from uremia caused by total obliteration of glomeruli. Characteristically, kidney size tends to be either normal or slightly enlarged, despite the chronic renal failure.

Bacterial endocarditis

Glomerular lesions occurring in the course of subacute bacterial endo-carditis have long been known as "focal embolic GN." It is now known, however, that these lesions are not embolic in nature but rep-resent a type of immune complex nephritis initiated by bacterial antigen–antibody complex. Clinically, hematuria and proteinuria of various degrees characterize this entity, but an acute nephritic presen-tation is not uncommon, and even rapidly progressive GN may occur in rare instances. The histologic lesions, when present, generally re-flect these clinical manifestations. Milder forms have a focal and seg-mental necrotizing glomerulonephritis, while the more severe ones ex-hibit a diffuse, proliferative GN; the rapidly progressive forms show crescentic glomerulonephritis.

Henoch-Schönlein purpura

This syndrome consists of purpuric dermal lesions involving the lower extremities and buttocks; abdominal pain, vomiting, and intes-tinal bleeding; nonmigratory arthralgia; and renal abnormalities. The disease is most common in children but also occurs in adults, in whom the renal manifestations are usually more severe. There is a strong background of atopy in about one-third of patients. The onset often follows an upper respiratory infection. Renal manifestations include gross or microscopic hematuria, proteinuria, or the nephrotic syn-drome. A small number of patients, mostly adults, develop a rapidly progressive form of glomerulonephritis.

Histologically, the renal lesions vary in severity from mild, focal mesangial proliferation to diffuse mesangial proliferation to rather typical crescentic glomerulonephritis. The prominent feature by fluo-rescence microscopy is the *deposition of IgA, sometimes with IgG and C3 in the mesangial region* in a distribution similar to that in IgA ne-phropathy (85). This has led to the belief that Berger's disease and Henoch-Schönlein purpura are perhaps spectra of the same disease.

The skin lesions consist of subepidermal hemorrhages and a necrotizing vasculitis involving the small vessels of the dermis.

Recurrences of hematuria may persist for many years after onset but most children follow a benign course. Patients with the diffuse lesions or with the nephrotic syndrome have a somewhat poorer prognosis and renal failure occurs in patients with the crescentic lesions (86).

Other systemic disorders

Goodpasture's syndrome, polyarteritis nodosa, and Wegener's granulomatosis are commonly associated with glomerular lesions which can be very similar. In the early or mild forms of involvement there is focal and segmental, sometimes necrotizing, GN and most patients have hematuria with rather mild decline in GFR. In the more severe cases associated with rapidly progressive GN, there are extensive necrosis, fibrin deposition, and the formation of epithelial crescents. These diseases, however, have different pathogenetic mechanisms. Goodpasture's syndrome is mediated by anti-GBM antibodies and exhibits linear fluorescence of immunoglobulin and complement, while polyarteritis nodosa and Wegener's granulomatosis are of somewhat more obscure etiology, although immune complexes are frequently present in the former. *Essential mixed cryoglobulinemia* is another rare condition in which deposits of cryoglobulins composed largely of IgG–IgM complexes induce cutaneous vasculitis, synovitis, and focal or diffuse proliferative glomerulonephritis (87).

Hereditary nephritis

Hereditary nephritis encompasses a group of hereditary renal diseases associated with glomerular injury. The most well-studied entity is so-called Alport's syndrome, in which nephritis is accompanied by nerve deafness and various ocular manifestations. Males tend to be affected more frequently and more severely than females and are more likely to progress to renal failure. The common presenting sign is gross or microscopic hematuria, frequently accompanied by erythrocyte casts. Proteinuria may occur and, rarely, the nephrotic syndrome develops. Symptoms appear at age 5 to 20 and the onset of renal failure is between ages 20 and 50 (88). The auditory defects may be subtle and require extensive hearing tests. The mode of inheritance in most kindreds is autosomal dominant. In some families a sex-linked dominant mode of genetic transmission is seen.

By light microscopy the early glomerular alterations are seen to consist of focal sclerosis and proliferation, but as the disease progresses there is increasing glomerulosclerosis, vascular narrowing, tubular atrophy, and interstitial fibrosis. With the electron microscope, characteristic basement membrane lesions are found in some (but not all) patients with hereditary nephritis. The basement membrane shows irregular foci of thickening or attenuation, with areas of splitting and lamination of the lamina densa. Similar alterations are found in the tubular basement membranes. Such basement membrane changes are seen focally in other diseases, but they are most widespread and pronounced in patients with this disorder (89). The nature of the basement membrane defect is unknown.

THE NEPHROTIC SYNDROME

In the preceding sections, it was noted that a number of categories of glomerulonephritis are characterized clinically by the nephrotic syndrome. Lipoid nephrosis and membranous glomerulonephritis present exclusively as the nephrotic syndrome, and the syndrome appears in many patients with focal sclerosis, membranoproliferative glomerulonephritis, and systemic lupus erythematosus. Thus the term does not imply a single disease entity, but a constellation of clinical findings dominated by heavy proteinuria. These conditions have in common the presence of glomerular damage and increased glomerular permeability to protein. Table 12-5 is a partial list of the many causes of the nephrotic syndrome. In addition to various types of glomerulonephritis, it includes generalized systemic disorders, circulatory disturbances, and infections. The most frequent of the secondary diseases are diabetes mellitus, amyloidosis, and lupus nephritis. This section is devoted to a brief discussion of the clinical features and pathophysiology common to all these conditions (90).

The nephrotic syndrome is characterized by heavy proteinuria, diminution of the level of plasma protein, generalized edema, and a rise in serum lipids.

Proteinuria

Many workers define the nephrotic syndrome by the finding of consistent proteinuria that exceeds 3.5 gm of protein per 24 hours. Most patients excrete amounts well in excess of that, and quantities exceeding 10 gm/24 hours are not uncommon. Protein loss in the urine may

TABLE 12-5 *Diseases Associated with the Nephrotic Syndrome*

---

1. Primary Glomerular Disease
    Lipoid nephrosis
        Focal sclerosis
    Membranous GN
    Membranoproliferative GN
    Other proliferative GN (focal; pure mesangial)

2. Systemic Diseases
    Diabetes mellitus
    Amyloidosis
    Systemic lupus erythematosus

3. Circulatory Disturbances
    Renal vein thrombosis (most cases secondary)
    Constrictive pericarditis (rare)

4. Toxins and Drugs
    Gold salts; mercurial diuretics; penicillamine

5. Infections
    Syphilis, malaria

6. Malignancy

---

occur in three ways: (1) diminished reabsorption by tubules of normally filtered protein, (2) increased secretion by tubules, and (3) increased filtration at the level of the glomerulus. It is now agreed that decreased reabsorption of the small amounts that are normally filtered cannot account for the massive quantities of protein found in most patients, and the evidence for tubular secretion is lacking. On the other hand, increased glomerular permeability is supported by the following findings:

1. In all patients with the nephrotic syndrome, there is structural evidence of glomerular injury. Even in lipoid nephrosis, where the light microscopic appearance is normal, there is a striking visceral epithelial lesion seen uniformly by electron microscopy.

2. Observations of relative clearance of serum proteins and dextran molecules in patients with the nephrotic syndrome suggest that proteinuria results from the molecular sieving action of an abnormally permeable glomerular filter. Similar conclusions can be derived from experiments in which human albumin was infused in nephrotic patients.

3. In a variety of experimental models of proteinuria, electron microscopy has shown that ultrastructural protein tracers injected intravenously are filtered in increased amounts across the capillary wall of glomeruli. Micropuncture studies in rats with aminonucleoside nephrosis, a model for minimal change disease, strongly suggest increased glomerular permeability as the cause of the proteinuria (reviewed in refs. 91–93).

The largest proportion of protein lost in the urine is albumin, but about one-third of the urinary proteins are the smaller globulins. In recent years there has been interest in the concept of "selectivity" of proteinuria in various cases of the nephrotic syndrome. A highly selective proteinuria is one that would allow loss only of the smaller molecular weight proteins, larger substances in the range of gamma globulin fractions being found in small amounts. A poorly selective proteinuria would contain larger molecular weight proteins in addition to albumin. In general, patients with lipoid nephrosis tend to have a highly selective proteinuria while those with membranous glomerulonephritis would have a poorly selective proteinuria; however, the value of selectivity as a clinically useful index in any one patient is questionable.

Hypoproteinemia

The hypoalbuminemia is mainly a reflection of the loss of urinary protein, since there is a relationship between the serum albumin level and the amount of protein lost. There is also a decrease in gamma globulin of the IgG type. However, IgM levels may be increased in patients with lipoid nephrosis but not in those with membranous glomerulonephritis (94). Studies have also shown that there is increased catabolism of protein, as in patients with the nephrotic syndrome (95).

Edema

Edema is frequently the first manifestation noted by the patient and can be so severe as to be incapacitating. The mechanism of edema formation is discussed in detail in Chapter 6. In brief, hypoalbuminemia causes loss of colloid oncotic pressure of the blood, which forces fluid into the interstitial spaces. There is also a decrease in the effective extracellular fluid volume, with increased aldosterone production, consequent retention of sodium and water, and further increase in edema.

The edema becomes generalized, and pleural and peritoneal effusions may occur.

Hyperlipidemia

The exact cause of the hyperlipidemia is unclear. Elevations of triglycerides, cholesterol, VLDL, and LDL are reported. The degree of hyperlipidemia is improved by albumin or dextran administration. Increased synthesis of lipoprotein by liver slices (96) has been demonstrated in experimental animals. The hypothesis is that hypoalbuminemia stimulates hepatic synthesis of albumin and this is associated with stimulation of the synthetic pathways for VLDL, which is converted by lipolysis to LDL. The hyperlipidemia increases the chance for development of atherosclerosis in patients with long-standing nephrotic syndrome, but a recent study has cast doubt on the magnitude of such increased risk (97).

Lipiduria

Lipiduria is manifested by oval fat bodies seen in the urine sediment; these represent excreted tubular cells containing lipoprotein filtered in the glomerulus and reabsorbed by tubules. Free fat is also seen as well as birefringent crystals of cholesterol esters having the appearance of a maltese cross.

Patients with the nephrotic syndrome are susceptible to infections; in the preantibiotic era mortality due to gram-positive bacterial infection (e.g., pneumococcal peritonitis) was not infrequent. There is also an increased incidence of venous thrombosis and consequent pulmonary embolism in these patients. This hypercoagulability is ascribed to loss of normal anticoagulant substances (such as antithrombin III) in the urine. In this regard, it has long been known that the nephrotic syndrome is associated with *renal* vein thrombosis, and the latter condition is routinely listed as a *cause* of nephrotic syndrome. However, it has been difficult to induce heavy proteinuria in experimental animals by obstructing the renal veins. Biopsies of patients with nephrotic syndrome and renal vein thrombosis show histologic and immunofluorescent findings suggestive of immune-complex nephritis; it has thus been argued that the renal thrombosis is not the *cause* of proteinuria but merely reflects the hypercoagulability of blood seen in nephrotic patients who have primary glomerulonephritis (98).

General references

R. H. Heptinstall. Pathology of the kidney, 2nd ed., Little, Brown, Boston, 1974.
B. M. Brenner and F. C. Rector, Jr. The kidney, Vols. 1 and 2, 2nd ed., W. B. Saunders, Philadelphia, 1980.
Strauss and Welt's diseases of the kidney, 3rd ed., L. Early and C. Gottschalk (eds.), Little, Brown, Boston, 1979.
C. M. Edelmann. Pediatric kidney disease, 1st ed., Little, Brown, Boston, 1978.
J. Hamburger, J. Crosnier, and J. P. Grünfeld (eds.). Nephrology. Wiley-Flammarion, New York, 1979.
J. Churg, B. Spargo, F. K. Mostofi, and M. Abell (eds.). Kidney disease—present status. Williams & Wilkins, Baltimore, 1979.
P. Kincaid-Smith, A. J. d'Apice, and R. C. Atkins (eds.). Progress in glomerulonephritis. Wiley, New York, 1979.

References

1. Wilson, C. B. and Dixon, F. J. The renal response to immunological injury. In The kidney, B. M. Brenner and F. C. Rector, Jr. (eds.). W. B. Saunders, Philadelphia, 1976, p. 838.

2. Wilson, C. B. and Dixon, F. J. Immunologic mechanisms in nephritogenesis. Hosp. Pract. 14:57, 1979.

3. Couser, W. G. and Salant, D. J. In situ complex formation and glomerular injury. Kidney Int. 17:1, 1980.

3a. Salant, D. J., Belok, S., Stilmant, M. M., Darby, C., and Couser, W. G. Determinants of glomerular localization of subepithelial immune deposits. Lab. Invest. 41:89, 1979.

4. Germuth, F. G., Jr. A comparative histologic and immunologic study in rabbits of induced hypersensitivity of serum sickness type. J. Exp. Med. 97:257, 1953.

5. Unanue, E. R. and Dixon, F. J. Experimental glomerulonephritis. Immunological events and pathogenetic mechanisms. Adv. Immunol. 6:1–90, 1967.

6. Dixon, F. J., Feldman, J. D., and Vasquez, J. J. Experimental glomerulonephritis: the pathogenesis of a laboratory model resembling the spectrum of human glomerulonephritis. J. Exp. Med. 113:899, 1961.

7. Oldstone, M. B. A. and Dixon, F. J. Immune complex disease in chronic viral infections. J. Exp. Med. 134(3, Pt. 2):32s, 1971.

8. Mellors, R. C. Autoimmune and immunoproliferative diseases of NZB/BL mice and hybrids. Int. Rev. Exp. Path. 5:217, 1966.

9. Dixon, F. J., Oldstone, M. B. A., and Tonietti, G. Pathogenesis of immune complex glomerulonephritis of New Zealand mice. J. Exp. Med. 134(3, Pt. 2): 65s–71s, 1971.

10. Houba, V. and Allison, A. C. Nephropathies associated with tropical parasitic diseases. In Nephrology, J. Hamburger, J. Crosnier, and J. P. Grünfeld (eds.). Wiley-Flammarion, New York, 1979, p. 791.

11. Hutt, M. S. R. (guest editor). The kidney in parasitism. Kidney Int. 16:1–74, 1979.

12. Cochrane, C. G. and Koffler, D. Immune complex disease in experimental animals and man. Adv. Immunol. 16:185–264, 1973.

13. Cochrane, C. G. and Hawkins, D. Studies on circulating immune complexes. III. Factors governing the ability of circulating complexes to localize in blood vessels. J. Exp. Med. 127:137, 1968.

14. Germuth, F. G., Jr. and Rodriguez, E. Immunopathology of the renal glomerulus: immune complex deposit and antibasement disease. Little, Brown, Boston, 1973.
15. Cochrane, C. G. Mechanisms involved in the deposition of immune complexes in tissues. J. Exp. Med. 134(3, Pt. 2):75s–89s, 1971.
16. Border, W. A. Immune complex detection in glomerular diseases. Nephron (in press).
17. Pussel, B. A., Scott, D. M., Lockwood, A. J., and Peters, D. K. Value of immune complex assays in diagnosis and management. Lancet 2:359, 1978.
18. Heymann, W., Hackel, D. B., Harwood, S., Wilson, S. G. F., and Hunter, J. L. P. Production of nephrotic syndrome in rats by Freund's adjuvants and rat kidney suspension. Proc. Soc. Exp. Biol. Med. 100:660, 1959.
19. Glassock, R. J., Edgington, T. S., Watson, J. I., and Dixon, F. J. Autologous immune complex nephritis induced with renal tubular antigen. II. The pathogenetic mechanism. J. Exp. Med. 127:573–588, 1968.
20. Van Damme, B. J. C., Fleuren, G. J., Bakker, W. W., Vernier, R. L., and Hoedemaeker, Ph.J. Experimental glomerulonephritis in the rat induced by antibodies directed against tubular antigens. IV. Fixed glomerular antigens in the pathogenesis of heterologous immune complex glomerulonephritis. Lab. Invest. 38:502–510, 1978.
21. Couser, W. G., Steinmuller, D. R., Stilmant, M. M., Salant, D. J., and Lowenstein, L. M. Experimental glomerulonephritis in the isolated perfused rat kidney. J. Clin. Invest. 62:1275–1287, 1978.
22. Golbus, S. and Wilson, C. B. Glomerulonephritis produced by the in situ formation of immune complexes in glomerular capillary wall. Kidney Int. 16:148, 1979.
23. Izui, S., Lambert, P. H., and Miescher, P. A.: In vitro demonstration of a particular affinity of glomerular basement membrane and collagen for DNA. A possible basis for local formation of DNA–anti-DNA complexes in systemic lupus erythematosus. J. Exp. Med. 144:428–443, 1976.
24. Unanue, E. R. and Dixon, F. J. Experimental glomerulonephritis. VI. The autologous phase of nephrotoxic serum nephritis. J. Exp. Med. 121:715, 1965.
25. Cochrane, C. G. and Janoff, A. The Arthus reaction. A model of neutrophil and complement-mediated injury. In The inflammatory process, B. W. Zweifach, L. Grant, W., and R. T. McCluskey (eds.). Academic Press, New York, 3:85–162, 1974.
25a. Kreisberg, J. I., Wayne, D. B., and Karnovsky, M. J. Rapid and focal loss of negative charge associated with mononuclear cell infiltration early in nephrotoxic serum nephritis. Kidney Int. 16:290–300, 1979.
26. Vassalli, P. and McCluskey, R. T. The pathogenetic role of the coagulation process in glomerular diseases of immunologic origin. Adv. Nephr. 1:47–63, 1971.
27. Naish, R. et al. The effects of defibrination with ancrod in experimental allergic glomerular injury. Clin. Exp. Immunol. 20:303, 1975.
28. Cotran, R. S. Monocytes, proliferation and glomerulonephritis. J. Lab. Clin. Med. 92:837, 1978.
29. Schreiner, G. F., Cotran, R. S., Pardo, V., and Unanue, E. R. A mononuclear cell component in experimental immunological glomerulonephritis. J. Exp. Med. 147:369–384, 1978.
30. Bahn, A. K., Schneeberger, E. E., Collins, A. B., and McCluskey, R. T. Evidence for a pathogenic role of a cell-mediated immune mechanism in experimental glomerulonephritis. J. Exp. Med. 148:246, 1978.

31. Bhan, A. K., Collins, A. B., Schneeberger, E. E., and McCluskey, R. T. A cell-mediated reaction against glomerular-bound immune complexes. J. Exp. Med. 150:1410, 1979.

32. Fillit, H. M., Read, S. E., Sherman, R. L., Zabriskie, J. B., and van de Rijn, I. Cellular reactivity to altered glomerular basement membrane glomerulonephritis. New Eng. J. Med. 298:861, 1978.

33. Zabriskie, J. B. The role of streptococci in human glomerulonephritis. J. Exp. Med. 134(3, Pt. 2):180s–192s, 1971.

34. Van de Rijn, I., Fillit, H., Brandeis, W. E., Reid, H., Poon-Kuig-T., McCarthy, M., Day, N. K., and Zabriskie, J. B. Serial studies on circulating immune complexes in post-streptococcal sequelae. Clin. Exper. Immunol. 34:318, 1978.

35. Glassock, R. J. Clinical aspects of acute, rapidly progressive and chronic glomerulonephritis. In Disease of the kidney, L. Earley and C. Gottschalk (eds.). Little, Brown, Boston, 1979, p. 691.

36. Baldwin, D. S. Poststreptococcal glomerulonephritis: a progressive disease? Am. J. Med. 62:1, 1977.

37. Kurtzman, N. A. Does acute poststreptococcal glomerulonephritis lead to chronic renal disease? New Eng. J. Med. 298:795, 1978.

38. Combes, B., Stastny, P., Shorey, J., Eigenbrodt, E. H., Barrera, A., Hull, A. R., and Carter, N. W. Glomerulonephritis with deposition of Australia antigen–antibody complexes in glomerular basement membrane. Lancet 2:234–237, 1971.

39. Boulton-Jones, J., et al. Renal lesions of acute infective endocarditis. Brit. Med. J. 2:11, 1974.

40. McCluskey, R. T. et al. Immune complex-mediated diseases. Human Pathol. 9:71, 1978.

41. Spargo, B. et al. The differential diagnosis of crescentic glomerulonephritis. Human Pathol. 8:187, 1977.

42. Teague, C. A., Doak, P. B., Simpson, I. J., Rainer, S. P., and Herdson, P. B. Goodpasture's syndrome: an analysis of 29 cases. Kidney Int. 13:492, 1978.

43. Willoughby, W. F. and Dixon, F. J. Experimental hemorrhagic pneumonitis produced by heterologous anti-lung antibody. J. Immunol. 104:28, 1970.

44. Wilson, C. B. and Smith, R. C. Goodpasture's syndrome associated with influenza A2 infection. Ann. Int. Med. 76:91, 1972.

45. Editorial. Hydrocarbon exposure and proliferative glomerulonephritis. Lancet 1:81, 1977.

46. Sternleib, I., Bennet, B., and Scheinberg, I. H. D-penicillamine-induced Goodpasture's syndrome. Ann. Int. Med. 82:673, 1975.

47. Briggs, W. A., Johnson, J. P., Teichman, S., Yeager, H. C., and Wilson, C. B. Anti-GBM antibody-mediated glomerulonephritis and Goodpasture's syndrome. Medicine 58:348, 1979.

48. Rees, A. J. et al. Strong association between HLA-DRW2 and antibody-mediated Goodpasture's syndrome. Lancet 1:966, 1978.

49. Lockwood, C. M. et al. Plasma exchange in nephritis. In Advances in nephrology, J. Hamburger et al. (eds.). Year Book Medical Publishers, Chicago, 1979, Vol. 8, p. 383.

50. Stilmant, M. M. et al. Crescentic GN without immune deposits. Kidney Int. 15:184, 1979.

51. Bierne, J. G. et al. Idiopathic crescentic glomerulonephritis. Medicine 3:49, 1977.

52. Morrin, P. A. F. et al. Rapidly progressive glomerulonephritis. A clinical and pathologic study. Am. J. Med. 65:446, 1978.

53. Atkins, R. C. et al. Tissue culture of isolated glomeruli from patients with glomerulonephritis. Lab. Invest. 17:515, 1980.

54. Cameron, J. S. Pathogenesis and treatment of membranous nephropathy. Kidney Int. 15:88, 1979.

55. Eagen, J. W. et al. Glomerulopathies of neoplasia. Kidney Int. 11:297, 1977.

56. Collaborative study of the adult idiopathic nephrotic syndrome. A controlled study of short-term prednisone treatment in adults with membranous nephropathy. New Eng. J. Med. 301:1301, 1979.

57. Habib, R. and Kleinknecht, C. The primary nephrotic syndrome of childhood: classification and clinicopathologic study of 406 cases, In Pathology Annual, S. C. Sommers (ed.). Appleton-Century-Crofts, New York, 1971, No. 6, pp. 417–474.

58. Habib, R. The idiopathic nephrotic syndrome. In Prevention of kidney and urinary tract diseases, C. H. Coggins and N. B. Cummings (eds.). DHEW Publ. No. (NIH) 78–855, 1978, p. 25.

59. Mallik, N. P. The pathogenesis of minimal change nephropathy. Clin. Nephrol. 7:87, 1977.

60. Brenner, B. M., Hostetter, T., and Humes, H. D. Molecular basis of proteinuria of glomerular origin. New Eng. J. Med. 298:826, 1978.

61. Seiler, M. W., Rennke, H. G., Venkatachalam, M. A., and Cotran, R. S. Pathogenesis of polycation induced alterations ("fusion") of glomerular epithelium. Lab. Invest. 36:48–61, 1977.

62. Andrews, P., Scanning electron microscopy of the nephrotic kidney. Virchows Arch. B. Cell Pathol. 17:195, 1975.

63. Churg, J. et al. Pathology of the nephrotic syndrome in children. A report for the international study of kidney disease in children. Lancet 1:1299, 1970.

64. Habib, R. Focal glomerular sclerosis. Kidney Int. 4:355, 1973.

65. Beaufils, H., Alphonse, J. C., Guedon, J., and Legrain, M. Focal glomerulosclerosis: natural history and treatment. A report of 70 cases. Nephron 21:75, 1978.

66. Cameron, J. S., Turner, D. R., Ogg, C. S., Chantler, C., and Williams, D. G. The long-term prognosis of patients with focal segmental glomerulosclerosis. Clin. Nephrol. 10:213, 1978.

67. Brown, C. B., Cameron, J. S., Turner, D. R., Chantler, C., Ogg, C. S., Williams, D. G., and Bewick, M. Focal segmental glomerulosclerosis with rapid decline in renal function ("malignant FSGS"). Clin. Nephrol. 10:51, 1978.

68. Llach, F., Descoeudres, C., and Massry, S. G. Heroin associated nephropathy: clinical and histological studies in 19 patients. Clin. Nephrol. 11:7, 1979.

69. West, C. D. et al. Hypocomplementemic and normocomplementemic persistent (chronic) glomerulonephritis: clinical and pathologic characteristics. J. Pediatr. 67:1089, 1965.

70. Ooi, B. S. et al. Classical complement pathway activation in membranoproliferative glomerulonephritis. Kidney Int. 9:1, 1976.

71. Davis, A. E. et al. Heterogeneity of nephritic factor and its identification as an immunoglobulin. Proc. Nat. Acad. Sci. 74:3980, 1978.

72. Simpson, I. J. et al. Prolonged complement activation in mice. Kidney Int. 13:467, 1978.

73. Peters, D. K. et al. Mesangiocapillary nephritis, partial lipodystrophy and hypocomplementemia. Lancet 2:535, 1973.

74. Noel, L. H. et al. HLA antigen in three types of glomerular nephritis. Clin. Immunol. Immunopathol. 10:19, 1978.

75. Habib, R. and Levy, M. Membranoproliferative glomerulonephritis. In Nephrology, J. Hamburger, J. Crosnier, and J. P. Grünfeld (eds.). Wiley-Flammarion, New York, 1979, p. 587.

76. Lamb, V. et al. Membranoproliferative glomerulonephritis with dense intramembranous alterations—a clinicopathologic study. Lab. Invest. 36:6, 1977.

77. Davis, A. E., Schneeberger, E. E., Grupe, W. E., and McCluskey, R. T. Membranoproliferative glomerulonephritis (MPGN Type I) and dense deposit disease (DDD) in children. Clin. Nephrol. 9:184, 1978.

78. Schwartz, M. and Cotran, R. S. Primary renal disease in transplant recipients. Human Pathol. 7:455–459, 1976.

79. Berger, J. IgA glomerular deposits in renal disease. Transplant Proc. 1:939, 1969.

80. Katz, A., Underdown, B., Minta, J., and Lepow, I. H. Glomerulonephritis with mesangial IgA deposits. Canad. Med. Soc. J. 7:209, 1976.

81. Appel, G. F., Silva, F. G., Pirani, C. L., Meltzer, J. I., and Estes, D. Renal involvement in systemic lupus erythematosus (SLE): a study of 56 patients emphasizing histological classification. Medicine 57:371, 1978.

82. Friend, P. S. and Michael, A. F. Hypothesis: immunologic rationale for the therapy of membranous lupus nephropathy. Clin. Immunol. Immunopathol. 10:35, 1978.

83. Bloodworth, J. M. B. A reevaluation of diabetic glomerulosclerosis 50 years after the discovery of insulin. Human Pathol. 9:439, 1978.

84. Brownlee, M. and Spiro, R. G. Glomerular basement membrane metabolism in the diabetic rat: in vivo studies. Diabetes 28:121, 1979.

85. Levy, M. et al. Anaphylactoid purpura nephritis in childhood: natural history and immunopathology. Adv. Nephrol. 6:183, 1976.

86. Sinniah, R., Feng, P. H., and Chen, B. T. M. Henoch-Schönlein syndrome: a clinical and morphological study of renal biopsies. Clin. Nephrol. 9:219, 1978.

87. Gamble, C. N. and Ruggles, S. W. The immunopathogenesis of glomerulonephritis associated with mixed cryoglobulinemia. New Eng. J. Med. 299:81, 1978.

88. O'Neill, W. M. et al. Hereditary nephritis: a re-examination of its clinical and genetic features. Ann. Int. Med. 88:176, 1978.

89. Bernstein, J. Hereditary renal disorders in renal disease. In Kidney disease—present status, B. Churg, B. Spargo, F. K. Mostofi, and M. Abell (eds.). Williams & Wilkins, Baltimore, 1979.

90. Earley, L. F. and Farland, D. Nephrotic syndrome. In Strauss and Welt's diseases of the kidney, 3rd ed., L. Early and C. Gottschalk (eds.). Little, Brown, Boston, 1979.

91. Glassock, R. J. The nephrotic syndrome. Hosp. Pract. 14:105, 1979.

92. Blantz, R. C., Hostetter, T. H., Brenner, B. M. Functional adaptations of the kidney to immunological injury. In Contemporary Issues in Nephrology, C. B. Wilson (ed.). Churchill-Livingston, New York, 1979, Vol. III.

93. Venkatachalam, M. A. and Rennke, H. G. Structural and molecular basis of glomerular filtration. Circ. Res. 43:337, 1978.

94. Giangiacomo, J., Clearly, T. G., Cole, B. R., Hoffsten, P., and Robson, A. M. Serum immunoglobulins in the nephrotic syndrome. A possible cause of minimal-change nephrotic syndrome. New Eng. J. Med. 293:8–12, 1975.

95. Gitlin, D., Janeway, C. A., and Farr, L. E. Studies on the metabolism of plasma

proteins in the nephrotic syndrome. I. Albumin, globulin, and iron-binding globulin. J. Clin. Inves. 35:44, 1956.

96. Radding, C. M. and Steinberg, D. Studies on the synthesis and secretion of serum lipoproteins by rat liver slices. J. Clin. Inves. 39:1560, 1960.

97. Wass, V. J., Jarrett, R. J., Chilvers, C., and Cameron, J. S. Does the nephrotic syndrome increase the risk of cardiovascular disease? Lancet 2:664, 1979.

98. Trew, P. A. et al. Renal vein thrombosis in membranous glomerulonephritis. Incidence and association. Medicine 57:69, 1978.

13

Vascular Diseases of the Kidney and Renal Hypertension

The blood supply of the kidney bears a special relationship to renal function. Blood flow to the renal cortex is about 500 ml/100 gm/ minute, a rate 5 to 10 times larger than that to such metabolically active organs as the heart, liver, and brain. Glomerular capillary pressure is the force promoting ultrafiltration in the glomerulus, and abnormal processes in the renal vessels which decrease renal cortical perfusion ultimately result in reduction of glomerular filtration (1). Such decreases in renal perfusion can occur due to functional changes in the vessel wall (e.g., vasoconstriction) or to organic abnormalities. Physiological alterations in arteriolar vessel tone has been alluded to in the sections dealing with the renal response to intravascular volume changes (Chapter 3); and pathologic vasoconstriction plays a role in the pathogenesis of some forms of acute renal failure (Chapter 8).

This chapter deals with the renal disorders that are caused primarily by *organic* abnormalities of renal vessels, mainly the arteries. These are among the most common diseases of the kidney and are related particularly to the problem of hypertension. In general, the morphologic and functional changes in the kidney are due to narrowing or occlusion of some part of the arterial system and to a reduction, therefore, in perfusion of the renal parenchyma supplied by the affected vessel. It is thus necessary to discuss, first, the *causes* of renal arterial narrowing and, second, the morphological *consequences*.

CAUSES OF RENAL ARTERIAL NARROWING

Arteriosclerosis

Arteriosclerotic changes in renal arteries of various sizes are by far the most common form of renal vascular pathology, since they occur to some extent in most normal individuals with aging, as do arteriosclerotic changes in other systemic arteries. The specific morphologic changes encountered depend on type and caliber of the artery, and include: (1) atherosclerosis, (2) hyaline arteriolar sclerosis, and, (3) fibroelastic hyperplasia.

ATHEROSCLEROSIS

Atherosclerosis involves the main renal artery and its larger branches and is identical in morphology and presumed pathogenesis to atherosclerosis seen in vessels elsewhere in the body. Together with changes in arterioles described below, atherosclerotic changes in the larger renal arteries account for the slight reduction in renal size that occurs with increasing age and the areas of ischemic atrophy and infarction seen in random postmortem examinations of elderly patients. In addition, some patients with atherosclerosis of one main renal artery develop renal artery stenosis and hypertension.

HYALINE ARTERIOLAR SCLEROSIS

This is a highly characteristic lesion of the smaller interlobular arteries and the afferent arterioles of the kidney. It consists of a thickening of the vessel wall due to deposition of an amorphous, eosinophilic hyaline material in the subendothelium. This thickening eventually impinges on and narrows the lumen. The lesion has received great attention because of its possible association with hypertension.

Hyaline arteriolar sclerosis occurs to some degree in normotensive individuals after the fifth decade, but its frequency and severity are increased in younger age groups in association with *hypertension* and *diabetes mellitus* (2). The nature of the hyaline material deposited in the intima is not completely known, but immunofluorescent and electron microscopic studies suggest that the hyaline is composed in large part of plasma proteins and lipids that have leaked out of the circulation, probably owing to the endothelial injury, and precipitated in the vessel wall (3, 4). Some studies have shown that the thickening is also a consequence of deposition of intimal basement membrane material. It is thought that hypertension accentuates endothelial damage and therefore, the severity of the sclerosis.

FIBROELASTIC THICKENING OF SMALL ARTERIES

This is a lesion of arcuate and interlobular arteries that consists of reduplication of the elastica and increased fibrous tissue in the media with consequent narrowing of the lumina. It often accompanies hyaline arteriolar sclerosis and increases in severity with age and in the presence of hypertension. Little is known of its pathogenesis, most workers including the changes together with those of smaller vessels. It should be differentiated from the hyperplastic arteriolitis characteristic of malignant hypertension, to be discussed on p. 348.

Vasculitis

The vasculitides are a group of diseases in which there is necrosis and inflammation of the vessel wall. These diseases often involve the kidneys, and the resulting narrowing of the lumen causes infarction, ischemia, hypertension, and renal failure. Examples are polyarteritis nodosa and hypersensitivity angiitis, two diseases that appear to be mediated by immunologic mechanisms (p. 351).

Embolism

Since the kidneys receive approximately one-fourth of the cardiac output, they are the most common sites of embolism from cardiac thrombi. Patients with mitral stenosis, bacterial endocarditis, and mural thrombi overlying myocardial infarcts are especially susceptible to developing embolism. Emboli are the most common cause of acute total occlusion, leading to renal infarction.

Thrombosis

Thrombi in renal vessels occur either: (1) Secondarily to atherosclerosis or vasculitis or (2) in association with disseminated intravascular coagulation, a serious disturbance of the coagulation mechanism complicating septicemias, intensive surgery, toxemia of pregnancy, and abruptio placentae. Intravascular coagulation in the kidney occurs principally in small arterioles and glomerular capillaries and results in focal infarction of cortex, or widespread renal cortical necrosis.

MORPHOLOGIC CONSEQUENCES OF REDUCTION IN RENAL PERFUSION

The morphologic consequences of arterial narrowing are determined by:

1. The arterial *level* at which the occlusion occurs. Renal arteries are end arteries, with little cross-communication and collateral circulation. Thus occlusion of the main artery affects the entire kidney, the interlobar artery, the lobes supplied by the vessel, and so on.

2. The *rate* at which reduction in blood flow occurs and the *degree* of reduction: thus acute total occlusion of an artery results in *renal infarction* distal to the occlusion, whereas more gradual, incomplete narrowing results in *ischemic atrophy*.

Renal infarction

Fresh infarcts are well demarcated areas of coagulation necrosis that appear yellow and usually wedge shaped on gross examination. Their size and localization are determined almost exactly by the caliber and location of the occluded vessel. The areas of coagulation necrosis are surrounded by an inflammatory reaction consisting of polymorphonuclear leukocytes and mononuclear cells in the first few days. With time, the infarcts become organized by granulation tissue, much of the necrotic material is resorbed, and the long-term result is a fibrotic scar that appears as a clear-cut depression on the cortical surface. Microscopically, such scars are composed of hyalinized glomeruli, collapsed or absent tubules, and interstitial fibrosis with varying degrees of chronic interstitial inflammation.

Most renal infarcts are clinically silent. Larger infarction may be associated with flank pain, hematuria, leucocytosis, and fever; and large infarcts in a solitary kidney may induce renal insufficiency.

Ischemic atrophy

Ischemic atrophy affects first and predominantly the tubular epithelium, especially that of the proximal convoluted tubules. Microscopically, the tubules become smaller and collapsed and have flattened epithelium and often thickened basement membranes. The glomerular changes are heterogeneous: the glomeruli are often crowded together, owing to atrophy of intervening tubules, but may be well preserved. Ischemic changes in the glomeruli do occur and should be differentiated from those that occur in glomerulonephritis. They include (1) thickening and wrinkling of the capillary walls, with a shrinkage of the glomerular tuft, which then appears more solid and compact; (2) deposition of collagen within Bowman's space between the glomerular tuft and Bowman's capsule, eventually leading to entire sclerosis of the glomerulus.

HYPERTENSION AND THE KIDNEY (5, 6)

The association of renal disease and hypertension has been appreciated since the time of Richard Bright, who recognized the coexistence of left ventricular hypertrophy and contracted kidneys even before blood vessel measurements were made. Subsequently, Tigerstedt and Bergman, in 1898, showed that a protein extracted from kidney tissue of the rabbit was able to cause a rise in blood pressure when injected into other rabbits; they termed this pressor substance renin (7). Renin was forgotten until 1934, when Goldblatt induced hypertension by causing renal artery stenosis and ischemia in the dog (8, 9). Since the work of Goldblatt the association between renal disease and hypertension has been investigated extensively, and various vasopressor and vasodepressor substances have been discovered; in addition, the important role of the kidney in affecting blood pressure by regulating sodium excretion and influencing aldosterone production has become apparent.

Hypertension is usually classified as essential or secondary, and the kidney is intimately involved in the pathogenesis of both types. Although secondary hypertension accounts for only 5–10% of all hypertensive patients, primary renal disease is by far the most common cause. Hypertension occurs, for example, in the course of (1) acute proliferative poststreptococcal glomerulonephritis; (2) almost all chronic renal diseases, such as chronic glomerulonephritis, chronic pyelonephritis, and polycystic kidney disease; (3) the necrotizing vasculitides, such as polyarteritis nodosa; (4) the connective tissue disorders such as lupus erythematosus and scleroderma; (5) the micro-

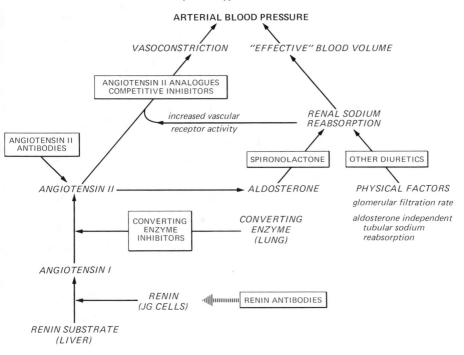

Fig. 13-1 The renin-angiotensin-aldosterone axis. The diagram also shows the inhibitors (in blocks) that can be used to block various steps of the sequence. (From Laragh, J. (10); slightly modified)

angiopathic hemolytic disorders; and (6) renal artery stenosis. The renal mechanisms responsible for hypertension are currently the subject of intensive study. Investigation in this area has been stimulated by improved methods of quantitating the various components of the pressor and depressor mechanisms and by the discovery of pharmacologic agents that can affect specific steps in the renin–angiotensin mechanism (Fig. 13-1). This section reviews only briefly the possible mechanisms involved and is devoted principally to a discussion of renal artery stenosis, benign nephrosclerosis, and malignant hypertension.

Mechanisms of renal hypertension

The level of arterial pressure depends on two hemodynamic variables: the cardiac output and the resistance offered by the blood vessels and blood to forward flow—*the total peripheral resistance* (11). Blood volume, through its effect on cardiac output, also influences blood pressure. For the most part, the total peripheral resistance is accounted for by resistance of the arterioles. Arteriolar resistance is determined by the relative thickness of the vessel wall in proportion to lumen size *and* the effect of neural and humoral substances that either constrict or dilate the vessel. Vasoconstrictor agents include norepinephrine, angiotensin II, and thromboxane, while the major vasodilators are the prostaglandins and kinins. Arterial hypertension results from an interplay of factors that may alter the relationship between the blood volume and the total arteriolar resistance.

The kidney participates in the control of blood pressure by affecting both peripheral resistance and blood volume. The mechanisms involved, which are deranged to various degrees in renal hypertension, can be grouped under three categories: (1) secretion by the kidney of vasoactive substances that increase blood pressure, (2) the maintenance of extracellular fluid volume (ECF), and (3) the elaboration by the kidneys of substances that normally lower blood pressure. These three mechanisms will be discussed separately but are clearly interrelated.

RENAL PRESSOR EFFECTS

The diseased kidney may form increased amounts of a substance that raises blood pressure. The renin–angiotensin–aldosterone axis is activated by (1) a decrease in afferent arteriolar pressure, (2) decreased sodium or chloride load in the macula densa and, (3) epinephrine and direct stimulation of nerves. The enzyme renin is formed and stored in the juxtaglomerular cells of the kidney, from which it is released into renal venous blood. Acting on a substrate in plasma called angiotensinogen, it intially splits off a large, inactive decapeptide, angiotension I, which is converted within the circulation into the octapeptide angiotensin II by a converting enzyme. Converting enzyme is synthesized by endothelial cells (12) and is present in large quantities in the lung, but is also found in the kidney, since experimental evidence indicates that the kidney may be capable of forming angiotensin II locally (13). Angiotensin II causes vasoconstriction, increases blood pressure, and stimulates the adrenal cortex to secrete aldosterone. (Further splitting of angiotensin II forms a heptapeptide known as angiotensin III, which is an important stimulus for aldosterone secretion in many species and does have a pressor effect, although less than that of angiotensin II.) Various peptidases (angiotensinases) within the circulation further degrade angiotensin into largely in-active peptide fragments. These relationships are summarized in Fig-ure 13-1, which also includes the effect of sodium concentration on arterial blood pressure and points the various steps in the renin–angiotensin–aldosterone mechanism where an inhibitory influence might be applied by a pharmacological or other agent. The system can, for example, be inhibited by renin antibodies, by inhibitors of the enzymes that convert angiotensin I to angiotensin II, by direct antibodies to angiotensin II, or by angiotensin II analogues and com-petitive inhibitors. From such studies the renin mechanism seems to play a role in hypertension initiated by renal artery stenosis (14, 15); in malignant hypertension, where extremely high levels of renin and aldosterone have been measured (16); in some of the vasculitides; in some patients with unilateral parenchymal disease (e.g., chronic pyelo-nephritis) (17); and in some patients with chronic renal failure of diverse etiologies (18).

It must be recalled (Chapter 5) that under normal conditions, any increased renin secretion is quickly corrected by negative feedback mechanisms that tend to suppress renin release and bring circulating renin levels back to normal. Thus, increased blood pressure will re-duce baroreceptor stimulation in the afferent arteriole and diminish renin secretion. Similarly, the increased ECF consequent to aldoste-rone secretion increases GFR, causing decreased sodium reabsorption and (through the sensors in the macula densa) diminished renin secre-tion. There is also evidence that angiotensin II itself directly sup-presses JG cell secretion. *Thus, in the presence of normal renal func-tion, plasma renin values are restored to normal.* In patients with chronic renal failure due to primary renal disease, these feedback con-trol mechanisms may be altered because (a) the patients are more likely to have sodium and water retention and (b) there is diminished restoration of renin secretion to normal by volume expansion (10).

SODIUM RETENTION

As should be well-known (Chapter 3) total body sodium is the main determinant of ECF volume and the latter in turn influences cardiac output and blood volume. Since the kidney is the principal organ re-sponsible for such sodium homeostasis, it is believed that sodium re-tention in renal disease is the most important factor responsible for hypertension in patients with end-stage kidney failure. Increased total exchangeable sodium and extracellular fluid volume are found in such patients, and there is marked improvement of blood pressure when these excesses are removed. Sodium retention is postulated to account also, at least in part, for the hypertension that occurs in acute glomerulonephritis.

RENAL DEPRESSOR EFFECTS

It has long been postulated that the diseased kidney may produce reduced amounts of a substance that lowers blood pressure either directly or by inactivating a hypertensive substance. This mechanism, known as "renoprival hypertension," was first suggested by experiments in which removal of both kidneys from one pair of parabiotic rats resulted in hypertension. It was suggested that the hypertension was caused by an inability of the remaining kidney to maintain a normal blood pressure, this being independent of the excretory function of the kidney (19, 20). At least three kidney-derived groups of antihypertensive agents are recognized:

1. Muirhead's renomedullary lipid. Muirhead and his co-workers (21) showed that transplants of renal medulla injected subcutaneously in the abdominal wall prevent hypertension induced by bilateral nephrectomy in the dog and rabbit and also the hypertension produced by clamping of the renal artery. They showed that the tissue that reversed the hypertension consisted entirely of renal medullary interstitial cells and, further, that a monolayer tissue culture apparently derived from such interstitial cells had an antihypertensive action. The antihypertensive principle in these extracts is a neutral lipid and appears to be distinct from the prostaglandins.

2. Prostaglandins. Prostaglandins (PG) are the most potent mediators of the antihypertensive activity of renal tissues. In early studies by Vane and his associates (22), it was found that the renal vasoconstrictor-antidiuretic action of angiotensin II was blunted by the release of PGE_2 intrarenally. When prostaglandin synthesis is prevented by indomethacin, an inhibitor of prostaglandin synthetase, the vasoconstrictor action of angiotensin II is substantially enhanced in the kidney.

In most species, prostaglandins decrease extracellular fluid volume, exert direct effects on vascular tone and reactivity, and blunt the renal vasoconstrictor and antidiuretic action of angiotensin II. In particular, the recently discovered *prostacyclin* causes an increase in renal blood flow, increased GFR, diuresis, natriuresis, and vasodilatation—all antihypertensive phenomena (23). It must be remembered, however, that *thromboxane*, another product of arachidonic acid metabolism, is a powerful vasoconstrictor and it, too, can be produced locally in the kidney.

3. Kinins. Evidence is accumulating that an intrarenal kallikrein–kinin system (similar to the plasma kinin system) exists, and that this normally serves as an antihypertensive principle, since kinins are profound vasodilators (24). Urinary kallikrein has been reported to be decreased in hypertensives suffering from renal parenchymal disease (24a).

There are poorly understood but obviously important relationships among the humoral systems operating in the kidney: renin–angiotensin, prostaglandins (including thromboxane), and kallikrein–kinin (25). For example, prostaglandins inhibit the actions of angiotensin II. Furthermore, converting enzyme, which converts angiotensin I to angiotensin II, is identical to kininase, which degrades the vasodilator agent bradykinin. It would appear that the hypertensive and hypotensive factors elaborated by the kidney are involved in some delicately balanced system controlling blood pressure. The contribution of these complex relationships to the development and sustenance of hypertension in human renal disease is still unclear but is now receiving intensive study.

Renal artery stenosis

Stenosis of one main renal artery or its larger branches may result in hypertension. This is a relatively uncommon cause of hypertension, responsible for 2–5% of cases but is of importance because (a) it is the most common, *curable* form of hypertension in man, since surgical treatment is successful in up to 90% of carefully selected cases and (b) much of our knowledge of the renal mechanism in hypertension has come from studies on experimental and human renal artery stenosis.

MECHANISM OF HYPERTENSION

That renal artery constriction can cause hypertension was clearly established as early as 1934 by the classical experiments of Goldblatt (8). He found that constriction of renal arteries in dogs, by application of a silver clamp, results in hypertension that begins in 24–72 hours and reaches its maximum level in about 1 week. The magnitude of the effect is roughly proportional to the amount of constriction, severe constriction causing marked elevations of pressure and renal failure similar to the course of malignant hypertension in man. The effect has been shown to occur in many mammalian species, and in the rat hypertension can be readily produced by constricting one renal artery while the other kidney remains intact (26). Further experiments in the rat with unilateral artery stenosis demonstrate that, when the constriction is sustained for many weeks, the opposite nonconstricted kidney shows arteriolar sclerosis, often with necrotizing lesions, while the ischemic kidney itself shows no vascular changes. Removal of the ischemic kidney results in a fall in blood pressure only if the contralateral nonischemic kidney does not exhibit the arterial lesions, or if the ischemic kidney is removed before arterial lesions develop in the contralateral kidney. These experiments led to the conclusions that the ischemic kidney is initially responsible for the hypertension and that it remains protected from the effects of hypertension by the clip on the renal artery; in contrast, the opposite kidney, not being protected, develops arterial changes that may then perpetuate the hypertension when the ischemic kidney is removed.

A large number of studies (reviewed in refs. 15 and 25), have been performed on the mechanism of hypertension in this experimental model, also called renovascular or ischemic hypertension. In spite of some conflicting results, the bulk of the evidence suggests that the renin–angiotensin mechanism is responsible for the initiation of this form of hypertension.

Renin is released in increased amounts from the experimentally ischemic kidney within minutes after renal artery constriction, and for the ensuing week or two; this has been shown in some, but by no means all, experimental models. It has been demonstrated that, in the acute stage of experimental renovascular hypertension, the elevated blood pressure can be prevented by prior treatment with a nonapeptide that blocks conversion of angiotensin I to angiotensin II (27); and also by antagonists of angiotensin II (28). Such findings support an important role for angiotensin in the acute phase of hypertension. But the results with regard to the more chronic sustained hypertension produced by long-term constriction or in the so-called one-clip kidney model are much less clear. Thus, more often than not, renin, angiotensin, and aldosterone levels are not elevated, or even decline while hypertension is sustained (29). Immunization against angiotensin or administration of antagonists neither protect rabbits from nor reduce the blood pressure rise in long-standing renovascular hypertension (30). Explanations for the sustenance of long-term renovascular hypertension are still speculative and include sodium retention (14), increased reactivity of vessels to subpressor concentrations of angiotensin II (31) (possibly due to disturbed sodium homeostasis in vascular smooth muscle), increased sympathetic stimulation and plasma norepinephrine levels induced by central neural mechanisms (32), inhibition of prostaglandin or kinin systems, involvement of other as yet unidentified pressor agents (33), or a combination of these factors (34).

PATHOLOGIC CHANGES

The most common cause of renal artery stenosis is atherosclerosis, most frequently occurring in the aorta in the form of a plaque occluding the origin of the renal artery. Alternately, the atheromatous process may involve the renal artery itself or one of its main branches. This lesion occurs more frequently in males, the incidence increasing with advancing age and diabetes mellitus. The lesion is usually eccentric but may be circumferential causing obliteration of the lumen. Superimposed thrombosis often occurs, and it may precipitate hypertension by reducing the blood supply even further.

The other major lesion leading to stenosis is *fibromuscular dysplasia* of the renal artery (35). This is a heterogeneous group of lesions characterized by fibrous or fibromuscular thickening that may involve the intima, the media, or the subadventitial area of the artery. The lesions are clearly nonatherosclerotic, can be bilateral, and may involve the distal part of the renal artery and one or more of its segmental branches. They are subclassified into intimal, medial, and adventitial dysplasias, with age and sex differences in incidence among the groups. By far the most common is so-called medial fibroplasia, which accounts for 65% of cases. Unlike atherosclerosis, the lesions as a whole are more common in females and tend to occur in the third and fourth decades. They can often be differentiated from atherosclerotic renal artery stenosis by arteriography, since they tend to be segmental, with alternating segments of thickening and thinning of the vessel. One characteristic arteriographic appearance is the so-called "string-of-beads" deformity seen especially in the medial type of dysplasia. The pathogenesis of the dysplasias is unknown, but they do represent an important group because they occur in younger people and can be corrected with surgery.

The *ischemic kidney* is usually reduced in size and shows signs of diffuse ischemic atrophy: crowded glomeruli with atrophic tubules, interstitial fibrosis, and focal inflammatory infiltrate. Areas of infarction are sometimes seen. Because a decrease in perfusion is a stimulus for renin secretion, examination of the juxtaglomerular apparatus shows hyperplasia and increased granularity. Because the arterioles in the ischemic kidney are usually protected from the effects of high blood pressure, arteriolar sclerosis is usually absent or mild. In contrast, a biopsy of the contralateral nonischemic kidney, which is not protected from the effect of hypertension, may show hyaline arteriolosclerosis, depending on the severity and duration of the hypertension.

PATHOPHYSIOLOGY AND CLINICAL COURSE

Few specific identifying features of renal artery stenosis are available from history and physical examination; as a general group, patients resemble those presenting with "essential" hypertension. The hypertension may be mild or very severe, and occasionally a *bruit* can be heard on auscultation over the kidneys. The diagnostic features are in the radiological examination, principally *arteriography,* and in the pathophysiological changes in the ischemic as opposed to the nonischemic kidney (36–38).

A single lesion that occurs in a major artery must produce a large decrease in luminal diameter to result in a significant hemodynamic effect, the development of a pressure gradient across the stenosis and reductions in blood flow and glomerular filtration rate. As the length of the stenotic lesion increases, a small reduction in lumen caliber is hemodynamically significant. Thus, for an atherosclerotic plaque about 1 cm in length, a 70% reduction in luminal diameter is likely to be significant. In the case of the fibromuscular dysplasias, which may be several centimeters in length, even smaller reduction in lumen caliber can reduce renal perfusion.

Measurements of function of the two kidneys separately (split function) by catheterization of the ureters reveal lower effective renal plasma flow and glomerular filtration rate on the ischemic side. The decrease in GFR results in increased reabsorption of sodium and water from the tubular fluid. This has been ascribed, at least in part, to slowing of the rate of tubular fluid flow, with increased transit time. There are decrease in the sodium concentration and increase in the concentration of solutes in the urine, the latter being reflected by an increase in urine osmolarity. Thus, bilateral ureteral catheterization reveals: (a) a *decrease* in GFR and plasma flow on the involved side, (b) a *decrease* in the sodium concentration, and (c) an *increase* in the osmolarity and creatinine concentration in the urine from the involved kidney.

The physiologic events also account for the characteristic changes in the intravenous pyelogram. The side with hemodynamically significant stenosis shows (a) a delay in the appearance of the contrast agent, owing to decreased blood flow and GFR; (b) a small kidney, owing to atrophy and decreased blood and tubular fluid volume; and (c) late hyperconcentration of contrast, owing to increased reabsorption of tubular fluid, leaving the nonreabsorbable contrast agent in high concentration.

A decrease in renal perfusion is also a stimulus for renin secretion, so that *increased renal vein renin concentration* is the best index of the hemodynamic significance of the stenotic lesion. Although many factors may influence observed renin levels in these patients, determination of renin levels from both renal veins (showing a renin ratio in the two renal veins of 1.5 : 1 or greater) allows prediction of a surgically correctable hypertension in 90% of patients (39). An antihypertensive response to angiotensin antagonists (e.g., Saralasin) is also used to assess those patients likely to benefit from surgical correction of the stenotic lesions, but the reliability of the technique is still controversial (40, 41). It must be stressed that patients who do not have overt evidence of renin–angiotensin activation may also respond to surgical correction, confirming that other mechanisms are involved in long-term renovascular hypertension (41a).

As the stenosis becomes more severe, it may result in extreme atrophy and nonfunction of the kidney unless an adequate collateral blood supply becomes available. A sudden decrease in luminal diameter due to thrombosis on an arteriosclerotic area produces renal infarction or, if the occlusion is partial, accelerated hypertension.

Benign nephrosclerosis

A certain degree of benign nephrosclerosis is seen in about 70% of random postmortem examinations of patients who die after the age of 60. It is defined as the form of renal disease associated with arteriolar sclerosis of the hyaline type. The frequency and the severity of the lesion are increased in younger age groups in association with hypertension and diabetes mellitus.

The relationship of essential hypertension to the hyaline arteriolosclerosis in the kidneys is not entirely clear. Earlier studies suggested that this may be a primary change perhaps leading to renal ischemia and activation of the renin–angiotensin axis. Autopsies and biopsies in essential hypertension have, however, shown a number of patients without arteriolosclerosis (2). The prevailing view is that high blood pressure results in accentuation of the vascular lesion; however, the possibility remains that the development of hyaline arteriolar sclerosis may sustain or aggravate the high blood pressure and may be responsible for the elevation of renin levels seen in both benign and malignant forms of essential hypertension.

PATHOLOGIC CHANGES

Grossly, the kidneys are slightly to moderately reduced in size to average weights of between 110 and 130 gm. The cortical surfaces show a fine and even granularity, and the kidneys are paler than normal. Histological examination reveals thick-walled, hyalinized afferent arterioles, and interlobular arteries with a modest to marked reduction in lumen caliber. In the interlobular and arcuate vessels there is often fibroelastic hyperplasia with elastic reduplication. Consequent to vascular narrowing, there is a patchy ischemic atrophy, which consists of (a) foci of tubular atrophy and interstitial fibrosis and (b) a variety of glomerular alterations; these include collapsed, wrinkled basement membrane; fibrous deposition within Bowman's space; and, finally, completely sclerosed glomeruli. In general, the severity of the ischemic atrophy parallels that of the vascular changes.

CLINICAL FEATURES

The clinical manifestations peculiar to the kidney are generally mild when benign nephrosclerosis is associated with aging or mild to moderate hypertension. There are modest reductions in renal plasma flow, and the glomerular filtration rates may remain normal or slightly reduced; hence, the filtration fraction is generally *increased*. Occasionally, there is a moderate loss of concentrating power, with mild proteinuria, and occasional hyaline and graular casts in the urine. In general, however, patients with more moderate degrees of benign nephrosclerosis appear to have lost an element of reserve and are thus more prone to develop azotemia in the face of volume depletion, surgical stress, or gastrointestinal hemorrhage.

More profound renal functional changes, including diminution of GFR and the development of the azotemia, do occur in certain patients with severe prolonged benign nephrosclerosis and hypertension. These patients are usually older patients, with both arterial and arteriolar sclerosis and with long-standing hypertension or diabetes mellitus. In the majority of patients with essential hypertension, however, when renal failure occurs, it is due to the development of the accelerated or malignant phase of hypertension.

Malignant nephrosclerosis

Malignant or accelerated hypertension is a dramatic complication of all forms of hypertension. The malignant phase is usually preceded by a benign one with a variable duration of 1–30 years but occasionally occurs *de novo,* being malignant from the start. This process also occurs as a complication of secondary forms of hypertension, including renal artery stenosis, glomerulonephritis, and pyelonephritis, and is a frequent cause of death from uremia in patients with scleroderma. The age of patients is lower in the malignant than in the benign phase of hypertension, and there is a high preponderance in males and in blacks.

PATHOLOGIC CHANGES

The kidney size depends on the duration of the preexisting benign phase, and in some patients the kidneys may be slightly larger than normal. The cortical surface exhibits small petechial hemorrhages, giving the kidney a peculiar "flea-bitten" appearance. The characteristic histological features are two:

1. *Fibrinoid necrosis* of arterioles. This is reflected by an eosinophilic granular change in the blood vessel wall, which stains positively for fibrin by histochemical and immunofluorescent techniques. In addition, there is often an inflammatory infiltrate within the wall, giving rise to the term *necrotizing arteriolitis.* Electron microscopic studies have shown that the material in the arteriolar wall consists of fibrin and other amorphous material and that there is conspicuous endothelial injury and leukocytic infiltration of the

arteriolar wall. Frequently, but not invariably, there is fibrinoid necrosis in the glomeruli, usually in continuity with the necrotic afferent arteriole.

2. In the interlobular arteries there is a characteristic intimal thickening caused by proliferation of elongated concentrically arranged cells, probably fibroblasts, together with fine concentric layering of collagen. The alteration, known as *hyperplastic arteriolitis,* is also referred to as "onion skin" layering of vessels and correlates well with renal failure in malignant hypertension.

The arteriolar and arterial lesions result in considerable narrowing of all vascular lumina, with ischemia and infarction distal to the abnormal vessels. There is also variable evidence of longstanding benign nephrosclerosis, with hyaline deposition in arterioles and fibroelastic hyperplasia of interlobular vessels.

PATHOGENESIS

The triggering mechanism for the development of malignant hypertension is unclear. High levels of renin and aldosterone have been reported, but the initial stimulus to hyperreninemia is obscure (42). Experimental studies of Giese suggest that the severe increases in blood pressure are responsible for the vascular necrosis that occurs in arterioles of the kidney and other organs (42). Such increase in blood pressure causes endothelial injury and leakage of fibrin and other plasma proteins into the wall of the arteriole, and the consequent development of luminal thrombi. Several authors (15, 42, 43) have stressed the similarity between the lesions of malignant hypertension and those seen in the microangiopathic disorders associated with intravascular coagulation. It has thus been proposed that malignant hypertension might be explained by sudden rises in vasoactive agents such as angiotensin, which cause vasoconstriction, endothelial damage, platelet thrombosis, and intravascular coagulation. By causing ischemia, the latter, in turn, may perpetuate the vicious cycle of hyper-reninemia and malignant hypertension (44). On the other hand, Linton (43) and Heptinstall (15) suggest that the intravascular coagulation may well *precipitate* the malignant phase of hypertension. The latter view is supported by the observation that intravascular coagulation and arterial intimal thickening often *precede* the development of hypertension in this group of microangiopathic hemolytic anemias, as discussed later. Whatever the mechanism of malignant hypertension, it is agreed that the cause of the renal insufficiency accompanying malignant nephrosclerosis is the profound ischemic change occurring consequent to the arterial and arteriolar narrowing.

CLINICAL FEATURES

The clinical features of malignant hypertension are related to the direct effects of very high intravascular pressure on a number of vital structures. Blood pressure can range from systolic pressures that may exceed 250 mm Hg to diastolic levels of 140 mm Hg or more. Patients complain of blurring of vision and show retinopathy, including hemorrhages, exudates, and papilledema. Headache and other signs of increased intracranial pressure, congestive heart failure, and uremia with its complex symptomatology complete this syndrome. The syndrome is a true medical emergency requiring the institution of aggressive antihypertensive therapy. It is in this group of patients that the first evidence for the efficacy of the new antihypertensive agents has become clear, but it is important to institute therapy promptly before the development of irreversible renal lesions. Before introduction of the new antihypertensive drugs, malignant hypertension was associated with a 50% mortality within 3 months of onset, progressing to a 90% mortality within a year. Recent data suggest that the majority of patients may now survive for over 5 years (45).

MISCELLANEOUS RENAL VASCULAR DISEASES

Microangiopathic hemolytic anemias

This term refers to a cluster of overlapping conditions which are characterized clinically by renal failure, microangiopathic hemolytic anemia, and thrombocytopenia; morphologically these syndromes result in thrombosis in the interlobular arteries, afferent arterioles, and glomeruli, together with necrosis and thickening of the vessel walls (46). The morphologic changes are similar to those of malignant hypertension, but in the hemolytic anemias they may *precede* hypertension and are sometimes seen in its absence. A common pathogenetic mechanism appears to involve endothelial damage, intravascular coagulation, and consequent ischemic injury (47). The diseases include: (1) childhood hemolytic uremic syndrome, (2) adult hemolytic uremic syndrome, (3) thrombotic thrombocytopenic purpura, and (4) scleroderma.

Childhood hemolytic uremic syndrome is a major cause of acute renal failure in children. It is characterized by manifestations of sudden bleeding (especially hematemesis and melena), oliguria, hematuria, a microangiopathic hemolytic anemia, and, in some children, neurological changes. Hypertension is present in about half the patients. Interlobular and afferent arterioles show fibrinoid necrosis and intimal hyperplasia and are often occluded by thrombi. If the renal failure is managed with diaylsis, mortality is limited to 10 and 15%. The etiology is unkown, but several bacterial, viral, and rickettsial agents have been implicated.

Adult hemolytic uremic syndrome occurs in adults under a variety of settings:

1. In pregnant women with septic abortion, or other complications of pregnancy.

2. In women in the postpartum period. This usually occurs after an uneventful pregnancy, one day to several months following delivery, and is characterized by microangiopathic hemolytic anemia, oliguria, anuria, and mild or absent hypertension (49).

3. In association with contraceptive agents. Both malignant nephrosclerosis and a typical hemolytic uremic syndrome develop with greater frequency in women taking contraceptives.

4. In association with infection, such as typhoid fever, *E. coli,* septicemia, viral infections, and shigellosis (50).

Thrombotic thrombocytopenic purpura is manifested by fever, neurologic symptoms, hemolytic anemia, thrombocytopenic purpura, and the presence of thrombi in glomerular capillaries and afferent arterioles. The entity differs from hemolytic uremic syndrome in that renal involvement occurs in only about 50% of patients, the picture being dominated by central nervous system and cardiac manifestations. Furthermore, evidence of overt intravascular coagulation is not easy to obtain.

Scleroderma, or progressive systemic sclerosis, is manifested by lesions in the arteries and connective tissue of a variety of organs, including the kidney (51). Renal involvement is common and is dominated by hypertension, which occurs in about 25–35% of cases of the disorder (52, 53). The chronic vascular lesions consist of intimal fibrotic thickening and elastic reduplication in the interlobular and arcuate arteries. About 10% of patients develop malignant hypertension and rapidly progressive renal failure; these show, in addition to the chronic lesions, prominent "mucoid" edema of vessel intima, thrombosis and fibrinoid necrosis of arterioles and glomerular capillaries, and overt evidence of intravascular coagulation, as seen in other microangiopathic disorders. It is noteworthy that many of the vascular changes, including the fibrinoid necrosis, may *precede* the development of hypertension in these patients (52). One hypothesis relates the vascular changes to the known increased vascular reactivity of patients with scleroderma to vasoconstrictor agents, particularly angiotensin and epinephrine. Localized vasoconstriction in the kidney could conceivably result in endothelial injury, which precipitates intravascular coagulation, and subsequent intimal thickening; the latter, in turn, may cause or aggravate hypertension (15, 52).

Atheroembolic disease

Fragmentation of atheromatous plaques in the aorta or renal artery leads to embolization into intrarenal vessels in elderly patients who have severe atherosclerosis, particularly after aortic surgery and aortography (54). These emboli can be recognized in arcuate and interlobular arteries by their content of cholesterol crystals which appear as rhomboid clefts. Frequently, they have no functional significance. However, cases of acute renal failure occur in elderly patients in whom renal function is already compromised, principally after surgery on atherosclerotic aneurysms.

Necrotizing vasculitis (polyarteritis)

The necrotizing vasculitides represent a heterogeneous group of disorders, with overlapping clinical and morphological manifestations, characterized by inflammation and necrosis of the vessel walls, predominantly arteries and arterioles but also veins and capillaries. Of the many subtypes of vasculitis (55, 56) three frequently involve the kidney: (1) *Classic or macroscopic polyarteritis nodosa,* (2) *hypersensitivity angiitis or microscopic* polyarteritis, and (3) Wegener's granulomatosis. Renal lesions are found in from 70 to 80% of such cases.

Classic polyarteritis nodosa involves mainly the small and medium-sized muscular arteries (e.g., coronary arteries and mesenteric arteries) and, in the kidney, affects primarily the segmental, lobar, and arcuate vessels. Early lesions are characterized by infiltration of polymorpho-nuclear leukocytes, eosinophils, and mononuclear cells, together with fibrinoid necrosis; later there is increasing fibroplasia progressing to dense fibrosis with narrowing of the arterial lumen. The lesions are focal in distribution and classically different stages in the progression of the lesions can be seen in a single kidney. Clinically, classic poly-arteritis is characterized by hypertension, gastrointestinal and hepatic involvement, neurological manifestations, the presence of subcutaneous nodules, and renal involvement in over 70% of cases; an allergic his-tory is relatively uncommon. In contrast, an allergic history is common in *hypersensitivity angiitis*. In the latter conditions, small interlobu-lar arteries and afferent arterioles are predominantly involved and, in the typical cases, most of the lesions appear to be of the same age. Hypersensitivity angiitis commonly affects the skin and can usually be traced to precipitating antigens such as a drug, a microorganism, or heterologous protein. Glomerular lesions occur in both forms, and run the gamut from focal necrotizing GN to severe crescentic GN. The latter is more common in hypersensitivity angiitis. The renal manifesta-tions vary from mild proteinuria or microscopic hematuria to rapidly progressive renal failure with severe oliguria. It must be emphasized that there is considerable overlap between these two forms of poly-arteritis, both in the clinical manifestations and in the morphological lesions. Some cases, principally of the macroscopic type, are domi-nated by hypertension.

Considerable clinical and experimental evidence suggests that both types of vasculitis are immunologically mediated. Most impressive is the demonstration of a high incidence of hepatitis-B antigenemia and circulating hepatitis-B antigen–antibody complexes in the sera of some patients with both forms of polyarteritis (57). Moreover, hepatitis-B antigen, immunoglobulins, and complement have been detected in the vascular lesions. It is thus assumed that this is a type of immune com-plex vasculitis. Drugs such as sulfonamides, penicillin, Dilantin, and iodides have also been associated with the development of vasculitis, principally of the microscopic type, but it must be confessed that the mechanism by which these substances cause the vasculitis is obscure. Autoimmune antibody or cell-mediated immunity against endogenous components of the vessel wall (a form of autoimmune vasculitis) has been postulated but the evidence for this is thus far equivocal.

Wegener's granulomatosis is a rare form of necrotizing vasculitis manifested by necrotizing granulomas of the upper and lower respiratory tract, focal necrotizing vasculitis, and renal disease in the form of focal or diffuse necrotizing glomerulonephritis, often with prominent crescent formation (58). Vasculitis is characterized by predominant localization of the inflammation in the adventitia and by the presence of granulomatous reaction with multinucleate giant cells. Because of its striking resemblance to polyarteritis and serum sickness, it is thought that the disease represents some form of hypersensitivity. The disorder responds dramatically to therapy with immunosuppressive drugs (such as cytoxan) suggesting an immunological mechanism, perhaps of the cell-mediated type (3). No specific etiological agent has so far been identified.

References

1. Hollenberg, N. K. Renal disease. *In* The microcirculation in clinical medicine, R. Wells, (ed.), Chapter 5. Academic Press, New York, 1973.
2. Bell, E. T. Renal diseases, 2nd ed. Lea & Febiger, Philadelphia, 1950.
3. Dustin, P., Jr. Arteriolar hyalinosis. *In* International review of experimental pathology, Vol. 1, G. W. Richter and M. A. Epstein, (eds.). Academic Press, New York, 1962, pp. 73–138.
4. Weiner, J., Spiro, D., and Lattes, R. G. The cellular pathology of experimental hypertension. II. Arteriolar hyalinosis and fibrinoid change. Am. J. Pathol. 47:457, 1965.
5. Kaplan, M. H. Clinical hypertension, 2nd ed. Williams & Wilkins, Baltimore, 1978.
6. Genest, J., et al. Hypertension: physiopathology and treatment. McGraw-Hill, New York, 1977.
7. Tigerstedt, R. and Bergman, P. G. Niere und Kreislauf. Skand. Arch. Physiol. 8:223–271, 1898.
8. Goldblatt, H., Lynch, J., Hanzal, R. F., and Summerville, W. W. Studies on experimental hypertension. I. The production of persistent elevation of systolic blood pressure by means of renal ischemia. J. Exp. Med. 59:347, 1934.
9. Goldblatt, H. The renal origin of hypertension. Charles C Thomas, Springfield, Ill., 1948.
10. Laragh, J. H. The classification and treatment of essential hypertension using the renin-sodium index for vasoconstriction-volume analysis. The Johns Hopkins Med. J. 137:184–194, 1975.
11. Frolich, E. D. Hemodynamics of hypertension. *In* Hypertension: physiopathology and treatment, J. Genest et al. (eds.). McGraw-Hill, New York, 1977, p. 15.
12. Hial, V., Gimbrone Jr., M. A., Peyton, M. P., Wilcox, G. M., and Pisano, J. J. Angiotensin metabolism by cultured human vascular endothelial and smooth muscle cells. Microvascular Res. 17:314–329, 1979.
13. Thurau, K. Modification of angiotensin-mediated tubulo-glomerular feedback by extracellular volume. Kidney Int. 8:s–202–s–207, 1975.
14. Ledingham, J. M. Experimental renal hypertension. Clin. Nephrol. 4:127, 1975.

15. Heptinstall, R. H. Hypertension and vascular diseases of the kidney. *In* Kidney disease: present status, J. Churg, B. H. Spargo, F. K. Mostofi, and M. R. Abell (eds.). Williams & Wilkins, Baltimore, 1979, pp. 281–294.

16. Hollenberg, N. K., Epstein, M., Basch, R. I., Couch, N. P., Hickler, R. B. and Merrill, J. P. Renin secretion in essential and accelerated hypertension. Am. J. Med. 47:855, 1969.

17. Delin, K., Aurell, M., and Graveus, G. Renin-dependent hypertension in patients with unilateral kidney disease not caused by renal artery stenosis. Acta Med. Scand. 201:345, 1977.

18. Peart, W. S. The place of renin in the mechanism of hypertension in chronic renal disease.

19. Grollman, A. and Rule, C. Experimentally induced hypertension in parabiotic rats. Am. J. Physiol. 138:587, 1943.

20. Grollman, A., Muirhead, E. E., and Vanatta, J. Role of the kidney in pathogenesis of hypertension as determined by a study of the effects of bilateral nephrectomy and other experimental procedures on the blood pressure of the dog. Am. J. Physiol. 157:21, 1949.

21. Muirhead, E. E., Rightsel, W. A., Leach, B. E., Byers, L. W., Pitcock, J. A., and Brooks, B. Reversal of hypertension by transplants and lipid extracts of cultured renomedullary interstitial cells. Lab. Invest. 35:162, 1977.

22. McGiff, J. C. and Vane, J. R. Prostaglandins and the regulation of blood pressure. Kidney Int. 8:s262–s270, 1975.

23. Hill, T. W. K. and Monocada, S. The renal hemodynamic and excretory actions of prostacyclin in anesthetized dogs. Brit. J. Pharmacol. 62:413, 1978.

24. Levinsky, N. G. Brief reviews: the renal kallikrein-kinin system. Circ. Res. 44(6):441, 1979.

24a. Mitas, J. A., III, Levy, S. B., Holle, R., Frigon, R. P., and Stone, R. A. Urinary kallikrein activity in the hypertension of renal parenchymal disease. New Eng. J. Med. 299:162, 1978.

25. Blumberg, A. L., Denny, S. E., Marshall, G. R., and Needleman, P. Blood vessel hormone interactions: angiotensin, bradykinin and prostaglandins. Am. J. Physiol. 232:H305–H310, 1977.

26. Wilson, C., Ledingham, J. M., and Floyer, M. A. Experimental renal and renoprival hypertension. *In* The kidney, Vol. 4, C. Rouiller and A. F. Muller (eds.). Academic Press, New York, 1971.

27. Miller, E. D., Jr., Samuels, A. I., Haber, E., and Barger, A. C. Inhibition of angiotensin conversion in experimental renovascular hypertension. Science 177: 1108–1109, 1972.

28. Macdonald, G. J., Boyd, G. W., and Peart, W. S. Effect of the angiotensin II blocker 1-Sar-8-Ala-angiotensin II on renal artery clip hypertension in the rat. Circ. Res. 37:640–646, 1975.

29. Woods, J. W. and Williams, T. F. Hypertension due to renal vascular disease, renal infarction, renal cortical necrosis, *In* Diseases of the kidney, 2nd ed., M. B. Strauss and L. G. Welt (eds.). Little, Brown, Boston, 1971, pp. 769–824.

30. MacDonald, G. J., Louis, W. J., Renzini, V., Boyd, G. W., and Peart, W. S. Renal-clip hypertension in rabbits immunized against angiotensin II. Circ. Res. 27:197, 1970.

31. Lupu, A. N., Maxwell, M. H., and Kaufman, J. J. Mechanisms of hypertension during the chronic phase of one clip two kidney model in the dog. Circ. Res. (Suppl. 1)40:57, 1977.

32. Dargie, H. J., Franklin, S. S., and Reid, J. L. Plasma noradrenaline concentra-

tions in experimental renovascular hypertension in the rat. Clin. Sci. Mol. Med. 52:477, 1977.

33. Haber, E. The renin-angiotensin system and hypertension. Kidney Int. 15:427, 1979.

34. Davis, J. O. The pathogenesis of chronic renovascular hypertension. Circ. Res. 40:439, 1977.

35. McCormack, L. J. Morphologic abnormalities of renal artery associated with hypertension. *In* Hypertension: Mechanisms and management, G. Onesti et al. (eds.). Grune & Stratton, New York, 1973, p. 707.

36. Foster, J. H. and Oates, J. A. Recognition and management of renovascular hypertension. Hosp. Practice 10:61–70, 1975.

37. Hunt, J. C. Renovascular hypertension. *In* Strauss and Welt's Diseases of the Kidney, 3rd ed., L. Early and C. Gottschalk, eds. Little, Brown, Boston, 1979, pp. 1357–1385.

38. Menard, J., Corvol, P., Plouin, P. F., and Lagnean, P. Renovascular hypertension. *In* Nephrology, J. Hamburger, J. Crosnier, and J. P. Grunfeld (eds.). Wiley-Flammarion, New York, 1979, pp. 197–210.

39. Marks, L. S. and Maxwell, M. H. Renal vein renin values and limitations in the prediction of operative results. Urol. Clin. N. Am. 2:311, 1975.

40. Marks, L. S., Maxwell, M. H., and Kaufman, J. J. Renin, sodium, vasodepressor response to saralasin in renovascular and essential hypertension. Ann. Intern. Med. 87:176, 1977.

41. Tegtmeyer, C. J., Latour, E. A., Vaughn, Jr., E. D. et al. Clinical experience with saralasin infusion in hypertensive patients. Invest. Radio. 12:496, 1977.

41a. Tucker, R. M., Strong, C. G., Brennan, Jr., L. A., Sheps, S. G., Brown, R. D., and Weinshilboum, R. M. Renovascular hypertension. Relationship of surgical curability to renin-angiotensin activity. Mayo Clin. Proc. 53:373, 1978.

42. Giese, J. Renin, angiotensin and hypertensive vascular damage: a review. Am. J. Med. 55:315–332, 1973.

43. Linton, A. L., Gavrad, H., Gleadle, R. I., Hutchison, H. E., Lawson, D. H., Lever, A. F., Macadam, R. F., McNicol, G. P., and Robertson, J. I. S. Micro-angiopathic haemolytic anaemia and the pathogenesis of malignant hypertension. Lancet 1:1277, 1969.

44. Kincaid-Smith, P. Participation of intravascular coagulation in the pathogenesis of glomerular and vascular lesions. Kidney Int. 7:242–253, 1975.

45. Pettinger, W. A. Recent advances in the treatment of hypertension. Arch. Int. Med. 137:679, 1977.

46. Churg, J. Coagulation and the kidney, *In* Kidney disease: present status, J. Churg, B. H. Spargo, F. K. Mostofi, and M. R. Abell (eds.). Williams & Wilkins, Baltimore, 1979, pp. 140–161.

47. Kaplan, B. S. and Drummond, K. N. The hemolytic-uremic syndrome is a syndrome (Editorial). New Eng. J. Med. 298:964, 1978.

48. Gianantonio, C. A. Hemolytic uremic syndrome, *In* Pediatric kidney disease, Ch. Edelman (ed.). Little, Brown, Boston, 1978, pp. 724–736.

49. Sun, N. C. J., Johnson, W. J., Sung, D. T. W., and Woods, J. E. Idiopathic postpartum renal failure. Review and case report of a successful renal transplantation. Mayo Clin. Proc. 50:395, 1975.

50. Koster, F. et al. Hemolytic uremic syndrome after shigellosis. Relation to endotoxemia and circulating immune complexes. New Eng. J. Med. 298:927, 1978.

51. Pirani, C. L. and Silva, F. G. The kidneys in systemic lupus erythematosus and other collagen diseases: recent progress. *In* Kidney disease: present status,

J. Churg, B. H. Spargo, F. K. Mostofi, and M. R. Abell (eds.). Williams & Wilkins, Baltimore, 1979, pp. 98–139.

52. Cannon, P. J. et al. The relation of hypertension and renal failure scleroderma (PSS) to structural and functional abnormalities of renal cortical circulation. Medicine 53:1240, 1974.

53. Oliver, J. A. and Cannon, P. J. The kidney in scleroderma. Nephron 18:141, 1977.

54. Kassirer, J. P. Atheroembolic renal disease. New Eng. J. Med. 280:812, 1969.

55. Fauci, A. S. et al. The spectrum of vasculitis. Clinical, pathologic, immunologic and therapeutic considerations. Ann. Int. Med. 89:660, 1978.

56. Paronetto, F. Systemic nonsuppurative necrotizing angiitis. In Textbook of immunopathology, Vol. III, P. A. Miescher and H. J. Muller-Eberhard (eds.). Grune and Stratton, New York, 1976, pp. 1013–1024.

57. Michelak, G. Immune complexes of hepatitis B surface antigen in the pathogenesis of periarteritis nodosa. Am. J. Pathol. 90:619, 1978.

58. Fauci, A. S. and Wolff, S. M. Wegener's granulomatosis and related diseases. Disease-a-Month 23:3, 1977.

14
Pyelonephritis and Other Tubulointerstitial Diseases

GENERAL DEFINITIONS

Pathologic changes in the renal interstitium are present to some degree in almost all renal diseases. We have seen, for example, that chronic interstitial inflammation and fibrosis occur in chronic sclerosing glomerulonephritis. However, a variety of chemical, bacterial, immunologic, and physical forms of injury to the kidney cause generalized or localized changes that affect *primarily* the interstitial tissues and tubules.

The terms *interstitial nephritis* and *tubulointerstitial* nephritis are used interchangeably to describe this group of disorders. Clinically these diseases are characterized by defects in tubular function; the latter include impaired ability to concentrate the urine, manifested clinically by polyuria and nocturia, salt wasting, diminished ability to excrete acids, or isolated defects in tubular reabsorption or secretion. In the chronic, advanced stages of these diseases, however, vascular and glomerular alterations may supervene, resulting in hypertension or proteinuria of varying degrees.

Table 14-1 lists some conditions and agents that produce significant interstitial renal changes. When the etiologic agent is known or the

TABLE 14-1   *Tubulointerstitial Diseases*

Bacteria
  Acute pyelonephritis
  Chronic pyelonephritis (including reflux
    nephropathy)

Drugs
  Acute hypersensitivity interstitial nephritis
    (e.g., methicillin)
  Analgesic nephropathy

Heavy metals
  Lead, cadmium

Metabolic diseases
  Urate nephropathy
  Nephrocalcinosis
  Hypokalemic nephropathy
  Oxalate nephropathy

Physical factors
  Vesicoureteral reflux
  Chronic urinary tract obstruction
  Radiation nephritis

Immunologic reactions
  Transplant rejection
  Tubulointerstitial disease associated with
    glomerulonephritis
  Sjögren's syndrome

Vascular diseases

Miscellaneous
  Balkan nephropathy
  Uremic medullary cystic disease
  Other rare diseases (sarcoidosis, toxoplasmosis)
  "Idiopathic" interstitial nephritis

---

associated disease is evident, interstitial nephritis is identified by cause (for example, analgesic nephropathy or irradiation nephritis), or by associated disease (for example, urate or gouty nephritis). In some chronic cases, however, the etiologic agents are unknown and there is no associated disease; the term *idiopathic chronic interstitial nephritis* has been used for such cases.

The pathologic landmark of acute interstitial nephritis is edema and cellular infiltration of the interstitium, and of *chronic* interstitial nephritis, infiltration with mononuclear cells, interstitial fibrosis, and tubular atrophy.

In this chapter, two diseases are discussed as prototypes of interstitial nephritis: pyelonephritis and analgesic nephropathy. In addition, reference is made to acute interstitial nephritis induced by drugs and to recent studies on immunologically mediated interstitial disease.

PYELONEPHRITIS (PN)

This is the most common of the interstitial nephritides and also one of the most common diseases of the kidney. There are two recognized forms. *Acute pyelonephritis* is a disorder of the kidney caused by bacterial infection and is thus the renal lesion associated with *urinary tract infection*. The pathogenesis of *chronic pyelonephritis* (CPN) is more controversial; while bacterial infection may play a dominant role, other factors are critically involved (e.g., vesicoureteral reflux and urinary tract obstruction).

Pathogenesis

BACTERIOLOGY

Certain considerations of bacteriologic features of the urinary tract are relevant to the pathogenesis of pyelonephritis.

1. In man, acute pyelonephritis is a component of the clinical syndrome of urinary tract infection, which also involves the lower urinary passages—mainly the bladder.

2. Human urine can support bacterial growth, and most bacterial species capable of causing pyelonephritis multiply well in urine except at certain pH and osmolality values (1).

3. Normal kidneys, bladder, and urine of humans (and experimental animals) are sterile, and it is only in the distal part of the urethra and in females the vaginal vestibule that organisms can be cultured under normal conditions (2). The most common species cultured in normal individuals are saprophytic species such as diphtheroids and *Staphylococcus albus*.

4. Most infections are caused by bacterial species that are normal inhabitants of the intestinal tract—*Escherichia, Enterobacter, Proteus*—and the evidence, at least for *E. coli*, indicates that the reservoir of infection is the patient's own fecal flora (3). These species

have a low order of virulence for most other tissues in the body. Gram-positive organisms, such as *Staphylococcus aureus* and *Streptococcus fecalis* (enterococcus) can also, however, produce infection.

In the pathogenesis of pyelonephritis, therefore, the first two main considerations are the manner by which such relatively avirulent normal inhabitants reach the kidney and the factors that enhance their pathogenicity for renal tissue.

Bacteria may reach the kidneys either by way of the bloodstream (hematogenous infection) or by ascension, via the ureters, from the lower urinary tract (ascending infection). Theoretically, bacteria can also reach the kidney via lymphatics, but this route has not been adequately demonstrated either experimentally or in man. Hematogenous infection does occur in the course of septicemia or endocarditis (e.g., in staphylococcal endocarditis), but the present evidence suggests that the ascending route is the one responsible for the majority of cases of pyelonephritis in man.

HEMATOGENOUS INFECTION

The kinetics of bacterial multiplication in the kidney have been well described in a series of experimental studies and are important in understanding the pathogenesis of renal infection (reviewed in Ref. 4).

When bacteria are introduced into the bloodstream from an infected focus (e.g., endocarditis or pneumonia), the majority are cleared by the phagocytic cells of the reticuloendothelial system, mainly the liver and the spleen. Only small numbers, about 1 out of every 10^4 bacteria, are trapped in the kidney, and these are usually destroyed by antibacterial mechanisms without the production of inflammation. A typical experiment is shown in Figure 14-1. If 5×10^8 *E. coli* are injected intravenously into a *normal* rat, only 10^4 bacteria reach the kidneys, their numbers remain stationary for up to 24 hours, and eventually they disappear. The bacteria are not filtered in the urine; no renal lesions develop, and the animal remains normal. Thus, the normal kidney is resistant to blood-borne infection with *E. coli*.

To cause infection in a kidney after hematogenous spread, it is necessary to injure the kidney before infection by some experimental means. The simplest of these is ureteral obstruction, and occluding the ureter for as short a time as 1 hour predisposes the normal kidney to infection. As seen in Figure 14-1, in the obstructed kidney the num-

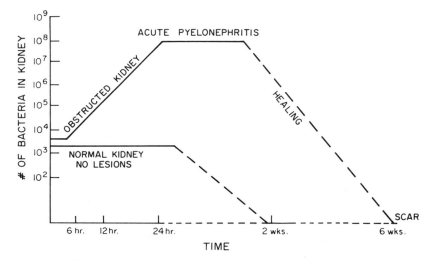

Fig. 14-1 Comparison of the time sequence of bacterial proliferation in the normal and obstructed kidney after intravenous injection of approximately 5×10^8 E. coli. The diagram is a schematic representation of data from different studies, and values for each curve are highly approximate (5).

ber of organisms initially trapped remains the same for 4 to 6 hours, but then multiplication occurs, and within 24–48 hours the numbers reach 10^8. Even if the occlusion is now removed, acute inflammation results from bacterial proliferation, and typical abscesses appear on the cortical surface. The obstruction that predisposes to infection can be either in the urethra (stricture), urinary bladder, ureters (stones or tumors), or the kidney proper, for example, renal scars. The mechanism by which obstruction increases the susceptibility of the kidney to infection is still unclear. Neither increased trapping of circulating bacteria nor simple "stagnation" of urine is responsible. Experimental evidence suggests that the main cause may be increased tissue pressure in the kidney, possibly interfering with the renal microcirculation during the obstruction phase (5).

In the course of experiments on hematogenous infection, it became apparent that in some experimental models, bacterial multiplication occurred first in the *medulla* and then spread to the cortex. In studies in which E. coli or Staphylococcus were injected directly either into the renal medulla or the cortex, it was found that as few as 10 bacteria can cause infection in the medulla and that more than 10^4 are needed to infect the cortex (6). This vulnerability of renal medulla is peculiar to some experimental species and is by no means absolute, but its mechanism has received considerable attention. The factors postulated to account for this phenomenon are many, but medullary hypertonicity seems to be the most important. The latter depresses phagocytosis by polymorphonuclear leukocytes. In addition, it has been shown that leukocytic exudation in response to local injury is both diminished and delayed in the medulla as compared to the cortex and that this difference can be largely negated if the medulla is made less hypertonic by water diuresis (4).

Whereas *E. coli* do not generally infect normal kidneys, *S. aureus* are capable of inducing pyelonephritis in the absence of obstruction. The outcome of experimental *E. coli* pyelonephritis is also depicted in Figure 14-1. The stage of acute pyelonephritis persists for 1–2 weeks, with continued acute inflammation and bacterial multiplication. Subsequently healing begins, and the numbers of organisms recovered decrease; by 6 weeks the kidneys become sterile and the areas of acute inflammation are replaced by scars. This sequence of events occurs spontaneously, without antibiotic therapy, correlates with a rise in serum titers of anti-*E. coli* antibodies, and is probably related to elimination of bacteria by specific immune mechanism (7). The sequence appears to be true also in uncomplicated human acute *E. coli* PN.

ASCENDING INFECTION

To explain how ascending infection can occur, one has to identify mechanisms by which pathogenic bacteria travel from the perineum and posterior one-third of the urethra to the urinary bladder, and from there on up the ureter, to the renal pelvis and medulla.

Urethral and introital colonization. Recent studies suggest that females susceptible to recurrent urinary tract infection are more likely to harbor potentially pathogenic bacteria (such as *E. coli*) in their posterior urethras and vaginal vestibules than are females not susceptible to infection (8). Furthermore, this "urethral and introital colonization" by bacteria appears to *precede* the development of overt bladder or kidney infection, and thus may be the initial determinant of urinary infection (8). The underlying basis for this colonization, now under intensive study (9), appears to involve the ability of bacteria to *adhere* to vaginal or urethral epithelial cells. Bacterial adherence, in turn, depends first on the surface properties of the bacteria themselves (presence of O or K antigens, or pili), and second on host factors (such as antibodies in vaginal secretions) which may increase or decrease bacterial sticking. Both bacterial and host factors have been implicated in increased adherence of bacteria seen in susceptible women (10). Despite this evidence, some workers doubt whether colonization plays more than a minor permissive role in the initiation of infection (11, 12).

From urethra to bladder. The only known mode of entry of organisms from urethra to bladder is by way of urethral instrumentation, as used in catheterization, cystoscopy, and urological surgery. Even with all precautions, catherization introduces organisms into the bladder, and long-term catherization, in particular, carries a high risk of infection (13). Whereas this mechanism certainly accounts for a great number of infections, a history of instrumentation cannot be obtained in many cases of PN. In the absence of instrumentation, urinary infections are much more common in females than males, and in the age group 15–40, the ratio of females to males affected is 8 : 1. This has been variously ascribed to the increased frequency of introital colonization described above, the shorter urethra in females, the absence of the antibacterial properties of prostatic fluid (14), and urethral trauma during sexual intercourse.

The latter point, in particular, has received much attention since it is common clinical experience that young women with urinary tract infection frequently relate their symptoms to sexual activity (e.g., honeymoon cystitis). Kunin (11) and Kass (12), however, caution that the association may be due simply to accentuation of an inapparent infection by urethral trauma or to a coincidental timing of events.

In the urinary bladder. In normal human beings and experimental animals, bacteria introduced into the bladder are usually cleared within a few days, with little evidence of inflammation (12). This so-called "antibacterial bladder defense mechanism" depends on three factors.

1. *Bacterial growth in the urine.* Although urine usually serves as a good culture medium, it has long been known that the growth of bacteria in the urine is dependent on pH and osmolarity. Asscher showed that first morning urine is actually not optimal for bacterial growth and that male urine supports bacterial growth far less than that of females (1). Nevertheless, sufficient bacterial mul-

tiplication occurs in most urine specimens, and a bacteriostatic action of urine would not alone be sufficient to sterilize the urine.

2. *Dilution of bacteria by voiding* continuously flushes bacteria out of the bladder and thereby maintains the number of organisms at a relatively low level. But a film of infected urine coats the surface of the bladder after micturition and supplies an innoculum for fresh supplies of urine entering from the ureter. Because bacteria may multiply at a rapid rate in the urine, dilution by voiding alone is not sufficient to account for sterilization except in unusual circumstances (16).

3. *Mucosal factors.* Because neither of the first two factors is sufficient to cause sterilization, an antibacterial mechanism residing in or very close to the bladder mucosa has been postulated and suggested by experimental studies in which exposure of bacteria to the isolated bladder mucosa resulted in inhibition of bacterial growth (17). The antibacterial substance(s) is not, however, known.

Whereas the *normal* bladder is able to clear bacteria readily, clearance mechanisms are interfered with in two clinically common situations: (1) the presence of a residual urine volume, in which the bladder cannot be emptied completely, and (2) existence of obstruction to urine flow. A residual urine predisposes to infection by increasing the volume of inoculum of bacteria to be diluted by noninfected ureteral urine. With bacterial multiplication, inflammation of the bladder develops, a condition to which the term *cystitis* is applied.

VESICOURETERAL REFLUX (VUR)

It is now well-established that vesicoureteral reflux (VUR) is the pathologic condition which causes ascension of infected urine into the kidney and, further, that VUR is the most important factor predisposing to acute and chronic pyelonephritis, particularly in infants and children (18, 19). In the normal urinary tract, VUR is prevented by virtue of the length of the intramural segment of the ureter, allowing for oblique insertion of the ureter into a tunnel in the bladder wall such that the intravesical part of the ureter is compressed during micturition (20). Failure of this valve mechanism is most commonly due to a shortening of the intravesical portion of the ureter, caused by congenital abnormal development of the ureteric bud, such that the ureteric orifices are displaced laterally (21). VUR is frequently familial, but the precise mode of inheritance is unknown.

VUR can be demonstrated by the voiding *cystourethrogram* in which the bladder is filled with opaque dye and the patient is instructed to void. When this condition is present, radioopaque dye can be seen refluxing into the ureter, often all the way into the pelvis. VUR is detected in 30–50% of infants and children undergoing radiographic studies for recurrent or persistent urinary tract infections, and it is also seen in adults with spinal cord injuries, bladder tumors, prostatic hypertrophy, and urinary stones. Vesicoureteral reflux varies from mild to severe and can be unilateral or bilateral. In the more severe cases between 30 and 60% of children exhibiting reflux eventually develop typical pyelonephritic renal scars (18, 22). In the severe forms of reflux, retrograde studies show that the injected dye fills the collecting ducts of some pyramids and fans out into the cortex in the shape of a V or a U. Such *intrarenal reflux* usually occurs in the poles of the kidney, a distribution which resembles that of the pyelonephritic scars in affected children (22).

The elegant studies of Ransley and Risdon (23, 24) provide a convincing anatomical basis for such intrarenal reflux. It appears that there are several anatomic types of papillae in normal human infants. The simple pointed type, depicted in most illustrations of normal papillae in textbooks, has slit-like papillary duct orifices which are occluded with a rise in pelvic pressure, and are thus nonrefluxing. Many "normal" papillae, however, have a concave valley-like or deeply indented tip with widened ducts of Bellini opening into the calyx. The orifices of such ducts cannot be occluded by a rise in pressure in the calyx, thus allowing retrograde entry of urine up the collecting ducts. In an autopsy study of infants dying from nonrenal causes, two-thirds of kidneys had at least one papilla of the potentially refluxing type, most being in the upper and lower poles of the kidneys, a distribution which corresponds to the usual distribution of pyelonephritic damage.

Thus, it is clear that vesicoureteral and intrarenal reflux are mechanisms by which bacteria can be delivered into the renal pelvis and renal parenchyma (25). Indeed, when cystourethrograms are done routinely on patients with pyelonephritic scars, the great majority of children and over 50% of adults exhibit VUR. Some workers thus would do away with the term chronic pyelonephritis and substitute for it "reflux nephropathy."

Acute pyelonephritis

PATHOLOGIC CHANGES

The development of the renal lesion in acute pyelonephritis has been studied in detail in the experimental animal, and the well-developed lesion in the human disease appears to have a similar morphogenesis (4). There is first deposition of bacteria in the glomerular and interstitial capillaries after hematogenous infection and in the presence of intrarenal reflux, ascending bacteria may reach the medulla or cortex directly. Bacterial multiplication occurs predominantly in the *interstitium* and tubules. Small colonies of organisms can be detected in the interstitium within 24 to 48 hours after infection. Typical acute inflammation then develops in the interstitium: There is edema, neutrophilic exudation, and deposition of fibrin. The renal tubules become necrotic, there is rupture of organisms in the tubular lumina, and then infection spreads to the cortex. The actions of bacterial toxins and enzymes from leukocytes result in gross abscess formation, so that the resulting lesion is a cortical abscess, which radiates into the medulla. After initial spread, hematogenous and ascending infections cannot be differentiated. In both types, glomeruli are spared of infection, except in some cases of fungal pyelonephritis and in massive infections.

It is important to realize that the lesions in acute pyelonephritis are focal and remain localized, often having a wedge-shaped appearance with the apex of the wedge in the medulla. In the presence of total ureteral obstruction, inflammatory reaction sometimes affects the entire kidney.

After the acute phase, healing occurs: Neutrophilic exudate is replaced by one that is predominantly mononuclear, with macrophages, and plasma cells, and later, lymphocytes. There are formation of granulation tissue, deposition of collagen, and eventual replacement of abscesses by scars that can be seen on the cortical surface as fibrous depressions. Such scars are characterized microscopically by atrophy of tubules, interstitial fibrosis and lymphocytic infiltration. Healing is associated with progressive diminution of the number of bacteria in renal tissue and eventual renal sterilization. The renal scars have a fairly nonspecific histologic appearance and may resemble scars produced by ischemic or other types of injury to the kidney. However, the pyelonephritic scar is typically associated with inflammation, fibrosis, and deformation of the underlying calyces and pelvis, reflecting the role of ascending infection and VUR in its pathogenesis.

CLINICAL FEATURES

Pyelonephritis occurs as an expression of diffuse urinary tract infection, which includes cystitis. Urinary infection may remain localized to the bladder; however, because the clinical manifestations of pyelonephritis are often those of the accompanying bladder infection, renal involvement is difficult to exclude on the basis of clinical features alone.

Pyelonephritis is often associated with specific predisposing conditions, some of which were covered in the discussion of pathogenic mechanisms. These include the following.

1. Urinary obstruction, either congenital (strictures, anomalies) or acquired (calculi, tumors in the urinary tract).

2. Instrumentation of the urinary tract, most commonly catheterization.

3. Vesicoureteral reflux (see earlier).

4. Pregnancy; 4–6% of all pregnant women develop bacteriuria some time during pregnancy, and 20–40% of these eventually develop symptomatic urinary infection if not treated (26).

5. Patients' sex and age. After the first year of life (when congenital anomalies of the urethra are common in males) and up to around age 40, urinary infections are much more common in females than in males. In the absence of obstruction and instrumentation, urinary tract infection in the age group of 15–40 is almost exclusively a disease of females. With increasing age, the incidence in males increases, this being related to prostatic hyperplasia and instrumentation.

6. Preexisting renal lesions, such as gouty nephropathy and analgesic nephropathy.

7. Diabetes mellitus. Whether diabetics have a higher incidence of urinary infection than nondiabetic controls is controversial. Increased rates of infection are probably related to more frequent

instrumentation, the general susceptibility to infection, and the neurogenic bladder dysfunction exhibited by such patients.

The symptoms of pyelonephritis include pain and burning on urination, frequency of urination, and in some cases, flank pain and fever. In the acute phase, the urine characteristically contains many leukocytes that derive from the inflammatory infiltrate. The presence of leukocytes in the urine (pyuria) does not differentiate upper from lower urinary tract infection. But the finding of leukocyte *casts* (pus casts) indicates renal involvement; pus casts are accumulations of leukocytes arranged in the shape of the renal tubule in which they have formed.

The diagnosis of urinary infection is established by culturing pathogenic bacteria from the urine. Contamination can be differentiated from true infection by quantitating the cultured bacteria; the studies of Kass (11, 27) have shown that culture of 10^5 organisms or more per ml of urine almost always signifies infection except under unusual circumstances.

It is frequently difficult to differentiate cystitis alone from pyelonephritis. As mentioned above, pus casts always indicate kidney involvement but are not always present. Recently it has been shown that bacteria in the urine of patients with pyelonephritis, when studied by immunofluorescent techniques, are coated with antibody (formed locally in the kidney), while those from patients with cystitis are usually not antibody-coated (28). The reliability of this *antibody-coated immunofluorescent test,* however, is controversial (29).

The course of uncomplicated acute pyelonephritis is usually benign and the symptoms disappear within a few days after institution of appropriate antibiotic therapy. Bacteria may, however, persist in the urine, the incidence of recurrence of urinary infection with new serological types of *E. coli* or other organisms being high, about 30% in some series (11, 30). Such bacteriuria then either disappears or persists sometimes for years.

In the presence of obstruction, vesicoureteral reflux, or other predisposing conditions, the response to treatment is less satisfactory, and repeated infections may occur. Antibiotic therapy often results only in the emergence of antibiotic-resistant organisms, or reinfection with less sensitive types. The likelihood of permanent renal damage and the development of chronic pyelonephritis in such a setting is greater in infancy and early childhood.

Chronic pyelonephritis (CPN)

Although there is some controversy regarding terminology, CPN is considered here as a chronic renal disorder in which *renal scarring is associated with pathologic involvement of the calyces and pelvis* (31). The specific criterion for pelvocalyceal involvement is important in that virtually all the conditions listed in Table 14-1 lead to chronic tubulointerstitial changes similar to those in CPN, but, with the exception of analgesic nephropathy, none significantly affects the calyces.

There are three variants of CPN:

Chronic PN with the vesicoureteral reflux (reflux nephropathy). As discussed earlier this is the most common type of CPN. Reflux may be unilateral or bilateral, thus the renal damage may cause scarring and atrophy of one kidney, or may involve both and lead to chronic renal insufficiency.

Chronic obstructive PN. Recurrent infections superimposed on diffuse or localized obstructive lesions lead to repeated episodes of inflammation and scarring resulting in a picture of chronic pyelonephritis. The effects of obstruction contribute to the parenchymal atrophy and, indeed, it is sometimes difficult to differentiate the effects of bacterial infection from those of obstruction alone. The disease can be bilateral, as in the congenital anomalies of the urethra (posterior urethral valves), resulting in fatal renal insufficiency unless the anomaly is reversed, or unilateral, such as occurs with urinary calculi and unilateral obstructive anomalies of the ureter.

Idiopathic chronic pyelonephritis. A small number of patients exhibiting the pathologic changes of chronic pyelonephritis give no history of recurrent urinary tract infection (32, 33) and do not exhibit overt evidence of VUR and obstruction. A number of possible explanations have been suggested for this type of CPN (34):

1. Vesicoureteral reflux may have caused the renal damage and then disappeared. Progressive damage may then be due to secondary hypertension, glomerulosclerosis, or immunologic injury.

2. Infection in the kidney may be present in the form of protoplasts or L forms. These bacterial forms lack part or all of their cell walls and can persist in the hypertonic environment of the renal medulla. They have been isolated from some patients with "sterile" pyelonephritis (35), but their exact role in the pathogenesis of renal damage is unknown.

3. Progressive damage occurs by immunologic mechanisms triggered by remote, forgotten, or asymptomatic urinary infections. Although this is an attractive hypothesis, experimental and clinical evidence for such a mechanism is not convincing (36).

We are thus left without a satisfying explanation for these—fortunately rare—cases.

PATHOLOGIC CHANGES

The most characteristic pathologic changes of chronic pyelonephritis are seen on gross, rather than microscopic, examination: the kidneys are irregularly scarred, the involvement is bilateral but usually asymmetrical. This contrasts with the gross appearance of kidneys with chronic glomerulonephritis, which are diffusely and symmetrically scarred. Because most chronic pyelonephritis is due to ascending infection and VUR, lesions affect the pelvis and calyces, which are deformed, blunted, and dilated. *The irregular scarring with underlying calyceal deformity is the hallmark of chronic pyelonephritis.*

Microscopically, there are varying degrees of interstitial inflammation and fibrosis both in the cortex and medulla. The tubules show atrophy in some areas, hypertrophy in others, and dilation. In the presence of active bacterial infection, neutrophils can be seen in the interstitium and in the tubules. The glomeruli may appear normal, except for periglomerular fibrosis, but in later stages, they may show ischemic changes, owing to secondary vascular and hypertensive alterations, or develop focal glomerulosclerosis (37) for as yet poorly understood reasons. None of the histologic changes described are specific for chronic pyelonephritis, since they can be mimicked by most of the interstitial diseases listed in Table 14-1. The diagnosis of chronic pyelonephritis on morphologic grounds thus rests on the gross appearance of the irregular scarring and pelvocalyceal deformity.

CLINICAL FEATURES

Patients with chronic pyelonephritis may present with the clinical manifestations of acute recurrent PN with back pain, fever, frequent pyuria, and bacteriuria, but more often exhibit a silent, insidious onset. Distinctive symptoms come to attention late in their disease because of the gradual onset of renal insufficiency and hypertension, or because of the discovery of pyuria or bacteriuria on routine examination. Loss of tubular function—in particular of concentrating ability—gives rise to polyuria and nocturia. Intravenous pyelography is necessary for accurate clinical diagnosis. Pyelograms show the affected kidneys to be smaller than normal, with characteristic coarse cortical scars with underlying blunted and deformed calyces. Significant bacteriuria may be present, but in the late stages it is sometimes absent. Some of these patients develop intractable hypertension which contributes to the progressive renal failure.

TUBULOINTERSTITIAL NEPHRITIS INDUCED BY DRUGS AND TOXINS

The kidney is particularly vulnerable to chemical injury because of its large blood supply, most of it to the cortex. Normal physiologic processes may increase the local concentrations of certain drugs or toxins in various segments of the nephron. For example, toxins that are reabsorbed by the proximal tubules cause predominant proximal damage, while those affected by concentrating mechanisms reach high levels in the medulla, predisposing it to injury. Chemicals which are insoluble in acid pH tend to precipitate in the distal tubules and collecting ducts, causing obstruction of tubular lumina.

Toxins produce renal injury by at least three mechanisms: (1) they may trigger an immunologic reaction, exemplified by the acute hypersensitivity nephritis induced by methicillin; (2) they may cause acute renal failure by direct tubular damage (such as in mercuric chloride poisoning) or by some other poorly understood mechanism (e.g., the antibiotic aminoglycosides, such as gentamicin); and (3) they may cause cumulative injury to tubules that takes years to become manifest, resulting in chronic renal insufficiency. The latter type of damage may be clinically unrecognizable until significant renal damage has occurred. Such is the case with analgesic abuse nephropathy, which is not usually detected until renal failure develops.

Here we shall discuss analgesic nephropathy and acute drug-induced interstitial nephritis as examples of these reactions.

Analgesic abuse nephropathy

This is a type of chronic renal disease caused by excessive intake of analgesic mixtures and characterized morphologically by chronic interstitial nephritis with *renal papillary necrosis*.

The association between renal disease and analgesic abuse was first noted in 1953 by Spühler and Zollinger in Switzerland (38); the renal damage was attributed to phenacetin, although the analgesic mixtures consumed often contained, in addition, aspirin, caffeine, and codeine. The association was subsequently confirmed in Sweden and other European countries and Australia. Patients who develop this disease usually ingest large quantities of analgesic mixtures (39), and consumptions of up to 30 kg of phenacetin over a 30-year period have been recorded, the average being 9.8 kg over a mean period of 13 years. The minimal amount of analgesic required for renal damage is thought to be between 2 and 3 kg. The disease occurs in all countries, including the United States, but the largest numbers of cases have come from Finland, Scandinavia, and Australia; it is clear that, even in these countries, factors other than simply the amount of analgesic consumed play a role in the pathogenesis. In the hotter climate of Queensland, Australia, for example, the incidence is particularly high, in part due to dehydration. The low reported incidence in the United States has been ascribed, at least in part, to patient denial of analgesic abuse. In a study of 101 patients with chronic interstitial nephritis, however, 20 gave a history of analgesic consumption of 3 kg or more (40, 41). In the southeastern United States 13.2% of patients seen in a major referral center for end-stage renal disease had analgesic nephropathy (42).

PATHOGENESIS

Although phenacetin was the agent first incriminated, most patients take a combination of analgesics, and experimentally, phenacetin, aspirin, and acetaminophen can cause papillary necrosis (43). In the rat, papillary necrosis is most readily induced by a mixture of aspirin and phenacetin, combined with water depletion (44). In man, however, cases that can be ascribed to intake of aspirin alone are rare. The evidence points to an additive effect of aspirin, phenacetin, and acetaminophen.

It is thought that, in the sequence of events leading to renal damage, papillary necrosis occurs first, and cortical scarring is a secondary phenomenon (45, 46). The cause of the papillary necrosis is unclear. The susceptibility of renal papillae to damage by phenacetin or its metabolite acetaminophen may be due to the establishment of a gradient (similar to that for urea), which produces a concentration in the papillae several times that in the cortex. Dehydration increases and overhydration reduces the concentration of acetaminophen in the kidney, findings which are consistent with a decreased and increased susceptibility to phenacetin under these respective conditions. Acetaminophen probably causes cell injury by its effect as an oxidant. By inhibiting prostaglandin synthesis, aspirin may induce its potentiating effect by inhibiting the vasodilatory effects of prostaglandin, thus producing renal tissue hypoxia.

PATHOLOGIC CHANGES

The hallmark of analgesic nephropathy is the presence of chronic interstitial nephritis and widespread bilateral papillary necrosis. Grossly, the kidney is either normal or slightly reduced in size, and the cortex exhibits depressed and raised areas, the depressed areas representing cortical atrophy overlying necrotic papillae. Microscopically, the papillary changes may take one of several forms: In the early cases, there is patchy necrosis and widening of the interstitium, but in the advanced form, the entire papilla is necrotic, often remaining in place as a structureless mass with ghosts of tubules and foci of dystrophic calcification. If segments or entire portions of the papilla have been sloughed and excreted in the urine, the underlying calyx appears dilated, accounting for some of the diagnostic radiological features of the disease. The cortical changes consist of loss and atrophy of tubules, and interstitial fibrosis and inflammation. These changes are almost certainly due to obstructive atrophy caused by the necrotic papilla. The glomeruli in the atrophic cortex may either be normal or show various degrees of hyalinization.

CLINICAL FEATURES

Analgesic nephropathy is much more common in women than in men and has been noted to occur predominantly in psychoneurotic women, factory workers, or individuals with recurrent headaches and muscular pains. The symptomatology is variable and may be minimal until chronic renal insufficiency occurs. If renal function tests are done, inability to concentrate the urine occurs early, as expected from lesions in the papillae. Recurrent urinary tract infections are frequent, and many patients develop colicky renal pain that can be caused by passing of a necrotic papilla or a stone through the ureter. Other findings include hypertension, renal failure associated with obstruction or sepsis, and the development of duodenal and gastric ulcers. The urine contains little protein, and the urinary sediment shows leukocytes and red cells; occasionally, entire tips of necrotic papillae may be recovered in the urine. Radiological examination may show papillary calcification, and diagnosis can often be established with the intravenous pyelogram, because of a characteristic deformity of the papillary and calyceal regions.

Although progressive impairment of renal function may lead to chronic renal failure, renal function may either stabilize or actually improve after withdrawal of analgesic intake; with proper therapy of the infection and drug withdrawal, analgesic nephropathy may represent one of the few types of recoverable chronic renal failure (47). Regrettably, patients with analgesic nephropathy who survive because of their discontinuance of the offending drug have a significantly increased risk of developing *transitional papillary carcinoma of the renal pelvis* (48).

Papillary necrosis

This is a serious and rather common renal condition, in which there is infarction necrosis occurring in the medulla, and particularly the papillae, usually affecting both kidneys.

The conditions associated with papillary necrosis are (1) pyelonephritis, (2) diabetes mellitus, (3) urinary tract obstruction, (4) analgesic nephropathy, and (5) sickle cell disease. Pyelonephritis is often but not always, present as a complication of diabetes or obstruction when papillary necrosis occurs. In the United States, about 50% of papillary necrosis is associated with diabetes, 40% with urinary tract obstruction, and 10% with other causes. In the diabetic and obstructive forms, both kidneys are usually affected, and virtually all papillae are necrotic, showing yellowish-green, sharply defined areas that involve the distal part of the renal pyramid. In the presence of pyelonephritis, there are also cortical and medullary abscesses. Microscopically, the necrotic tissue is rather sharply defined and is separated from the non-necrotic areas by a rim of leukocytes. Clinically, the development of papillary necrosis is an ominous sign in patients with diabetes or obstruction, and acute renal failure rapidly supervenes, followed by death from uremia. In the small number of patients that do not succumb, necrotic papillae may either calcify or slough, leaving a dilated, blunted calyx. Papillary necrosis accompanying analgesic nephropathy has been described above.

Papillary necrosis is also seen in sickle cell disease, but here the necroses are more patchy and rarely involve the entire papilla. Other associated conditions are alcoholic cirrhosis and severe vascular renal disease.

Acute interstitial nephritis induced by drugs

This is a form of acute interstitial reaction in the kidney that occurs as a hypersensitivity response to a variety of drugs, especially penicillin derivatives. The incidence of this adverse reaction to therapeutic agents is increasing. First reported after the use of sulfonamides, the most frequent reactions are ascribed the antibiotic methicillin (49), although ampicillin, rifampin, penicillin, the antiepileptic drug phenindione, the thiazides, and furosemide have also been implicated (see review in ref. 50). The clinical manifestations include fever, a skin rash, eosinophilia, and evidence of renal disease. The latter includes hematuria, mild proteinuria, and a rising serum creatinine. In some patients, a typical syndrome of *acute renal failure* develops, usually about 2 weeks after antibiotic therapy. It is important to consider antibiotic-induced renal hypersensitivity in the differential diagnosis of acute renal failure because cessation of the offending drug is usually followed by recovery, although irreversible damage has been reported.

Histologically, the glomeruli are normal. The principal change is in the interstitium: there are edema and infiltration with polymorphonuclear leukocytes, lymphocytes, plasma cells, and, in some cases, large numbers of eosinophils. There is, in addition, evidence of tubular necrosis and tubular regeneration, common to other forms of acute tubular necrosis.

Several points suggest that this is an immunologically mediated reaction: (1) The clinical manifestations, including the latent period, the lack of correlation with the dose of antibiotic, the eosinophilia, and the rash, have always pointed to a hypersensitivity reaction. (2) Immunofluorescent studies in some patients have shown linear staining of IgG and C3 as well as antibody directed against the haptenic group of methicillin, along the tubular basement membrane (TBM). It has been suggested that the drug hapten, which is secreted by the proximal tubules, conjugates with the TBM, thus stimulating anti-TBM antibody production, with ensuing damage to the tubules and secondarily to the interstitium (51). While this is an attractive hypothesis, the vast majority of patients with drug-induced hypersensitivity nephritis fail to show anti-TBM antibody staining by fluorescence microscopy or anti-TBM antibodies in their serum (52). (3) IgE serum levels are increased in some patients with drug-induced nephritis, and IgE-containing plasma cells and basophils are present in the infiltrate, suggesting an allergen-reaginic type reaction in the pathogenesis of the lesion (52). (4) The occurrence of cross-sensitivity to other drugs after discontinuation of methicillin therapy also supports the theory of a hypersensitivity reaction. (5) The mononuclear infiltrate and the demonstration of cell-mediated immunity to the drug hapten in some patients suggest a delayed hypersensitivity-type reaction. Despite this evidence, however, the precise immunologic sequence of events leading to renal damage is unknown.

IMMUNOLOGICALLY MEDIATED INTERSTITIAL AND TUBULAR DISEASE

Table 14-1 gives known causes of acute and chronic interstitial diseases of the kidney; however, there are instances of interstitial nephritis in which the etiology is not apparent, and the term *idiopathic interstitial nephritis* is often used to describe such cases. It is possible that these represent a heterogenous group of conditions with variable etiologies, either infectious or environmental. The possibility, however, that the renal interstitium and tubules can be damaged by immunologic reactions similar to those that occur in glomerulonephritis has received a great deal of attention recently (54). Experimentally, it has been possible to induce two types of immune nephritis in tubules and interstitium.

Tubular immune-complex disease

In experiments in rabbits and rats, injections of homologous renal tissue in Freund's adjuvant result in tubular damage, interstitial fibrosis, and mononuclear cell infiltration, with minimal changes in the glomeruli. Immunofluorescence microscopy reveals *granules* containing immunoglobulin and complement along the tubular basement membranes, very reminiscent of the granules seen in immune-complex glomerulonephritis. Electron microscopy confirms the presence of electron-dense deposits along the tubules. The sequence of events suggested for this type of nephritis is the following: Immunization with homologous renal tissue results in the production of circulating antibodies to *cytoplasmic* component of tubular cells. Such circulating antibodies diffuse across the peritubular capillaries and combine with a tubular cytoplasmic antigen that leaks out of the epithelial cell to form an immune complex. Peritubular granular deposits in humans are found most frequently in patients with lupus nephritis usually associated with glomerulonephritis, and in other forms of glomerulonephritis (cryoglobulinemia, MPGN) but their occurrence in idiopathic interstitial and tubular disease has been limited to rare case reports (55).

Antitubular basement membrane antibody disease

This type of disease can be induced in certain strains of guinea pigs and rats by injections of tubular basement membrane preparations with adjuvant (56–58). The animals develop an interstitial infiltration with mononuclear cells and tubular cell damage. Immunofluorescence microscopy reveals smooth, continuous *linear* accumulations of immunoglobulins and complement along the basement membranes of the proximal tubules. When antibody is eluted from these kidneys, it reacts *in vitro* with normal tubular basement membrane, and the lesions can be transferred by serum, supporting the importance of antitubular basement membrane antibodies in the pathogenesis of renal disease in experimental animals. There are genetic differences in the susceptibility of strains of experimental animals to this disease; for example, the Brown/Norway strain of rats is especially susceptible, but the usual Sprague-Dawley strain is not. In man, anti-TBM antibodies have been shown to occur in Goodpasture's syndrome, in association with anti-GBM antibodies, in renal allografts, in rare cases of interstitial nephritis due to methicillin or chronic idiopathic interstitial nephritis (59). Thus, whereas immunologic lesions in both of these models do resemble those seen in chronic interstitial nephritis, it is not clear that they play a major role in the pathogenesis of primary interstitial and tubular diseases of the kidney in man (60).

General references and reviews

R. S. Cotran. Interstitial nephritis, *In* Kidney disease: present status, J. Churg, B. H. Spargo, F. K. Mostofi, and M. R. Abell (eds.). Williams & Wilkins, Baltimore, 1979, pp. 254–280.

R. S. Cotran and J. Pennington. Urinary tract infection, pyelonephritis, and reflux nephropathy, *In* The kidney, 2nd ed., B. M. Brenner and F. C. Rector (eds.). W. B. Saunders, Philadelphia, 1980.

R. S. Cotran. Tubulointerstitial diseases, *In* The kidney, 2nd ed., B. M. Brenner and F. C. Rector (eds.). W. B. Saunders, Philadelphia, 1980.

L. R. Freedman. Interstitial renal inflammation, including pyelonephritis and urinary tract infections, *In* Strauss and Welt's diseases of the kidney, 3rd ed., L. Early and C. Gottschalk (eds.). Little, Brown, Boston, 1978, pp. 817–877.

R. H. Heptinstall. Interstitial nephritis. A brief review. Am. J. Pathol. 83:214–236, 1976.

R. H. Heptinstall, ed. Urinary tract infection and pyelonephritis, *In* Pathology of the kidney, 2nd ed., Vol. II. Little, Brown, Boston, 1974, pp. 837–875.

C. J. Hodson and P. Kincaid-Smith. Reflux nephropathy. Masson, New York, 1979.

P. Kincaid-Smith (guest editor). Analgesic nephropathy. Kidney Int. 13:1–113, 1978.

C. M. Kunin. Detection, prevention and management of urinary tract infections, 3rd ed. Lea & Febiger, Philadelphia, 1979.

K. Kuhn and J. Brod. Interstitial nephropathies, *In* Contributions to nephrology. S. Karger, Basel, 16:1–167, 1979.

R. T. McCluskey and R. G. Colvin. Immunological aspects of renal tubular and interstitial diseases. Ann. Rev. Med. 29:21, 1978.

References

1. Asscher, A. W., Sussman, M., Waters, W. E., Davis, R. H., and Chick, S. Urine as a medium for bacterial growth. Lancet 2:1037–1041, 1966.
2. Stamey, T. A. Urinary infections. Williams & Wilkins, Baltimore, 1972.
3. Gruneberg, R. N., Leakey, A., Bendall, M. J., and Smellie, J. M. Bowel flora in urinary tract infection: effect of chemotherapy with special reference to cotrimoxazole. Kidney Int. 8:122, 1975.
4. Cotran, R. S. Experimental pyelonephritis, *In* The kidney, Vol. 2, C. Rouiller and A. F. Muller (eds.). Academic Press, New York, 1969, pp. 269–361.
5. Freedman, L. R. Experimental pyelonephritis. XII. Changes mimicking chronic pyelonephritis as a consequence of renal vascular occlusion in the rat. Yale J. Biol. Med. 39:113–118, 1966.
6. Freedman, L. R. and Beeson, P. B. Experimental pyelonephritis. IV. Observations on infections resulting from direct inoculation of bacteria in different zones of the kidney. Yale J. Biol. Med. 30:406, 1958.
7. Sanford, J. P., Hunter, B. W., Akins, L. L., and Barnett, J. A. Immunity and obstructive uropathy as determinants in the pathogenesis of experimental pyelonephritis with observations on the distribution of antibody in hydronephrotic kidneys, *In* Progress in pyelonephritis, E. H. Kass (ed.). Davis, Philadelphia, 1965, pp. 255–271.
8. Stamey, T. A. and Sexton, C. C. The role of vaginal colonization with enterobacteriacea in recurrent urinary infections. J. Urol. 113:214, 1975.
9. Stamey, T. A., Whener, N., Mihara, G., and Condy, M. The immunologic basis of recurrent bacteriuria: role of cervicovaginal antibody in enterobacterial colonization of the introital mucosa. Medicine 57:47, 1978.
10. Svanborg-Eden, C. S. Attachment of *E. coli* to human urinary tract epithelial cells. Acta Microbiol. Scand. Suppl. 1978.
11. Kunin, C. M. Detection, prevention and management of urinary tract infections, 3rd ed. Lea & Febiger, Philadelphia, 1979.

12. Kass, E. H. An approach to the management of resistant urinary tract infections. Kidney Int. 16:204, 1979.
13. Beeson, P. B. The case against the catheter. Am. J. Med. 24:1, 1958.
14. Fair, W. R., Timothy, M. M., and Churg, H. D. Antibacterial nature of prostatic fluid. Nature 218:444, 1968.
15. Kunin, C. M. Sexual intercourse and urinary infections. New Eng. J. Med. 298:376, 1978.
16. Cox, C. E. and Hinman, F., Jr. Factors in resistance to infection in the bladder. I. The eradication of bacteria by vesical emptying and intrinsic defense mechanisms, In Progress in pyelonephritis, E. H. Kass (ed.). Davis, Philadelphia, 1965, pp. 563–570.
17. Hand, W. L., Smith, J. W., and Sanford, J. P. The antibacterial effect of normal and infected urinary bladder. J. Lab. Clin. Med. 77:605–615, 1971.
18. Smellie, J., Edwards, D., Hunter, N., Normand, I. C. S., and Prescod, N. Vesicoureteric reflux and renal scarring. Kidney Int. 8:65s–72s, 1975.
19. Hodson, C. J. Reflux nephropathy. Med. Clin. N. Am. 62:1201, 1978.
20. Retik, A. B. Vesicoureteral reflux. In Pediatric kidney disease, C. M. Edelman (ed.). Little, Brown, Boston, 1978.
21. Stephens, F. D. Cystoscopic appearance of ureteric orifices associated with reflux nephropathy, In Reflux nephropathy, C. J. Hodson and P. Kincaid-Smith (eds.). Masson, New York, 1979, pp. 119–125.
22. Rolleston, G. L., Shannon, F. T., and Utley, W. L. Follow-up of vesicoureteral reflux in the newborn. Kidney Int. 8:S59, 1975.
23. Ransley, P. G. and Risdon, R. A. The pathogenesis of reflux nephropathy. Br. J. Radiol. 14(suppl.):1, 1978.
24. Ransley, P. G. and Risdon, R. A. Renal papillary morphology in infants and young children. Urol. Res. 3:111, 1977.
25. Hodson, C. J., Maling, T. M., McManamon, P. J., and Lewis, M. J. The pathogenesis of reflux nephropathy (chronic atrophic pyelonephritis). Br. J. Radiol. 13(suppl.):1, 1975.
26. Norden, C. W. and Kass, E. H. Bacteriuria of pregnancy—a critical appraisal. Ann. Rev. Med. 19:431–470, 1968.
27. Kass, E. H. Chemotherapeutic and antibiotic drugs in the management of infections of the urinary tract. Am. J. Med. 18:764, 1955.
28. Thomas, V., Shelokov, A., and Forland, M. Antibody-coated bacteria in the urine and site of urinary tract infection. New Eng. J. Med. 290:588, 1974.
29. Rubin, R. and Cotran, R. S. Immunological aspects of pyelonephritis with a critical survey of antibody-coated bacteria test. Fourth International Symposium on Pyelonephritis, H. Losse and A. W. Asscher (eds.). Georg Thieme Verlag, Stuttgart, 1980.
30. Freedman, L. R. Natural history of urinary infection in adults. Kidney Int. 8:96s–100s, 1975.
31. Heptinstall, R. H. The enigma of chronic pyelonephritis. J. Infec. Dis. 120:104, 1969.
32. Angell, M. E., Relman, A. S., and Robbins, S. L. "Active" chronic pyelonephritis without evidence of bacterial infection. New Eng. J. Med. 278:1303, 1968.
33. Schwartz, M. M. and Cotran, R. S. Common enterobacterial antigen in human chronic pyelonephritis and interstitial nephritis. An immunofluorescent study. New Eng. J. Med. 289:830, 1973.
34. Heptinstall, R. H. Interstitial nephritis. Am. J. Pathol. Vol. 83, 1:213, 1976.

35. Fairley, K. F., Becker, G. J., Butler, H. M., McDowell, D. R. M., and Leslie, D. W. Diagnosis in the difficult case. Kidney Int. 8:12s–19s, 1975.

36. Cotran, R. S. Pathogenesis of chronic pyelonephritis: the role of humoral and cell-mediated reactions to bacterial and renal antigen. Sixth International Congress of Nephrology, Florence, Italy, 1975. Karger, Basel.

37. Kincaid-Smith, P. Glomerular lesions in atrophic pyelonephritis (RN). In Reflux nephropathy, J. Hodson and P. Kincaid-Smith (eds.). Masson, New York, 1979, pp. 268–272.

38. Spuhler, O. and Zollinger, H. U. Die chronish-interstitielle nephritis. Z. Klin. Med. 151:1, 1953.

39. Grimlund, K. Phenacetin and renal damage at a Swedish factory. Acta Med. Scand. 174 (suppl. 405):3, 1963.

40. Murray, T. and Goldberg, M. Chronic interstitial nephritis: etiologic factors. Ann. Int. Med. 82:453–459, 1975.

41. Murray, T. G. and Goldberg, M. Analgesic-associated nephropathy in the U.S.A. Kidney Int. 13:64–71, 1978.

42. Gonwa, T. A., Hamilton, R. W., and Buckle, W. Importance of analgesic nephropathy in the etiology of end-stage renal disease in Northwest North Carolina. Kidney Int. 16:930, 1979.

43. Murray, T. and Goldberg, M. Analgesic abuse and renal disease. Ann. Rev. Med. 26:537–550, 1975.

44. Molland, E. A. Experimental renal papillary necrosis. Kidney Int. 13:5, 1978.

45. Burry, A. F. The evolution of analgesic nephropathy. Nephron 5:185, 1967.

46. Gloor, F. J. Changing concepts in pathogenesis and morphology of analgesic nephropathy as seen in Europe. Kidney Int. 13:27–33, 1978.

47. Kincaid-Smith, P., Nanra, R. S., and Fairley, K. F. Analgesic nephropathy: a recoverable form of chronic renal failure, In Renal infection and renal scarring, P. Kincaid-Smith and K. F. Fairley (eds.). Mercedes, Melbourne, 1970, p. 384.

48. Bengtsson, U. et al. Malignancies of the urinary tract and their relation to analgesic abuse. Kidney Int. 13:107, 1978.

49. Ditlove, J., Weidmann, P., Bernstein, M., and Massry, S. G. Methicillin nephritis. Medicine (Baltimore) 56:483–491, 1977.

50. Kleinknecht, D., Kanfer, A., Morel-Maroger, L., and Mery, J. Ph. Immunologically mediated drug-induced acute renal failure. Contr. Nephrol. 10:42–52, 1978.

51. Border, W. A., Lehman, D. H., Egan, J. D., Sass, H. J., Glode, J. E., and Wilson, C. B. Antitubular basement-membrane antibodies in methicillin-associated interstitial nephritis. New Eng. J. Med. 291:381–384, 1974.

52. Ooi, B. F., Ooi, Y. M., Mohini, R., and Pollak, V. E. Humoral mechanisms of drug-induced interstitial nephritis. Clin. Immunol. Immunopathol. 10:330, 1978.

53. Van Ypersele de Strihou, C. Acute oliguric interstitial nephritis. Kidney Int. 16:751, 1979.

54. McCluskey, R. T. and Colvin, R. G. Immunological aspects of renal tubular and interstitial diseases. Ann. Rev. Med. 29:21, 1978.

55. Andres, G. A. et al. Immunologically mediated interstitial disease. Fogarty International Center monograph on the Prevention of Kidney and urinary tract disease. C. H. Coggins, and N. B. Cummings (eds.). DHEW Publ. No. (NIH) 78-855, Washington, D.C., 1978, pp. 251–263.

56. Steblay, R. W. and Rudofsky, U. Renal tubular disease and autoantibodies

against tubular basement membrane induced in guinea pigs. J. Immunol. 107:589–594, 1971.

57. Sugisaki, T., Klassen, J., Milgrom, F., Andres, G. A., and McCluskey, R. T. Immunopathologic study of an autoimmune tubular and interstitial renal disease in Brown Norway rats. Lab. Invest. 28:658–671, 1973.

58. Lehman, D. H., Wilson, C. B., and Dixon, F. J. Interstitial nephritis in rats immunized with heterologous tubular basement membrane. Kidney Int. 5:187–195, 1974.

59. Bergstein, J. and Litman, N. Interstitial nephritis with anti-tubular basement-membrane antibody. New Eng. J. Med. 292:875–878, 1975.

60. Levy, M., Guesry, P., Loirat, C., Dommergues, J. P., Nivet, H., and Habib, R. Immunologically mediated interstitial nephritis in children. Contr. Nephrol. 16:132, 1979.

Appendix: Membrane Transport

Many substances cross cell membranes. The uptake of substrates by cells for energy metabolism and growth and the release of waste products from cells produce a large traffic of solutes and water across plasma membranes. In general, substances may be transported across cell membranes either passively or actively. "Transport" refers to movement of matter across a permeability barrier, a plasma membrane in the case of the individual cell or a layer of cells in the case of transporting epithelia (intestinal mucosa, renal tubular epithelia, etc.). This transport is regarded as "passive" if it occurs without any direct coupling to the energy metabolism of the transporting cell and as "active" when an energy supply from cell metabolism is necessary.

Passive transport may occur by simple diffusion or may be carrier mediated. In both cases the substance transported moves down a chemical or electrochemical potential gradient. With diffusion the flux, J, across the permeability barrier is linearly proportional to the activity or potential gradient of the substance across the barrier. Carrier-mediated transport shows saturation kinetics; the rate of transport reaches some limiting value as the concentration of the transported solute increases, because reactive sites on the permeability barrier through which or on which the solute may cross the barrier become fully occupied by the solute in question. The movement in both instances is "downhill"; down a chemical potential gradient or, in the case of charged solutes, such as ions, down an electrochemical gradient. Active transport shares the saturation kinetics of carrier-mediated transport, but the solute in question may be moved "uphill" against an electrochemical potential gradient; the energy for such "uphill" transport is supplied by the energy metabolism of the cell.

Figure A-1 depicts the forces that may affect transport across a permeability barrier. In Figure A-1a, solute at two different concentrations, $C_2 > C_1$, is added to a vessel divided into two chambers by a membrane. If the membrane is permeable to the solute, there is a net transfer of solute from the higher, C_2, to the lower, C_1, concentration

Fig. A-1 Forces driving solute and solvent transport.

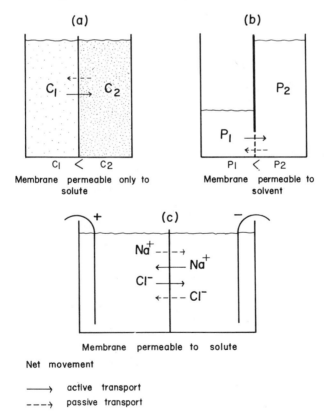

until the concentrations on the two sides of the membrane become equal. Net transfer of solute from the low concentration C_1 to the higher concentration C_2 could occur only if energy were supplied to move the solute up its concentration gradient.

Figure A-1b depicts the simple effects of a hydrostatic pressure difference $P_2 > P_1$ on the movement of solution through a barrier permeable to the liquid. Net transfer of fluid from P_2 to P_1 would occur spontaneously or passively, but net transfer of liquid from P_1 to P_2 would require energy and thus would be an active process. If the liquid contained a dissolved solute to which the membrane were also permeable, then, as solvent moved from left to right, solute would be swept along through the membrane with it. This so-called "solvent drag" effect is an additional driving force that can affect the net movement of solute across a permeability barrier.

Figure A-1c depicts the effect that an electrical potential imposed by two charged, reversible electrodes dipping into the solution on opposite sides of the permeability barrier has on the transport of charged species, Na^+ and Cl^-, across the membrane. A net transport of Na^+ ions to the electrically negative side of the membrane and a movement of Cl^- in the opposite direction would be expected if the membrane has a finite permeability for Na^+ and Cl^-. Net movements of these ions in the opposite directions would require their active transport, for the transfers would be "uphill" against the electrical driving forces.

Having pictured the kinds of driving forces that move solutes or solvent across a permeability barrier, we can consider the quantitation of these forces. The three driving forces diagrammed in Figure A-1 may be expressed in differential form (1). The diffusion force per mole is $- RT\, d \ln a / dx$ in which $d \ln a / dx$ is the gradient of chemical activity of the diffusing species, and $a = fc$ with f the activity coefficient and c the concentration. The electrical driving force is $- zF\, (d\Psi / dx)$ in which z is the charge of the diffusing species, F is the Faraday, and $d\Psi / dx$ is the gradient of electrical potential through the membrane. An expression for the force acting on the diffusing molecules or ions consequent to the flow of solvent across the membrane may be obtained (1). For a dilute solute the rate of flow of solution may be regarded as equal to the rate of flow of solvent (water) across the membrane. The force acting on a mole of water in the direction of flow is $- dp / dx$, which is the gradient of hydrostatic or osmotic pressure across the membrane. With g_w, the frictional force acting on 1 mole of water at unit velocity, $-(dP/dx)(1/g_w)$ must be the linear rate of flow across the membrane. The force arising from solvent flow that acts on 1 mole of solute is, therefore, $-(dP/dx)(G/g_w)$ where G is the frictional force between 1 mole of solute and water at unit velocity.

The total external forces acting on a solute that can penetrate the membrane is thus:

$$\frac{d\bar{\mu}}{dx} = -\left(RT\frac{d\ln c}{dx} + RT\frac{d\ln f}{dx} + zF\frac{d\Psi}{dx} + \frac{G}{g_w}\frac{dP}{dx}\right) \tag{1}$$

where c is the concentration and f the activity coefficient of the solute.

By analogy with Ohm's law the driving forces, potentials, may be divided by appropriate resistance terms to obtain the rate of flow or the flux of matter across the barrier. The flux, J_i, of the ith solute across a unit area of membrane is proportional to the force per mole, to the concentration, and to the fraction A of the total membrane area available to penetration by the solute in question. It is also inversely proportional to the frictional resistance g which is the friction on one mole of solute at unit velocity. J_i is thus,

$$J_i = -\frac{A}{g} \cdot c \cdot \frac{d\bar{\mu}}{dx} \tag{2}$$

$$J_i = -\frac{A}{g}c\left(RT\frac{d\ln c}{dx} + RT\frac{d\ln f}{dx} + zF\frac{d\Psi}{dx} + \frac{G}{g_w}\cdot\frac{dP}{dx}\right) \tag{3}$$

$$J_i = -\frac{d\bar{a}}{dx}\frac{ART}{gf}\cdot\exp\left[-\frac{zF\Psi + \int\frac{G}{g_w}\left(\frac{dP}{dx}\right)dx}{RT}\right] \tag{4}$$

in which $\bar{a}$, the electrochemical activity, is defined

$$RT\ln\bar{a} = \mu - \text{const.} = RT\ln c + RT\ln f + zF\Psi + \int\frac{G}{g_w}\left(\frac{dP}{dx}\right)dx \tag{5}$$

This expression clearly cannot be solved expicitly, since the gradients as well as A, g, and c are all unknown functions of x, the distance through the membrane. Though no solution for J_i is possible, considerable information may be gained by examining the ratio of the fluxes of the ith solute in the two opposite directions across the membrane. If the ith solute crosses the membrane through the same pathways in the two opposing directions, then it is evident that nearly all the unknowns cancel in the expression for the flux ratio

$$\frac{J_{i_{1 \to 2}}}{J_{i_{2 \to 1}}} = -\frac{(d\bar{a}_{i_1}/dx)}{(d\bar{a}_{i_2}/dx)} = \frac{\bar{a}_{i_1}}{\bar{a}_{i_2}} \tag{6}$$

or taking the logarithm of both sides and introducing the definition of electrochemical activity from Equation (5):

$$\ln \frac{J_{i_{1 \to 2}}}{J_{i_{2 \to 1}}} = \ln \frac{c_1}{c_2} + \frac{zF}{RT} d\Psi + \frac{G}{RT} \int_0^x \frac{1}{g_w} \left(\frac{dP}{dx}\right) dx \tag{7}$$

This flux ratio, though still somewhat cumbersome, can be informatively applied in situations where there is no significant net volume flow across the membrane. For example, when a cell is in a steady state, it undergoes no volume change, and the flux of any penetrating solute into the cell must just equal its flux out of the cell, so that solvent drag $= 0$ and

$$J_{i_{1 \to 2}} = J_{i_{2 \to 1}} \tag{8}$$

or

$$0 = \ln \frac{a_1}{a_2} + \frac{zF}{RT} \Delta\Psi \tag{9}$$

$$\Delta\Psi = -\frac{RT}{zF} \ln \frac{a_1}{a_2} \tag{10}$$

which is the familiar Nernst equation. Note that it is derived, and thus strictly valid, only for the condition of no net movement or transference of the penetrating ion across the permeability barrier.

What is the source of the membrane potential difference $\Delta\Psi$? This may be appreciated by considering the following example. A container is divided by a semipermeable membrane into two compartments, A and B. The membrane has the property of being permeable only to the cation K^+, but not to the anion Cl^-, of the 0.1 molar aqueous potassium chloride solution filling compartments A and B. It is also impermeable to water. Such permeability characteristics could be approximated by a very finely porous membrane with a high concentration of fixed negative charges along the porous channels. The density of fixed negative charges, for example, $-COO^-$ or $-SO^=_4$, in the membrane will repel the negative chloride ions of the solution but expedite the passage of the positive potassium ions through the membrane. With equal concentrations of KCl in compartments A and B (Fig. A-2) there will be zero membrane potential difference across the membrane as measured by the two balanced, reversible electrodes, usually two calomel half cells, and recorded on the potentiometer, V. If the concentration of KCl in compartment B is reduced to 0.01 M (Fig. A-2b), however, then conditions across the membrane are no longer symmetrical; a chemical concentration difference now exists across the membrane such that KCl will tend to diffuse from its higher concentration in A to its lower concentration in B. But the membrane separating the compartments is permeable to the K^+, but not the Cl^-. Thus, a slight movement of K^+ will occur from B to A. But this results in a separation of charge. Hence, compartment B becomes electrically positive to compartment A, owing to the slight excess of

Fig. A-2 Chemical gradients as the source of membrane potential.

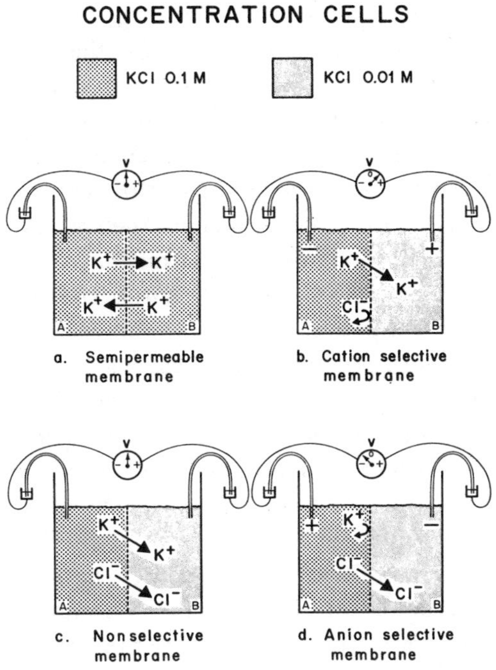

CONCENTRATION CELLS

KCl 0.1 M   KCl 0.01 M

a. Semipermeable membrane

b. Cation selective membrane

c. Nonselective membrane

d. Anion selective membrane

positive potassium ions in B and the residual surplus of negative chloride ions in A. This potential difference, or membrane potential, will be just large enough to counterbalance the tendency of potassium ions to diffuse from A to B. Clearly, the greater the concentration difference between compartments A and B, the greater the diffusion force tending to drive K^+ from A to B, to increase the separation of charges, and hence, to increase the membrane potential. It is this potential difference that is precisely defined by the Nernst equation, just derived,

$$\Delta\Psi = -\frac{RT}{zF} \ln \frac{K^+{}_B}{K^+{}_A}$$

With a tenfold concentration difference between the solutions in compartments A and B and at 25°C, $d\Psi$ should equal 58 millivolts (mV).

If the membrane dividing compartments A and B were replaced by a semipermeable anion-selective membrane (Fig. A-2d), the direction of the electrical potential would be reversed. Now only Cl^- ions could penetrate the fine channels lined with fixed positive charges, and this would exclude the K^+ ions. Chloride would diffuse from A to B until a membrane potential developed that just balanced the force of diffusion. The resulting separation of charges would render compartment B electrically negative to compartment A. The Nernst equation would give the same numerical value for the membrane potential, $\Delta\Psi$, but with the sign or polarity reversed. The actual excess of K^+ in the first case or Cl^- in the second that moves from compartment A to B is far too small to be measured by the most sensitive chemical methods. But the consequence of this separation of charges is readily detectable electrically as the membrane potential.

Most real membranes, including plasma membranes, are not so perfectly ion selective as the hypothetical charged membranes used in our example. It is informative to see how the relationships just described are modified in leaky membranes. As the porosity of the aqueous channels becomes coarser (Fig. A-2c), chloride ions will begin to leak across the barrier from compartment A to B. The passage of Cl^- ions from A to B will tend to short-circuit out the membrane potential established by the diffusion of potassium ions. The value for $\Delta\Psi$ measured in the potentiometer will fall accordingly. Its value will depend on the relative mobilities of K^+ and Cl^- across the membrane. If the membrane becomes so leaky as to afford no greater restraint on the movement of Cl^- ions than it exerts on the potassium ions, then clearly no separation of charges will occur as KCl diffuses from its higher concentration in compartment A to compartment B. The potentiometer will record zero potential difference across the membrane, so that $\Delta\Psi = 0$. Furthermore, once both ions, K^+ and Cl^-, can penetrate the membrane, equilibrium conditions no longer hold; transference of solute across the membrane will occur until the concentration of solute, KCl, is equal in compartments A and B. To use the Nernst equation to calculate the membrane potential of such nonsteady-state conditions is a misapplication of the equation; however, it is often done to see how closely the measured membrane potential approximates the observed concentration distribution of various ionic species on the two sides of a permeability barrier. When combined with additional information regarding the system, such measurements can yield important information. Table A-1 shows how they may be applied to the distribution of Na and K between the intracellular and extracellular fluids of muscle.

From this application of the simplified flux ratio equation we see that the distribution of sodium ions between intracellular and extracellular phases of muscle is far from the expected steady-state value and that potassium is distributed so that its electrochemical potential is nearly equal on the two sides of the muscle cell membrane. The large discrepancy between the calculated and measured membrane potential in the case of sodium is consonant with other information indicating that Na^+ is actively transported out of the cell. Moving Na^+ against both a chemical and electrical potential gradient must be an "uphill," active process. By contrast the slight discrepancy between the calculated equilibrium potential for potassium and the measured

TABLE A-1 *Application of Nernst Equation to the Distribution of Na and K in Frog Muscle (2)*

	CONCENTRATION		MEMBRANE POTENTIAL[a]	
	C_o	C_i	Calculated	Measured
	(mEq/kg water)		(------ mV ------)	
Na	140	15	+57	
				−92
K	2.5	139	−100	

[a] The sign (+ or −) refers to the electrical potential within the cell relative to that of the extracellular fluid surrounding the cell.

membrane potential exists because the muscle's plasma membrane has a finite permeability to other ions, and the potassium ion is itself accumulated in muscle by an active transport process probably coupled with active extrusion of Na^+ via the Na–K-dependent adenosine triphosphatases of the plasma membrane.

One very debatable aspect of making a calculation such as this is the assumption that the activity coefficients for Na^+ and K^+ within the cell are the same as in the extracellular fluid and close to 1.0, actually 0.75 at the ionic strength of extracellular fluid. If a significant fraction of either ion were in fact "bound" within the cell interior, as in an ion exchange resin, then the calculation would be invalid. Moreover, if significant portions of cell water are structured or "bound," the water within the cells that is available to dissolve solutes will be less than the total water content of the cells. Finally compartmentation of water and solutes within cells may be present. All these complicating possibilities make our assumption that the water and ions within cells are in simple, uniform aqueous solution a gross oversimplification.

With the development of glass electrodes sensitive to, and specific for, potassium or sodium, and of improved micropuncture techniques, the activity of intracellular potassium and sodium has been estimated by inserting electrodes into single cells of several tissues (listed in reference 5). Early measurements in skeletal muscle (3) and nerve fibers (4) suggested that most of the intracellular potassium is in a free state. In mammalian heart muscle (5) the activity coefficient for intracellular potassium was 0.612, compared with 0.745 in extracellular fluid (Tyrode's solution). Thus, though the activity coefficient of intracellular potassium may be the same or slightly, but significantly, less than that of a simple aqueous solution of uni-univalent salts, it is perhaps less depressed than one might have anticipated in the presence of the polyvalent intracellular anions. The activity coefficient of sodium in the same study was found to be much more depressed (0.175) than that of potassium, but the uncertainties in measuring the low concentrations of sodium in cells bathed by a sodium-rich extracellular fluid make the resulting activity coefficients (γ_{Na}) very uncertain ($\gamma_{Na} = a_{Na}/C_{Na}$), in which a_{Na} is the activity of intracellular sodium as estimated with a sodium-sensitive microelectrode and C_{Na} is the estimated concentration of intracellular sodium determined as the difference between total tissue sodium and the extracellular fluid content of sodium estimated with the aid of a presumed extracellular marker, e.g., inulin, sulfate. Furthermore, nuclear magnetic resonance studies that had earlier been thought to indicate that some two-thirds of tissue sodium was "bound," were reexamined and found to have been misinterpreted; the findings more likely reflect tumbling of sodium ions within an anisotropic medium or rapid exchange between free sodium ions and a minute fraction of bound sodium ions (6).

Since the estimate of intracellular ion concentration depends also on determination of the intracellular water content, the chemical activity of the water is an important factor affecting ion activities. To the extent that water may exist in some "bound" or ice-like, structured form, it will exclude ions, and the activity of the particular ion will be relatively high when compared with its apparent intracellular concentration. Though some nonsolvent water must exist in apposition to the complex interfaces within cells, nuclear magnetic resonance studies seem to indicate this does not constitute a major phenomenon (7).

The complex intracellular structure revealed by electron microscopy raises the further expectation that compartmentation of ions and water may occur within subcellular organelles.

The effects of these several factors may be to augment or diminish the differences between overall apparent intracellular ionic concentrations and activities. Considerable clarification in the complex area of cellular electrophysiology may be expected when precise ion or salt activities can be substituted for the rough estimates of concentration used today. In the study of intracellular activity of potassium in heart muscle (5), for example, a much better agreement between the measured plasma membrane potential and that calculated from the ratio of intracellular to extracellular potassium was obtained when measured intracellular potassium activity was substituted in the Nernst equation for the estimated concentration of that ion intracellularly.

Some of the complexities that can be introduced into the simplistic consideration of "active" or "passive" transport, which may occur when carrier molecules are present in the cell membranes, deserve mention. By "carrier molecule" we mean a component of the plasma membrane that has the ability to bind the solute in question and in this complexed state to move the solute molecule across the membrane, permitting its liberation on the opposite side. This "ferry boat" concept has been useful in explaining the great specificity characteristic of some cellular transport systems and the phenomena of *counter-transport* and *exchange diffusion.*

If a sugar, for example, is capable of being transported across a cell membrane on a carrier molecule, then a high concentration of this sugar within the cell would result in its leakage from the cell via the carrier molecule. But if the medium surrounding the cell contained a structurally similar sugar that could also be transported on the carrier molecule, this second sugar might be accumulated simultaneously within the cell. The diffusion potential for the first sugar, causing its exit from the cell via the carrier molecule, would provide the driving force to draw the second sugar into the cell. Such "uphill" accumulation of the second sugar is called counter-transport. The high initial concentration of the first sugar within the cell must have resulted from either active transport of that sugar or its synthesis within the cell.

By "exchange diffusion" we mean the traffic of a solute across a membrane in combination with a carrier molecule that can move across the membrane in either direction only when its binding sites are saturated with the specific solute. Thus, exchange diffusion cannot produce a net movement of solute across a membrane, but it can increase the traffic in both directions so that the flux equation may no longer apply. It can also lead to rapid isotopic equilibration of a solute across a membrane without this indicating any net movement of solute. If the specific solute is removed from one side of a membrane and there results a decrease in the flux of the solute from the opposite side, then presumably, exchange diffusion was involved in the traffic of that solute across the membrane.

In one of the classic experiments in biology, Ussing applied the flux ratio equation, which he had derived, to a study of ion transport across the isolated frog skin (8). In this experiment a sheet of abdominal skin from a frog, or the histologically simpler toad bladder, is held as a membrane separating two halves of a lucite chamber (Fig. A-3). A Ringer's solution bathes each side separately, and a spontaneous electrical potential is measured with balanced calomel electrodes across the skin or bladder. The potential may be 10 to 170 mV and is directed so that the outside or mucosal surface is electrically negative relative to the inner or serosal bathing medium. If an external potential source is applied across the two ends of the lucite chamber and directed so as just to nullify the spontaneous membrane potential, an electrical current is observed to flow in the external circuit. This

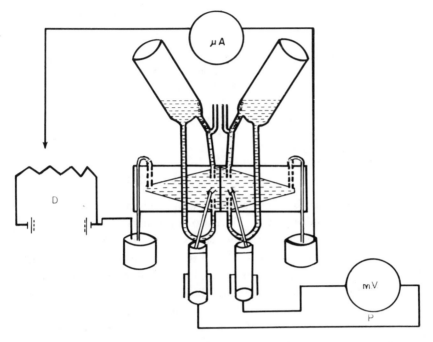

Fig. A-3 Apparatus for short-circuit current measurement.

"short-circuit current," which may be measured with a microammeter, is the current necessary to keep the electrical potential across the tissue at zero when the tissue is bathed on both sides by a Ringer's solution of identical composition. The flow of current through the solution indicates an asymmetric movement of some ion or ions across the tissue. To ascertain which ion or ions were moving asymmetrically, Ussing labeled the sodium in one bathing medium with ^{22}Na and the other with ^{24}Na, so that the separate fluxes of sodium could be measured simultaneously in the two directions across the epithelium. The results of such a double isotope-labeling experiment are shown for the isolated urinary bladder of the toad in Table A-2 (9).

Note that the movement of sodium from the mucosal to serosal medium is greater than its movement from serosa to mucosa; the difference is the net transport of sodium from urinary surface to serosa. Furthermore, when the net sodium reabsorption is compared with the short-circuit current and both are expressed in the same units, there is excellent agreement between the two values. Clearly, the electrical ac-

TABLE A-2 *Comparison of Sodium Flux and Short-Circuit Current through Isolated Toad Bladder (9)*

NO. OF 30-MIN PERIODS	MEAN Na FLUX		MEAN NET Na TRANSPORT	MEAN SHORT-CIRCUIT CURRENT	MEAN DIFF
	M → S[a]	S → M[a]			
	(----------------- μ Amps/cm^2 ----------------------)				
14	24.4	3.1	21.3	20.1	1.2 ± 1.1

[a] M → S mucosal to serosal
S → M serosal to mucosal

tivity of the isolated bladder is totally and solely accounted for by the net transport of sodium ions. Since no asymmetric movement of any ion is expected across a membrane bathed on both surfaces with media of identical chemical composition and in the absence of a transepithelial electrical potential, it is evident that the asymmetry of sodium flux must be the result of activity of the bladder epithelium. In fact, when Ussing and Zerahn performed this experiment in 1951, it was the first time that we had clear proof of active ion transport and knowledge of which ionic species was actually transported.

Since the asymmetric and specific movement of sodium is an active process, it must be coupled to a source of energy in the bladder. When the oxygen consumption of isolated, paired half bladders is measured with one half bathed in a sodium-containing medium and the other in sodium-free choline or magnesium Ringer's solution, a reduced oxygen consumption is observed in the absence of sodium (see Table A-3A). Furthermore, when the oxygen consumption of isolated toad bladders is measured for three successive hours and the results are expressed as microliters of oxygen consumed per milligram of dry weight, the Q_{O_2}, the value remains quite constant over the 3-hour period (see Table A-3B). If, however, all sodium is removed from the bathing medium so that there is none to transport, the rate of oxygen consumption is again seen to be quite low. After a 1-hour period of measurement, adding sodium back to the choline or magnesium Ringer's solution resulted in an increased Q_{O_2}. From other observations we know that factors that can stimulate sodium transport in this tissue, such as vasopressin or aldosterone, also stimulate increased energy metabolism—increased oxygen and substrate utilization (9).

The relationship between transport process and metabolic reactions

TABLE A-3

A. *Comparison of Q_{o_2} of Toad Bladder in the Presence and Absence of Sodium*

	Na RINGER	Mg RINGER	ΔQ_{o_2}	Na RINGER	CHOLINE RINGER	Q_{o_2}
MEAN	1.28	0.63	−0.65	1.58	0.97	−0.61
S.E. mean diff.			±0.06			±0.14
P			<0.001			<0.01
		(7 paired experiments)			(8 paired experiments)	

B. *Effect of Added Sodium on Q_{o_2} of Toad Bladder in Sodium-free Ringer*

	1	2	3	MEAN Δ (HOURS 2–1)	S.E. MEAN Δ	P
No sodium	0.88	0.81	0.73	−0.07	±0.04	0.1
Sodium added[a]	1.04	1.21	1.23	+0.17	±0.02	<0.001

[a] Sodium added at end of first hour to choline or Mg Ringer (Q_{o_2} = μl O_2/mg dry tissue/hr, 8 experiments on 8 paired half bladders).

in biological systems has been stated in phenomenological terms by Kedem (10, quoted), who assumed that active transport involves a metabolically dependent chemical reaction taking place within the transporting cells. If all flows are considered interdependent, the phenomenological relations may be written:

$$\Delta \bar{\mu}_i = \sum_{k=1}^{n} R_{ik} J_k + R_{ir} J_{ch} \tag{11}$$

$$A_r = \sum_{k=1}^{n} R_{rk} J_k + R_{rr} J_{ch} \tag{12}$$

in which $\Delta \bar{\mu}_i$ is the difference in electrochemical potential on the two sides of the membrane for the ith component; J_k is the flow of matter; J_{ch} the rate of metabolic reaction; the R's the resistances or coupling coefficients between the flows of the various molecular species crossing the membrane (R_{ik}), between matter and metabolism (R_{ir} and R_{rk}), and to the flow of the metabolic reaction (R_{rr}); and A_r is the driving force or affinity of the chemical reaction. The rate of oxygen consumption or of CO_2 production of the metabolic reactions that drive the transport process may be a measure of J_{ch}. Since chemical reactions are scalar (nondirectional), the orientation of the transport process is implicit in the coefficient R_{ir}, which must be a vector, and the reactions must occur in an anisotropic medium—hence the function of cell membrane to give direction to scalar reactions.

When the bladder or frog skin is short-circuited, sodium is transported from one surface of the epithelium to the other without a difference in electrical or chemical potential. Thus, the work of transport is solely to overcome the internal resistance to sodium movement through the epithelium. For each sodium ion that moves from mucosal bathing medium to serosal bathing medium, an anion must move in the same direction or a cation in the opposite direction to maintain electrical neutrality. During short circuiting, of course, a chloride ion is precipitated from the mucosal medium as silver chloride when a silver atom gives up its electron to the silver:silver chloride electrode. The liberated electron travels to the silver:silver chloride electrode in the serosal medium via the external circuit, where a silver ion is reduced to metallic silver and its associated chloride is liberated into the serosal medium to balance the sodium. Thus, the external circuit is the route by which chloride ions accompany the transported sodium from mucosal to serosal media. *In vivo* or in the open-circuit state, the transport of sodium renders the serosal medium positive to the mucosal bath. This membrane potential draws chloride ions with the sodium ions or other cations in the opposite direction (see Fig. 2-12). The net result of the sodium transport is thus to effect reabsorption of sodium chloride from urine to body fluid or secretion of cation—hydrogen or potassium—into the urine. Of course, in other tissues the transport species may differ; hydrochloric acid by gastric mucosa, sodium chloride by the ion-pair "pump" in gallbladder epithelia, potassium by the midgut of cecropiae (silkworm), and so on.

Little is known yet about the molecular mechanisms of active ion transport, though there are now several promising leads. The transport process must have two definite features. It must have specificity, i.e., the ability to recognize specifically sodium ions in the case of frog skin, toad bladder, and renal tubule; and it must be able to transduce metabolic energy into the translocation of sodium ions across the permeability barrier imposed by cell membranes.

At least one transduction system has been identified as the membrane-bound, sodium–potassium-dependent adenosine triphosphatase that was first observed by Skou (11) in nerve tissue but has subsequently been shown to be ubiquitous in animal tissues. This enzyme is capable of being phosphorylated by the gamma phosphate of ATP in the presence of sodium ions and dephosphorylated on exposure to potassium ions. Whittam (12) has shown that the enzymatic process in red cell ghosts is directional insofar as it is stimulated by sodium ions within the cell and potassium ions outside the cell, i.e., on the appropriate sides of the plasma membrane, to effect sodium transport out of the erythrocyte and potassium transport into the cell. The details of how the splitting of phosphate by this enzyme from ATP results in transport of sodium out of the cell and of potassium into the cell are not understood. The enzyme is a protein that is located within the lipid membrane of the cell and possibly penetrates the lipid permeability barrier. Being a complex lipoprotein it has until recently resisted isolation and purification, but apparently Kyte (13) has accomplished this now from kidney tissue, which is rich in this enzyme.

Insight into how ions could be recognized with the specificity that characterizes transport processes of biological membranes has come from studies initiated in Russia on the mode of action of certain natural antibiotic substances. Valinomycin, the first of such compounds to be studied, has a remarkable specificity for potassium ions. Figure A-4 shows that the valinomycin added to the sodium chloride solution bathing the two surfaces of a lipid bilayer membrane prepared from lipids extracted from red blood cell membranes had no effect on the very high electrical resistance of this artificial membrane (14). When the lipid bilayer membrane was bathed by a potassium chloride solution, the addition of valinomycin reduced the initial high resistance of 10^8 to 10^3 ohms, a change of five orders of magnitude in the permeability of the lipid bilayer to potassium ions! Valinomycin is a doughnut-shaped macrocyclic molecule composed of repeating lactate and amino acid molecules (Fig. A-5). Its outer hydrophobic surface penetrates a lipid membrane or phase readily, while its centrally oriented carbonyl oxygens are apparently positioned effectively to form ligands for potassium. In fact, they appear to replace the hydration shell of aqueous potassium with little energetic or stearic hindrance. The aqueous potassium ion seems to mistake the interior of a valinomycin molecule for its ever-present but ever-changing shell of water molecules. In this comfortable berth it apparently can be ferried across the

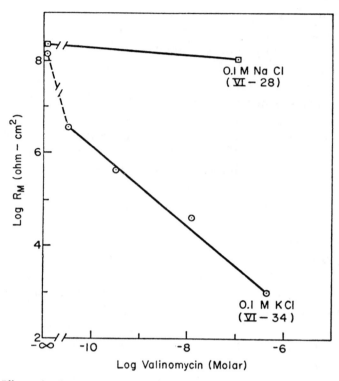

Fig. A-4 Effect of valinomycin on the electrical resistance of a bimolecular lipid membrance in the presence of NaCl or KCl. Reprinted from (14) with permission of the *Journal of General Physiology*.

lipid bilayer. The somewhat smaller sodium ion (Table A-4) cannot fit the valinomycin interior so well and thus cannot be transported. Interestingly, valinomycin bears no electrical charge until its interior is occupied by a K^+ ion. Thus, all the earlier efforts to base the specificity of biological ion transport systems on electrostatic binding with components of the membranes failed to appreciate the specificity and binding affinity of multiple weaker forces when stearic factors were favorable to make the binding forces additive.

Today many natural products are known to bind small ions as valinomycin does. Some are charged and some are uncharged. Some are linear molecules, like the nonactin series, which apparently can wrap around an alkali metal ion and carry it through a lipid bilayer. Some, such as alomethicin, are composed entirely of naturally oc-

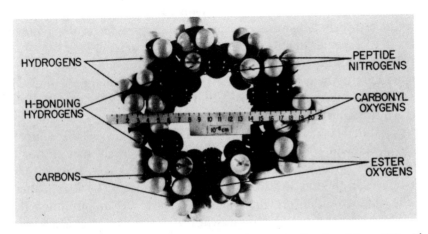

Fig. A-5 Corey-Pauling space-filling model of valinomycin. Reprinted from (15) with permission of the *Journal of General Physiology*.

curring amino acids. Some, like amphotericin B, form ligands for anions, Cl^-, rather than cations. Some, like valinomycin, appear to serve as carriers for their ion load, and others like amphotericin B again, seem to join together to form pores across the lipid bilayer through which the appropriate ion can move.

Almost simultaneously with these discoveries of properties in naturally occurring molecules, Pedersen, at duPont, synthesized a family of heterocyclic organic molecules that have the ability to carry small

TABLE A-4   *Estimated Diameters in Ängstrom Units of Univalent Cations*[a]

	CRYSTAL-LOGRAPHIC (PAULING)	STOKES–EINSTEIN (17)	CORRECTED HYDRATED (17)	CORRECTED HYDRATED (16)
Li	1.20	4.74	7.4	6.80
Na	1.94	3.66	6.5	5.52
K	2.66	2.50	5.0	4.62
Rb	2.96	2.36	4.7	4.56
Cs	3.38	2.38	4.8	4.56
$N(CH_3)_4^+$	6.94	4.08	6.94	—
$N(C_5H_{11})_4^+$	10.58	10.58	10.58	—

[a] This table shows values for ionic diameters taken from the literature (16, 17). The values designated as taken from reference 16 are from Table 17 of that work. Reprinted from (15) with permission of the *Journal of General Physiology*.

ions into nonpolar liquid environments (18). Pedersen's compounds also have hydrophobic outer surfaces and oxygen molecules pointed toward their center that form ligands with small ions.

Most natural and synthetic compounds bind potassium with a higher affinity than sodium; in a few, however, this affinity is reversed, though in none to the degree required for the specificity to sodium of known transport process in cell membranes.

Attempts to find small molecules in cells that may be the counterpart of valinomycin and serve as ion carriers have not met with success. On the other hand, at least two molecules have been isolated that seem to meet the specifications of carrier substances. The first of these is the sulfate-binding protein isolated by Parde (19) from salmonella. This protein, induced by the presence of sulfate in the culture medium, can be obtained in good yield by simply shocking the bacteria osmotically. The protein is not present in salmonella that have not been induced to elaborate the carrier system. The second carrier protein has been isolated and characterized by Wasserman (20). When rachitic chicks are treated with vitamin D, a new protein can be extracted in large amounts from their intestinal mucosa. This protein specifically binds calcium ions, but its actual role in intestinal absorption of calcium is still undefined.

With appreciation of the ion-binding properties of the natural and synthetic ionophores and the presence of proteins within cell membranes, it is easy to speculate about the nature of the specific ion transport systems. A membrane protein with an alomethicin-like head at one end might serve as a "carrier" molecule. Simple thermal motion might move the ion-binding portion of the molecule backward and forward across the plasma membrane. In active transport by such carrier molecules, phosphorylation and dephosphorylation at some active but remote site on the protein might produce allosteric changes in the protein that would alternately increase and decrease the affinity of the carrier portion of the molecule to an ion. Exposure of the carrier portion of the phosphorylated molecule to sodium on the inside of a cell might cause it to bind sodium ions. With this carrier portion exposed at the outside surface, the presence of extracellular potassium might induce dephosphorylation of the protein. This would produce a conformational change in the carrier that would decrease its affinity for sodium, and the sodium would be discharged outside the cell. Repeated cycling of this process would yield an ion pump that uses the metabolic energy of ATP to phosphorylate and dephosphorylate the carrier and thus move sodium up a chemical and electrical potential gradient. Obviously, this crude speculation will need testing, but at long last, techniques to make such tests are becoming available.

References

1. Ussing, H. H. The alkali metal ions in biology. I. The alkali metal ions in isolated systems and tissues. Springer, Berlin-Gottingen-Heidelberg, 1960.

2. Adrian, R. H. The effect of internal and external potassium concentration on the membrane potential of frog muscle. J. Physiol. 133:631–658, 1956.

3. Lev, A. A. Determination of activity coefficients of potassium and sodium ions in frog muscle fibers. Nature (Lond.) 201:1132, 1964.

4. Hinke, J. A. M. The measurement of sodium and potassium activities in the squid axons by means of cation-selective glass micro-electrodes. J. Physiol. (London) 156:314, 1961.

5. Lee, C. O. and Fozzard, H. A. Activities of potassium and sodium ions in rabbit heart muscle. J. Gen. Physiol. 65:695–817, 1975.

6. Shporer, M. and Civan, M. M. Nuclear magnetic resonance of sodium-23 linoleate-water. Basis for an alternative interpretation of sodium-23 spectra within cells. Biophys. J. 12:114–122, 1972.

7. Civan, M. M. and Shporer, M. ^{17}O nuclear magnetic resonance spectrum of $H_2{}^{17}O$ in frog striated muscle. Biophys. J. 12:404–413, 1972.

8. Ussing, H. H. and Zerahn, K. Active transport of sodium as the source of electric current in the short-circuited isolated frog skin. Acta Physiol. Scand. 23:110–127, 1951.

9. Leaf, A. Transepithelial transport and its hormonal control in the toad bladder. Ergebnisse der Physiologie (Reviews of Physiology) 56:216–263, 1965.

10. Katchalsky, A. and Curran, P. F. Nonequilibrium thermodynamics in biophysics. Harvard University Press, Cambridge, 1965, pp. 88–89.

11. Skou, J. C. Enzymatic basis for active transport of Na^+ and K^+ across cell membrane. Physiol. Revs. 45:596–617, 1965.

12. Whittam, R. The asymmetrical stimulation of a membrane adenosine triphosphatase in relation to active cation transport. Biochem. J. 84:110–118, 1962.

13. Kyte, J. Properties of the two polypeptides of sodium- and potassium-dependent adenosine triphosphatase. J. Biol. Chem. 247:7642–7649, 1972.

14. Andreoli, T. E., Tieffenberg, M., and Tosteson, D. C. The effect of valinomycin on the ionic permeability of thin lipid membranes. J. Gen. Physiol. 50:2527–2545, 1967.

15. Tosteson, D. C., Cook, P., Andreoli, T. E., and Tieffenberg, M. The effect of valinomycin on potassium and sodium permeability of HK and LK sheep red cells. J. Gen. Physiol. 50:2513–2525, 1967.

16. Stern, K. H. and Amis, E. S. Ionic size. Chem. Rev. 59:1–64, 1959.

17. Robinson, R. A. and Stokes, R. H. Electrolyte solutions. Butterworth, London, 1955, p. 121.

18. Pedersen, C. J. Cyclic polyethers and their complexes with metal salts. J. Am. Chem. Soc. 89:7017–7036, 1967.

19. Pardee, A. B. Purification and properties of a sulfate-binding protein from Salmonella typhimurium. J. Biol. Chem. 241:5886–5892, 1966.

20. Wasserman, R. H., Corradino, R. A., and Taylor, A. N. Vitamin D-dependent calcium-binding protein. J. Biol. Chem. 243:3978–3986 and 3987–3993, 1968.

Index